Good Pharn

Good Pharma

The Public-Health Model of the Mario Negri Institute

Donald W. Light and Antonio F. Maturo

palgrave
macmillan

First published in 2015 by PALGRAVE MACMILLAN® in the United States—a division of St. Martin's Press LLC, 175 Fifth Avenue, New York, NY 10010.

Where this book is distributed in the UK, Europe and the rest of the world, this is by Palgrave Macmillan, a division of Macmillan Publishers Limited, registered in England, company number 785998, of Houndmills, Basingstoke, Hampshire RG21 6XS.

Palgrave Macmillan is the global academic imprint of the above companies and has companies and representatives throughout the world.

Palgrave® and Macmillan® are registered trademarks in the United States, the United Kingdom, Europe and other countries.

ISBN: 978-1-137-38833-9

Library of Congress Cataloging-in-Publication Data

Light, Donald, Jr., 1942– , author.
    Good pharma : the public-health model of the Mario Negri Institute / Donald W. Light, Antonio F. Maturo.
        p. ; cm.
    Includes bibliographical references and index.
    ISBN 978-1-137-38833-9 (hardback)
    I. Maturo, Antonio, author.   II. Title.
    [DNLM: 1. Istituto di ricerche farmacologiche Mario Negri.
2. Academies and Institutes—history—Italy.   3. Ethics, Pharmacy—Italy.   4. History, 20th Century—Italy.   5. Pharmaceutical Preparations—Italy.   6. Research—Italy. QV 24]
    RS67.I82
    615.10945—dc23

                                                            2014047429

A catalogue record of the book is available from the British Library.

Design by Amnet.

First edition: July 2015

10 9 8 7 6 5 4 3 2 1

Dedicated to Mario Negri
a bold, imaginative philanthropist who contributed to Italian and
international science

Contents

List of Illustrations

Foreword

In January 2008, I was the guest of Silvio and Anny Garattini at their home in Umbria. I had never previously visited this part of Italy, and the Garattini's treated me to a guided tour of some spectacular sites in nearby Montefalco, where the Church of San Francesco was particularly memorable. Just as memorable, however, were the many people who stopped us to greet Silvio and his wife affectionately as we were walking round the town. How come the director of a pharmacological research institute was known to and clearly appreciated by so many people?

As we set off to return home, Anny Garattini explained that Silvio was widely known and appreciated by the Italian public because he believes scientists supported by public funds should ensure that they tell the public about their work. Silvio does this by writing regularly in newspapers and magazines, and by contributing to radio and television broadcasts. The consequence is that he had become a very trusted national figure.[1] Although Silvio comments on real advances in research for patients, he also exposes features of medical research and practice that do not serve the best interests of the public. Drawing attention to these concerns and addressing them have long been features of the Mario Negri Research Institute, which Silvio and a group of like-minded young colleagues founded in 1961.

After we returned home, I asked Silvio and Anny whether anyone had written a history of this remarkable research institute, driven as it is by an ethical imperative to do "patient-oriented" rather than "patent-oriented" pharmacological research? No one had, although there had been occasional talk about a biography of Silvio. I suggested that, given the extensively documented corruption and inefficiency in a research enterprise currently shaped by commercially driven pursuit of patents, a history of the Institute would provide a needed moral beacon. An account of the Mario Negri Institute could make clear that there is a successful alternative to the patent-oriented model of drug discovery and evaluation.

The following day, Silvio and I set off to the Rome Science Festival to urge that patients and the public deserve big changes in how drugs are evaluated.[2] The idea of a history of the Institute buzzed in our heads. Resources

---

[1] Wagstaff A. The people's pharmacologist. *Cancer World*. 2008; May/June:28–33.

[2] Garattini S, Chalmers I. Patients and the public deserve big changes in evaluation of drugs. *BMJ*. 2009;338:804–806.

would be needed for the necessary research, and most of all, to secure the time of skilled analysts and writers in both English and Italian. Seven years later, this excellent book written by Donald Light and Antonio Maturo is the result.

Since its inception, the mission of the Mario Negri Institute has been:

> to do research of international quality to improve people's health, based on independent, transparent science, openly used to educate doctors and patients about how best to address their health needs.

This mission has been reflected in over 12,000 articles published in scientific journals and about 5,000 articles published in the lay press, and in @ParticipaSalute, a website, newsletter, and organization to bring patient, medical, and nursing associations together with researchers, to discuss key issues about health care and to promote patient empowerment.[3]

The community orientation of the Institute is reflected in the way that it sees clinical trials as a way to make clinicians and patients aware of uncertainties about the effects of treatments, and to take collective responsibility for addressing the most important among these.

> Research is an expression of care. It cannot be separate, parallel or occasional (as it is for commercial testing) and yet still be clinically real. The greatest risk in clinical medicine is to dissociate care from research about how effective that care is. Yet this is what usually happens. Rather, research into treatments must be nested within practice.[4]

In a plea published in the *Lancet* shortly before his untimely death, Alessandro Liberati, a senior member of the Institute's staff, put it well:

> I have had the opportunity to consider from more than one perspective the mismatch between what clinical researchers do and what patients need. I am a researcher; I have responsibility for allocating funding for research; and I have had multiple myeloma for the past decade. A few years ago I stated publicly that several uncertainties I faced at the beginning of my disease were avoidable . . .
>
> If we want more relevant information to become available, a new research governance strategy is needed. Left to themselves, researchers cannot be expected to address the current mismatch. Researchers are trapped by their own internal competing interests—professional and academic—which lead them to compete for pharmaceutical industry funding . . . An essential component of any new governance strategy would be to bring together all the stakeholders,

---

[3] Mosconi P, Colombo C, Satolli R, Liberati A. PartecipaSalute, an Italian project to involve lay people, patients' associations and scientific-medical representatives in the health debate. *Health Expectations.* 2007;10:194–204.

[4] Tognoni G, Caimi V, Tombesi M, Visentin G. Italian general practitioners of the Rischio e Prevenzione Study Project. primary care as a permanent setting for research. *Primary Care Research and Development.* 2012;13:1–9.

starting from an analysis of existing and ongoing research, produced independently of vested interests.[5]

In 2009, Paul Glasziou and I estimated that over 85 percent of the massive worldwide investment in pharmaceutical and medical research was being wasted.[6] Our analysis led to the preparation of a series of *Lancet* papers, in which the sources of waste were analyzed in more detail (www.researchwaste .net). The introductory paper in the series[7] called for systems of oversight and regulation to be developed that would protect the integrity of the scientific process. It referred specifically to the Mario Negri Institute as providing an inspiring role model, and listed its many commendable features:

1. Institutional and economic independence from government, industry, and academia.
2. Absolute transparency-accountability in research planning, implementation, and publication—from basic research to clinical trials; and from epidemiology to environmental projects and technology assessments.
3. Rejection of patenting of discoveries made by the Institute.
4. Exclusive control of all steps in research and all data from the clinical trials in which it is involved, whether sponsored by the Institute, by industry, or by anyone else.
5. Promotion of research as an integral component of health care through building networks of hospitals and clinicians interested in and committed to participating in research on a voluntary and long-term basis.
6. Development of large-scale clinical trials based on the population of patients who will actually use the medicines being evaluated, encouraging these to become seen as a "normal" component of responsible clinical care and an effective tool for continuing professional development.
7. Promotion of public policies to support research for unmet needs, rather than for marketing and the need for profits.
8. Monitoring the transferability of research evidence into clinical practice, taking advantage of the professional networks described above.
9. Continuous promotion of broad scientific literacy through the mass media, and educating the public about the principles and realities of pharmacological and pharmaceutical research.

These principles are made explicit in the "Chart of values and ethical conduct" of the Mario Negri Institute.

---

[5] Liberati A. Need to realign patient-orientated and commercial and academic research. *The Lancet*. 2011;378:1777–78.

[6] Chalmers I, Glasziou P. Avoidable waste in the production and reporting of research evidence. *The Lancet*. 2009;374:86–89.

[7] Macleod MR, Michie S, Roberts I, Dirnagl U, Chalmers I, Ioannidis JPA, Salman RA-S, Chan A-W, Glasziou P. Biomedical research: increasing value, reducing waste. *The Lancet*.2014;383:4–6.

In giving us *Good Pharma: The Public-Health Model of the Mario Negri Institute*, Donald Light and Antonio Maturo will help the world to see how there can be a renaissance in research oriented—above all—to serving the interests of patients and the public.

Iain Chalmers
Oxford, August 2014

Preface and Acknowledgments

Although this book began as a commissioned history of how a few, young, Italian scientists designed and built a new kind of research institution that became internationally famous and attracted researchers from around the world for advanced training, the relevance of how the Mario Negri Institute kept its moral integrity and its science unsullied by worldwide forces that were compromising research, publications, and medical practice led us to carry out an extended case study of the Institute as a model for reforming how medicines are developed for humanity.

Before starting, we read other books about distinguished labs—Scripps, Lawrence Labs, Oak Ridge, Bell Labs, and Rutherford. But none of them had developed an ethos of research in the service of people, especially those with serious or rare medical conditions, in the service of the downtrodden community where Mario Negri researchers worked, in the service of the nation through developing environmental pharmacology, and in the service of all patients in fighting against tainted regulations that put too many risky drugs on the market with little evidence of added benefit. And none of them had developed a coherent set of strategies for keeping the research process transparent and independent of pressures from funders.

Through the rules and practices developed largely by the founding director, Silvio Garattini, the Mario Negri Institute became a model that, together with the many researchers it trained, has elevated Italian science and international pharmacological research. Given the ways in which commercial research fails to come up on its own with significant clinical advances, biases clinical trials, and compromises medical knowledge, we need a paradigm shift from the Bad Pharma that Goldacre and others have detailed to the Mario Negri model of research, evaluation, and the production of scientific knowledge for the public and patients everywhere.

As two medical sociologists with broad interests in health, society, and comparative health policy, we corresponded in 2010 and met in Princeton in June 2012. We have worked closely on this institutional history ever since. Besides having the advantage of being bilingual and teaching medical sociology at both the University of Bologna and Brown University, Antonio Maturo was a coauthor with Giuseppe Remuzzi, one of the Institute's most celebrated researchers who has served on the editorial boards of both the *New England Journal of Medicine* and the *Lancet*. During 2012–2014, Donald Light spent about 40 days on site, sleeping and eating at the Institute in Milan or visiting its labs in Bergamo and Ranica, and doing 2–4 hour interviews in person or by phone. Maturo spent about 20 days at labs on the Milan and Bergamo campuses and doing in-depth interviews. Altogether we interviewed about 60 past and present researchers and administrators, some two or three times. We shared and compared notes, as well as meals and walks. We both read piles of the research papers by those we interviewed.

Research on the Institute was deepened by Light winning a research fellowship at the Edmond J. Safra Center for Ethics at Harvard University, where he joined half a dozen current and former fellows doing policy research on how the pharmaceutical industry has compromised the US Food and Drug Administration, the publication of medical research, and the practice of medicine. (Other groups studied institutional corruption in banking, university research, big audit firms, environmental protection, and especially Congress.) Constant exposure to how institutions are being corrupted underscored the need for a book on institutional integrity, in this case, a research institute that has figured out how to thrive without succumbing to compromising pressures, as many labs have who depend on industry funding. The Institute has also spoken out against the conflicts of interest and compromises that impair pharmaceutical research from helping patients. During Light's year at the Center, Maturo visited him and worked further on the book.

Drafting began in 2013, and Light had principal responsibility for supervising and writing the book; but Maturo was specifically responsible for Chapters 2, 4, and 7. In all our work, we sent drafts back to the researchers interviewed as a validity check, and many of them offered corrections, criticisms, and further material on their research. Nevertheless, how we wrote up work at the Institute is our responsibility alone. At all times, despite the pressures of grants and contract research, Mario Negri researchers took time to respond promptly and helpfully.

We are first indebted to Sir Iain Chalmers and Professor Garattini for conceiving this project and inviting us to do it. The ARMR Foundation, an association at the forefront for the research on rare diseases based in Bergamo, generously supported the research. We are indebted to our chairs and deans for supporting our work on this book and giving us the time to work on it. Our families and loved ones both spurred us on and put up with numerous incursions into personal spaces. Among the researchers at the Institute, Ariela Benigni, Vittorio Bertele', Maurizio Bonati, Maria Benedetta Donati, Maurizio D'Incalci, Roberto Fanelli, Giovanni de Gaetano, Enrico Garattini, Giuseppe Remuzzi, Gianni Tognoni, and many others have provided historical and critical perspectives in their generous comments on drafts. Most generous has been Professor Garattini in digging up historical materials, arranging for interviews with past members of the Institute, commenting on drafts, and challenging us in this work. He and we have been greatly assisted by Elvira Carcano and Flavia Boniardi. Judith Baggott, the Institute's long-time English editor, shared her long memory of people and events as well as her editorial skills to the book, especially to Chapter 4. Isabella Bordogna provided valuable assistance on several occasions, and Vanna Pistotti was invaluable in pulling together the illustrations for the book. We hope readers find the final results rewarding.

List of Abbreviations

ADHD	Attention Deficit and Hyperactivity Disorder
AIFA	Italian Medicines Agency
AKF	Acute Kidney Failure
ANMCO	(Italian) Association of Hospital Cardiologists
ARMR	(Foundation for) Help for Research on Rare Diseases
CCU	Coronary Care Units
CINP	International College of Neuropsychopharmacology
CNR	(Italian) National Center for Research
CPMP	Committee for Proprietary Medicinal Products
CQI	Continuous Quality Improvement
CTEP	Cancer Therapy Evaluation Program
CUF	Italian Unified Committee on Pharmaceuticals
EORTC	European Organization for Research and Treatment of Cancer
EMA	European Medicines Agency
EPAR	European Public Assessment Report
EPO	Erythropoietin
ESRD	End Stage Renal Disease
FDA	Food and Drug Administration
GISEN	Italian Network of Nephrology Centers
GISSI	Italian Group for the Study of the Survival of Streptokinase in Myocardial Infarction
GiViTI	Group for the Evaluation of Interventions in Intensive Care Medicine
GMOs	Genetically Modified Organisms
GSK	GlaxoSmithKline
HUS	Hemolytic Urenic Syndrome
ICU	Intensive Care Unit
IRCCS	Italian Scientific Institutes for Recovery and Treatment
ISN	International Society of Nephrology
ISN-GO	Commission on Global Advancement of Nephrology at the International Society of Nephrology
KHDC	Detection and Management of Chronic Kidney Disease, Hypertension, Diabetes and Cardiovascular Disease
MI	Myocardial Infarction
NCI	National Cancer Institute

NHS	National Health Service
NIH	National Institutes of Health
NNH	Number Needed to Harm One Patient
NNT	Number Needed to Treat to Make One Patient Better
PETA	People for the Ethical Treatment of Animals
RCT	Randomized Clinical Trials
REIN	Renal Insufficiency Study
SK	Streptokinase
SSRI	Selective Serotonin Reuptake Inhibitors
TCDD	Tetrachlorodibenzo-p-dioxin
TPA	Tissue Plasminogen Activator
TTP	Thrombotic Thrombocytopenic Purpura
VCR	Vaccine Research Center
WHO	World Health Organization

Introduction

Beneficence through Principled Research for Patients

Forty years ago, Phil Lee, the chancellor of a world-class medical university, joined Milton Silverman in describing the distorting effects of drug companies on the goal of medicine—to prevent, cure, or manage disease and serious risks.[1] They followed up with books on how companies continued to sell drugs regarded as dangerous in rich countries to millions of hapless victims in Africa, Latin America, and Asia.[2]

Thirty years ago, John Braithwaite synthesized a wide range of evidence about corporate crimes in the pharmaceutical industry.[3] These crimes have only increased, it seems, at least in the United States, where avarice keeps driving the premier-brand global companies like GSK (GlaxoSmithKline), Pfizer, Merck, Lilly, and others to go beyond misleading tests and marketing to criminal (or rather, allegedly criminal) acts that risk or harm millions of patients. They then deny any wrongdoing as they pay half a billion, a billion, or more in penalties and fines.[4]

Twenty years ago, Thomas Moore described how one of the most deadly drugs ever, Tambocor, was approved by the modern FDA and used widely by cardiologists, killing at least 50,000 patients. An authority on drug safety, Moore has explained how drugs are developed, approved, and promoted with minimal attention to safety because of perverse incentives.[5]

Ten years ago, Marcia Angell, the former editor-in-chief of the *New England Journal of Medicine*, pulled together research that she and another distinguished editor-in-chief, Arnold Relman, had undertaken for an influential bestseller, *The Truth about the Drug Companies: How They Deceive Us and What to Do about It*.[6] Many well-researched articles and books have followed that detail unethical and even criminal acts that harm patients on a large scale.[7]

Recently, Ben Goldacre, a doctor and expert in science, published the global bestseller, *Bad Pharma*.[8] In readable, graphic prose, Goldacre tells readers why they cannot trust their doctors or the medicines they prescribe because of unethical science:

Medicine is broken . . . We like to imagine that doctors are familiar with the research literature, when in reality much of it is hidden from them by drug companies . . . We like to imagine that regulators let only effective drugs onto the market, when in reality they approve hopeless drugs, with data on side effects casually withheld from doctors and patients.

Drugs are tested by people who manufacture them, in poorly designed trials, on hopelessly small numbers of weird, unrepresentative patients, and analysed using techniques which are flawed by design, in such a way that they exaggerate the benefits of treatments.

Goldacre specifies and references every word like "broken," "weird," and "flawed." He draws on years of research about the "ghost management" of medical knowledge through behind-the-scenes invisible "publication planning corporations" that shape medical knowledge on which doctors rely to prescribe effective drugs for their patients. His chapter, "Bad Regulators" describes the ways in which they do not protect the public from harmful or ineffective drugs but rather protect drug companies through layers of secrecy and hide the risks of harmful side effects. He devotes 100 pages to deceptive and distorting forms of marketing that get doctors to prescribe drugs of unproven benefit (because regulators do not require real evidence that new drugs are better).

Although companies have developed a small, steady number of clinically superior new drugs that help millions and add to a large medicine chest of effective drugs discovered over previous years and decades, they devote most of their research budget to turning out scores of clinically minor drugs in order to replenish their product lines.[9] Entire classes of what we have been led to believe were breakthrough innovations in medical science, like hormone replacement therapy for postmenopausal women or SSRI drugs for depression, now lie discredited, but only after millions of people have swallowed billions of doses, with harmful side effects.[10]

Through documents discovered in litigation and through policy research, details have emerged about the ways in which the major companies have denied, dismissed, or suppressed evidence of harmful side effects and exaggerated how beneficial new drugs are for patients.[11] An outpouring of industry-crafted articles or new stories in medical journals, newspapers, popular magazines, on the Web, and on television exaggerate the benefits and understate the harms of new drugs. An epidemic of harmful side effects have resulted, about 80 million a year in the United States alone that includes 2.7 million hospitalizations and 128,000 deaths from drugs when properly prescribed.[12] Few "innovative" drugs have offsetting advantages over better-established postpatent drugs. Thus prescription drugs themselves, even when properly prescribed, have become the fourth leading cause of death, tied with stroke. Drugs we take to get better are a greater cause of death than diabetes, or Alzheimer's disease, or pneumonia. They are an especially high risk for the elderly. Medical sociologists and anthropologists overlook prescription drugs as a major health risk tied into the organization and financing of health care.

People want Good Pharma, not Bad Pharma, but don't know how to restore research integrity and the search for better, safer drugs. They will find some answers in this book about the Mario Negri Institute for Pharmacological

Research and its commitment not only to research integrity, despite being surrounded by biasing and compromising practices, but also to a social mission and ethos centered on compassion and outreach, especially to the vulnerable, sick, and suffering.

Imagine a highly successful, independent, nonprofit research institute where no discoveries are patented because patenting corrupts the scientific process and impedes research by keeping methods and results secret as one decides which research strategy is most likely to lead to patents and profits. The Mario Negri practices open science—full transparency, especially of things that don't work out so everyone can learn from them.

Imagine a research institute that never drops a promising drug-candidate because its profit potential is too low. Imagine a research institute that investigates seriously any promising cure, even if it cannot be patented because the mission of research is patients, not profits. All patent-oriented research labs and companies claim they are dedicated to better drugs for patients, but not if they can't be patented. And, in fact, as we just showed, about 90 percent of all drugs they discover offer few or no clinical advantages for patients, even though they get approved as "safe and effective." In Mario Negri trials, which test for clinical superiority as few commercial trials do, these drugs would fail because they would be proven of little advantage to patients based on patient-oriented outcomes. Doctors and patients volunteer to participate in Mario Negri trials with little or no pay because Mario Negri organizes their trials to be like a shared social mission to get answers to a question of clinical importance. Commercial trials are well known to be designed to produce marketing messages for profit and results that meet regulators' low bars for approval without evidence of clinical superiority. None of the Institute's 12,000 scientific articles has been ghost-managed or ghostwritten, as articles from commercial trials so often are. The "impact factor" or measure of citation by other scientists of its articles is high (see Figure 0.1). Some of its senior researchers are among the thousand most cited in the world, and Giuseppe Remuzzi served on the boards of the *New England Journal of Medicine* and *The Lancet*.

Scientific Publications – the Mario Negri Institute

- More than 12,000 publications in peer-reviewed journals
- About 230 scientific books
- More than 58,178 citations in peer-reviewed, scientific journals; 13.23 citations per publication/H index 94 (2006-2013)
- 18 researchers with H index higher than 30
- 4 of the 51 'highly cited' Italian researchers (ISI)
- In the last ten years:

2,499 articles with impact factor higher than 3

1,217 articles with impact factor higher than 5

371 articles with impact factor higher than 10

Figure 0.1   Institute publications

This is the Mario Negri Institute for Pharmacological Research in Italy (IRFMN–Istituto di Ricerche Farmacologiche "Mario Negri"). Not *pharmaceutical* research, which seeks patents and profits, but *pharmacological* research, devoted to finding clinically more effective drugs for patients regardless of patents in open, transparent ways that maximize collaborative efforts. Under the leadership of Silvio Garattini, the Mario Negri Institute has figured out how to be what Erik Olin Wright calls a "real utopia,"[13] a working solution to the many forms of scientific and intellectual corruption so prevalent in patent-driven research that leading medical journals have spent the past 20 years trying to protect themselves and their reputations against them. The Institute has figured out how to contract with Big Pharma[14] while keeping control of its research design, data, methods, results, and publications. The Mario Negri public-health model can show the way that research teams in universities and elsewhere can take back their scientific integrity.[15] But to do so, they must not seek patents and profits from royalties, because that pursuit compromises good science in too many ways, and too many potentially beneficial medicines or new uses get ignored.

This book tells how one institute developed research principles of medical ethics and a research community grounded in trust, open science, and collaboration. It suggests a paradigm shift. Patent-driven research has proven to be largely medically and morally bankrupt. As one study after another attests, we live in a world of biased and intentionally misleading medical knowledge about our drugs, and medical practice has lost its moral integrity through commercial influences. Millions of patients are harmed and diseases of the world's poor are not even considered. While the Bayh-Dole Act in 1980 may have launched "30 years of patent-driven innovation" in other fields, in pharmaceuticals it has transformed the great pharmaceutical companies of the post–World War II era from centers of in-depth searches for breakthrough drugs to global marketing machines that search for any new development that can be patented for profits from government-protected high prices.

It is time to consider a paradigm shift to patient-driven research free of commercial biases in methods and medicine. As we will indicate at the end of this story, it's not hard to achieve—except that most of the stakeholders are profiting or hope to profit. The Mario Negri Institute is not only a working model for developing better medicines but also a model of how drugs should be marketed and prescribed: (1) full disclosure of how the risks of harm compare to the chances of benefits, (2) cautions against taking drugs unless one has to, and (3) advice to take the lowest dose possible for the shortest time needed. Why ingest toxic though beneficial chemicals any more than one has to? As Vittorio Bertele' a physician and head of the Mario Negri Health Policy Laboratory said, *If one starts with what is best for the patient, all else follows easily and clearly.* Conversely, if one starts with what is best for marketing, patents, and profits, very different consequences follow.

Once you starting thinking about what is best for patients, it takes you places you did not expect. Readers will learn where it has taken the Mario Negri and wonder, "Why don't other research institutes undertake similar initiatives to protect patients from harmful drugs or train patient groups to separate the wheat from the chaff? Why don't they too advocate for regulatory rules and procedures that lead to clinically better medicines and actively monitor the one in five chance of serious adverse reactions from new drugs?" Like all researchers, those at the Mario Negri have to endlessly apply for grants and do their research within budget. But they pool funds to support each other when grants are thin and to do outreach projects for patients. In Chapter 7, readers will learn how the Mario Negri waged war on dangerous and ineffective drugs, taking substantial losses as companies punished them. These campaigns went well beyond policy recommendations and partial fixes, like the current campaign for transparency of clinical trial results. The Institute's leaders developed and implemented another "real utopia," a fully operating model of a regulator bent on protecting patients from harmful and useless drugs and on reducing the unnecessary costs to taxpayers and patients.

The Mario Negri Institute provides a model for how emerging countries can develop superior, transparent biomedical research to improve their people's health and help their economies grow. The Institute is the paragon of science and social mission that can inspire creative governments and philanthropists because it does original research on unmet needs of seriously ill patients, with no consideration of profits. With the right strategies and investments, other countries can foster similar first-class research institutes, independent of commercial or political influence, in order to develop cost-effective medicines and more real clinical advances than the patent-driven research practiced by Big Pharma. The Mario Negri approach also means far fewer but better-designed clinical trials, as explained in Chapter 6, at much lower cost than the tens of thousands of commercial trials that provide little valid information of clinical use. If one starts with what is best for the patient, what follows easily and clearly is a very different approach to clinical trials, grounded in a shared desire to improve patient outcomes.

Historically, the founder of the Mario Negri Institute, Silvio Garattini, drew inspiration from the National Institutes of Health and other distinguished examples in the 1950s, such as the Rockefeller Institute, in order to minimize both commercial and political/governmental influence on its scientific research. As described in Chapter 1, he witnessed the many ways in which dependency on academic hierarchies and commercial or even government funding could slant research, cut off promising lines of investigation, threaten dissenting researchers, or suppress findings not to their liking. He was determined to create an institute independent of universities, government ministries or politicians, and companies—a private, nonprofit institute devoted to research-based contributions to society and patients. As countries like India, China, and Brazil struggle to reward true innovation and avoid patent manipulation for pseudoinnovation,[16] they might consider taking their arguments to their logical conclusions and institute a new paradigm for research integrity, good pharma, and low costs.

The Institute's policy of not patenting its discoveries reflects a time-honored tradition when for decades medicines were regarded as a societal good meeting a societal need and therefore were exempted from patents. Researchers at the Institute receive no pay beyond their regular, modest salaries. The Institute feels like a community of graduate students. One would be hard-pressed to tell in the cafeteria or at one of the many seminars when researchers present their work, who is the director of a department or chief of a lab and who is a staff researcher. Some leave for much higher paying jobs with pharmaceutical companies but most do not.

When the Mario Negri Institute opened in 1963, it represented an unusual kind of organization, independent of the winds of political factions, of the stifling bureaucratic and hierarchical controls in Italian universities, or of the corporate priorities for profit and market power. When Silvio Garattini made a formative visit to the United States in 1957 to some of the leading medical research centers, he saw that research could be a full-time career, rather than something one did on the side to get promoted in the academic hierarchy. He admired the hands-on, egalitarian, open-door character of productive research teams in "America," as he and many Europeans like to call the United States. He instituted open discussions and debates among junior and senior staff about the strengths and weaknesses of an idea or an experiment in order to realize the shared goal of finding the best scientific approach to a question or problem. His warmth and informality replaced standing on ceremony when a director enters a room.

While many American institutes were part of government or a university, Garattini realized neither would work in Italy, and so he sought funding outside of both and linked to an international scientific community by making the unheard-of requirement that all publications would be in English. This history describes the determination and risks involved in founding the Institute and how it grew through the decades. Chapters 4, 7, and 8 describe its service to patients and their doctors, and its public actions against drugs or other remedies that lacked good scientific evidence of benefit to patients. Garattini established principles, rules, and practices that have enabled the Institute to keep the integrity of its research intact, despite political and commercial pressures that now have so deeply compromised much pharmaceutical research elsewhere.[17]

The Institute's principles and norms can be organized into the classic bioethics framework of beneficence, respect for autonomy, and nonmaleficence, only rethought in terms of research integrity to address illness and suffering.[18] Beneficence perhaps comes first, and respect for autonomy is really part of beneficence, an important principle that enables beneficence to be achieved. Reducing the incapacitating effects of illness enhances individual autonomy.[19] Nonmaleficence is part of, or complements, beneficence. The key to beneficial research is institutional autonomy, freedom from possibly corrupting influences from corporations, government officials, or sponsoring institutions who may bias the research, its analysis, or its publication as the medical science on which doctors and patients rely. With this introduction, let us turn to the normative and practical ethics of the Mario Negri Institute for Pharmacological Research that make it such a timely exemplar for science policy in the twenty-first century.

Beneficence

A boyhood imbued with Catholic social ethics and years helping his disabled mother and brother influenced Garattini's emphasis on dedicating the Institute to helping the sick and suffering through research. Of course, almost every pharmaceutical company and research enterprise makes a similar claim. For example, knowledgeable readers will recall that Merck's motto was "Putting Patients First," as it redoubled its sales efforts to get millions more patients to take the high-priced painkiller, Vioxx (refocoxib), even after a front-page article in the *New York Times* and an FDA report emphasized its high risks of cardiovascular trauma.[20] It emphasized so-called beneficence by marketing Vioxx as better and safer, though the drug was no more effective than other anti-inflammatories, and reduced stomach bleeds that pertain to only 4 percent of patients. Even those patients could be given a proton pump inhibitor. According to Merck marketing materials submitted to the US Congress, its special marketing staff were trained to dodge critical questions about the drug's cardiovascular risks, and they succeeded in persuading doctors to put 80 million patients on Vioxx, which led to one of the worst drug disasters in history. Other major companies claiming beneficence have also promoted their drugs in harmful, even criminal ways.[21] So one must be careful about who claims to put patients first.

Multiple Implications of Beneficence

This history of how the Mario Negri institutionalized medical ethics provides readers with various ways in which the Mario Negri Institute has implemented beneficence in several ways. It led to a reconceptualization of what the field of clinical pharmacology means and how it contributes to society. It guided the Institute in its care of the rats and mice that are used to investigate pathways and identify mechanisms of action in diseases for which no effective treatment exists. Another implication of beneficence for the Institute has been to integrate cellular or subcellular bench research with bedside care, and to create valuable feedback loops in both directions for better science. The Institute achieved full bench-to-bedside integration much earlier than elsewhere, in the late 1970s. Integrating laboratory with clinical research began early through comparisons of pharmacokinetics in animals and humans and in clinical trials. Discovering how renal failure occurs and learning how to stop it is an example of bench-to-bedside integrated research described in Chapter 3.

Beneficence has also meant a dedication from the beginning to train graduate and postgraduate students. Chapter 4 describes the Institute's hands-on, applied method of training researchers, in contrast to a university approach centered on courses and exams. The Institute has trained more than 6,000 postuniversity scientists, including 800 foreign research fellows who chose the Institute for postdoc training. These advanced graduates have populated distinguished institutes and centers throughout the world. In a similar vein, the Mario Negri Institute has dedicated itself to developing ways to educate and inform patients and providers, using its research knowledge.

Beneficence is also evident within the Institute's own organizational culture, described in Chapter 2, of a supportive community, an extended family that leads to many marriages and children. In interviews, many senior scientists referred to it as "the family." Despite below-market pay, many stay on for years (though only if they can keep winning grants in head-to-head competition).

"Let me introduce you to one of our younger staff," said Flavia Boniardi, an administrator who married one of the researchers years ago. "By younger," she added parenthetically, "I mean someone who's been here less than 30 years."

"How many years have you been here?" we asked our new, middle-aged acquaintance.

"29 years." Everyone laughed.

This moment brought home what we found in interviews about why so many do not want to leave the beneficent family or community, despite low salaries. No one punched a time clock for decades, until a new law required it. "Self-motivation is everything," Garattini told us. Employees could stay home to look after their sick child, or cat, or parent, and arrange their research around personal needs, including after hours.

Clinical Trials for Better Patient Care

"Any trial should be designed to provide the best information for doctors and patients," Professor Garattini told us as we talked about the Institute and its ethics. Yet what even physicians do not know is that few commercially funded trials today provide any useful information to help make better prescribing decisions. To him, this is obvious—why would a clinical trial be designed with any other goal than to benefit patients? Yet some readers may know that nearly all trials are not, and regulators even require them not to be, as explained in Chapter 8.[22] Several chapters will describe the Institute's exemplary approach to trials and its vigorous critiques of trials of no use to patients, resulting in new drugs with no clinical advantages to offset their risks of harm.[23]

"No trial should be approved as 'safe and effective' without information that it is safer and more effective than existing therapies," Garattini continued. Yet regulators routinely approve drugs as "safe and effective" without such evidence. "No data on the clinical performance should be confidential or subject to protection as proprietary information," Garattini told us. "Ethically doing so violates the rights of subjects in the trials, unless it is fully explained to them in advance that they are volunteering for a trial whose results will not be disclosed to them or other patients and doctors."

In order to benefit patients, "All trials must use hard clinical end points unless there are good reasons for not doing so." Based on years of hands-on experience reviewing trial evidence for the European Medicines Agency (EMA), Garattini continued:

Quality of life, morbidity, and mortality should be the outcome measures of clinical trials. Publishing trials with surrogate end points that are not necessary is an unethical practice . . . used to persuade doctors to prescribe a new drug as "superior." Any ethical journal should therefore refuse to publish such articles. This should be added to the ethical standards of medical journal editors.

"Non-inferiority trials are usually unethical," Garattini explained, because they test whether or not new drugs are *worse* than a drug already in use by a certain percentage.[24] Instead, one should test to see if a new drug has a superior balance of efficacy and safety as measured by patient outcomes. He continued:

No ethics committee should approve such a trial, on ethical grounds. Informed consent must make clear to patients that they are being asked to volunteer in a trial that will test the hypothesis that the new drug is not more than a certain percentage *worse* than an existing therapy. And if the new drug is superior, the trial will not be able to prove it. Not informing patients who are putting themselves at risk of harm is unethical.

"Placebo-controlled trials are also unethical when an effective therapy already exists," Garattini added, "because they violate the Declaration of Helsinki by keeping patients in the control arm from receiving an effective therapy."

The Mario Negri Institute conducts about 80 clinical trials at any one time involving about 70,000 patients using these ethical standards of beneficence and receives funding from a variety of sources. Because a trial is not started until a complete review of all evidence is carried out and a clear hypothesis is formulated with a strong end point, Mario Negri trials are clinically more important and less costly than industry trials. Figure 0.2 summarizes the key features of a Mario Negri trial. Any nation's legislators or regulators could follow Mario Negri's example and require clinical trials that prove a new drug effectively improves patient-oriented outcomes before approving it.Figure 0.2. Features of a Mario Negri trial.

Unlike most pharmaceutical research centers, the Mario Negri Institute urges patients not to take drugs unless safer, healthier alternatives are insufficient. "People should be given drugs that improve their health at the lowest effective dose possible for the shortest time, because all drugs are toxic." By contrast, commercially funded and designed trials often use high doses to generate evidence of their effectiveness more quickly, even though the high dose usually means there will be stronger toxic reactions, too. If trials are kept short, they will not pick these up, and then the drug is approved as "safe and effective" at an unsafe, high dosage that goes into the label as the recommended dose. A substantial percentage of label changes involve lowering the high dose used in trials, after experience in practice shows that a lower dose is better. The Mario Negri Institute thus represents a radically safer, less costly, and more sensible alternative to the commercial goal of getting as many people on patented drugs as possible.

1. Research trials conceived as an integral part of health care by developing networks of providers as planners, recruiters, and co-authors of the trials, based on practice-relevant questions.[64-66]

2. Designed to reliably measure its impact on patients and public health, based on systematic reviews of evidence regarding existing therapy and the proposed intervention,

3. Tests how much better or worse an intervention is in clinical, patient-oriented terms. Superiority designs. Active comparators and no surrogates, if possible. Appropriate duration of treatment and follow up.

4. Registered in a public register before inclusion of the first participant.

5. Recruits a population representative of those likely to be treated in current clinical practices, minimizing disturbance of their care. Unpaid patient volunteers. Informed of the trial's purposes and importance.

6. The independent trial team controls the design, the data, the analysis, and publication, which happens as soon as possible, irrespective of findings. Raw anonymized data sets are made available to the scientific community upon legitimate request once the trial is completed.

Complete transparency and accountability of research design, implementation and publication.

Figure 0.2   Features of a Mario Negri trial

Scientific or technical innovation, Garattini notes, usually does not translate into better clinical outcomes. The industry defines "innovation" in terms of new molecules; but almost half of them do not prove to be clinically superior to using previously new drugs that have become generic. "We learn a great deal about the science of a given disease every year; but very little that actually helps patients," Garattini said. Only about 10 percent of new medicines in the past decade have been judged by independent review teams of experts as clinically superior,[25] a pattern supported by Le Fanu's history of modern medicine and Healy's recent review of how pharmaceutical companies have invented new diagnostic categories representing new diseases and risks to compensate for running out of sick patients.[26]

Institutional Autonomy for Research Integrity

From an institutional point of view, autonomy has been the most fundamental and radical principle of the Institute. Few European and Italian research institutes had ever been independent of the swings of politics and governments

- No patents will be sought, because patenting distort research, create corrupting dependencies, and build silos of secrecy.

- No contract or grant will be accepted for work not already of interest to the research staff and in their areas of competence. All protocols for research will be supervised by the project's principal researchers.

- With advice from department heads and the director, researchers in each lab will decide what research they want to do and seek funding for it.

- Researchers control their data, its analysis, and its publication. Transparency is essential for good scientific research. All data of a project belong to the Institute and are publicly available. While leading-edge policy is only now discovering how essential access to the raw data is,[64] researchers at the Institute understood this decades ago.

- Self-motivation and self-discipline are key. People manage their own time.

- To maintain independence, no funding from any source will exceed ten percent of the Institute's income. Donations with strings attached are not accepted.

- Expenditures are not to exceed available funds.

- All findings will be published in English, and all articles will be written by the researchers who did the work - no ghost-management or ghost-writing.[11,19,20] The in-house translator/editor works for the Institute and the researchers, not for any third party.

Figure 0.3   Rules for integrity

or from political patronage for favors, and free from what Garattini and the other pioneers experienced as the self-protecting academic fiefdoms of chairs and deans that controlled what young researchers could investigate. In Chapter 1 on the early years, we shall draw on the sociological studies of Renée C. Fox and other scholars to portray the institutional barriers to research integrity and innovation faced by the young researchers as they dreamed of having their own institute.

Institutional autonomy for research integrity meant creating a new kind of institution, inspired by American exemplars but going some steps further. Garattini even sold the shares in the pharmaceutical company that made up most of the initial endowment from the imaginative Mr. Negri, because being dependent on the fortunes of the company or executive pressures might compromise the Institute. Before Garattini had founded the Mario Negri Institute, no one had thought through so fully the organizational principles of institutional independence. They are summarized in Figure 0.3.

No Patents

The logic of institutional autonomy for research integrity applies especially to patents. When the longtime exemption of medicines from patents as a societal good fell under intense industry pressure in the 1970s, the Institute decided after much debate that no discoveries would be patented. Patents and their prospects for revenue can distort research toward what is patentable and most attractive to investors instead of what is most beneficial for patients. Garattini adds, "If you start patenting, your research activities will take a certain pathway." By engendering concerns about who might steal the ideas or discoveries of another, patents can also stifle collaboration, open science, and fruitful synergies across projects. "Patents are an obstacle to collaboration and an incentive to hide data or methods," Garattini wrote us. They discourage team efforts over time, or working on several interrelated approaches to solving a scientific problem.

Sheila Jasanoff, the international authority on science policy at Harvard University, points out that patents also ignore the social construction of innovations. They "presume the existence of identifiable inventors and a single moment of invention."[27] They ignore the "interpretative flexibility" and room for creative modification usually inherent in new discoveries or medicines.[28]

Jasanoff points out that patents bracket unexpected uses and failures once tried, and so can patent holders bent on profiting from them. They also ignore the contingencies built into complex technologies and their interactions with different patients. Sociological studies find that patents "create and naturalize the very objects and rights that [they] claim to protect."[29] While people attribute thinglike properties to inventions, thereby taking them out of the political realm, they "inevitably are repositories of human values, beliefs, imagination, power." Patents "create and maintain property rights in specific forms that are anything but preordained."[30]

There is a deeper effect that patenting has on independent research to find more effective medicines that science and technology studies illustrate, though they have not researched. Laboratories are globally powerful places where medical facts and accounts are more constructed than found. To do that successfully, one needs allies and alliances, including nonhuman elements or contributors.[31] The deep point of science and technology studies is that "facts" are events, or features, reactions that get singled out, defined, and measured as "facts" more than other reactions, events, or features, in negotiated ways.[32] They result from what gets measured and how, what model of reality is used or constructed to put those measurements together, what gets dismissed as "noise" or irrelevant, and what networks or institutions or journals legitimate a presented "fact" as a fact. This involves considerable tacit knowledge and tinkering, not what people normally think of as science.

Researchers negotiate within a lab and then with the outside world how to "see" when something meaningful is happening (pushing aside other things that are happening) and how to represent what is happening through models, an account, and measurements.[33] How, then, do researchers imbued with the potential to patent and profit choose how to model, pursue, measure, and construct accounts differently from researchers imbued with the desire to find a clinically better drug without the potential to patent and profit? To take the infamous example of Vioxx (refocoxib), an anti-inflammatory and pain pill that reduced stomach bleeds in the small percentage of patients with that problem but had several times the risk of thrombotic events, the chief scientist knew early that the deadly risk was built into the mechanism of action.[34] But he and colleagues constructed a scientific account of Vioxx that highlighted the reduced risk of stomach bleeds to characterize Vioxx as the safest Cox-2 drug, while hiding or downplaying its deadly risk.[35] A special sales force was trained to fan out and persuade doctors to switch to Vioxx. Their distortions of good pharma and good science are disturbing.[36] The profit-bent constructions of research made billions, while tens of thousands of patients died. Had independent research teams with no interest in profits run trials like those described in Figure 0.2 that measure all negative as well as positive effects on patients and publish all outcomes, the traumatic effects would have been known at least five years before Vioxx was withdrawn.[37]

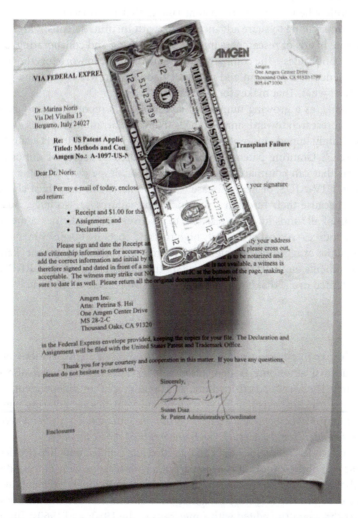

Photo 0.1   Patent rights "sold" for $1 bill, even for a drug priced at $3,600 a dose

For such reasons, the Mario Negri Institute has not applied for patents on any of the many techniques, methods, and drugs that its research teams have developed. There is no Technology Transfer Office because there is no technology to "transfer" since it's all transparent. For example, Amgen asked the Institute to patent the discovery in animal research that EPO (erythropoietin) could reduce rejection in kidney transplantations. Amgen already sold EPO for anemia for about $3,600 per injection and wanted to create a monopoly market where it could charge as much or more by getting a use patent for kidney transplantation. The Institute explained its policy, and we discovered the results, displayed on a bulletin board in the corridor outside a lab: a letter from Amgen's senior patent coordinator confirming the purchase of intellectual property (IP) rights, with a one-dollar bill pinned to the letter as payment in full.

Another benefit of the no-patent rule is that pharmaceutical companies have been willing to share advanced work with Institute scientists, knowing it is in safe hands of researchers interested in sharing and collaborating. Scientists on both sides—the company and the Institute—can work together on the real science of a problem and not worry about who will control the patentability of what. That makes for much better science.

Patents, as a growing number of law professors report, not only redirect medical research toward small changes that can warrant high prices, but they increasingly impede innovation by creating barriers and thickets against new research.[38] Granting patents liberally has resulted in scores of minor innovations that can command very high prices for desperately ill patients with cancer, HIV-AIDS, or heart disease.[39] Companies claim they must charge so much because their research costs, including failures, are so huge. But 84.6 percent of all funds for basic research to discover new medicines comes from public sources so most of the early high risk and costs are borne by taxpayers.[40] Companies exaggerate their high costs for research and development (R&D).[41] Governments and citizens pay about six times more than alleged R&D costs for patented drugs that have few new benefits 90 percent of the time.[42]

Autonomy for Beneficence

The deeper implication of no patents and the other manifestations of real institutional autonomy is that *autonomy serves beneficence and also good research*. The Mario Negri Institute, as a "real utopia" of independent, rigorous, open science exists to serve society and help sick or suffering patients. *Autonomy is not an end in itself to carry out one's mission, but rather a necessity to serve patients and society through uncorrupted medical science.*

For decades, medicine has been regarded as a public good, like fire departments or public schools. It is even part of a conservative view of a good society that fosters the flourishing and autonomy of individuals.[43] Patents are not needed to fire the scientific imagination, and one can see this in the early books that Garattini edited with Americans in the 1950s and 1960s: The eager curiosity and energy of inquiry among the researchers is palpable. In the 1965 preface of a book of excellent new papers on serotonin, Irving Page from the Cleveland Clinic exuded about the unstoppable zeal of researchers at the Mario Negri Institute and many other centers, unrelated to the prospects of patenting or profits:

> People are most extraordinarily ingenious; what they will discover! Serotonin in walnuts and bananas and in jelly-fish and in carcinoids . . . Study of serotonin has occupied thousands of scientists the world over which illustrates perfectly the unifying and cohesive power of [open] research itself.[44]

Such shared and unfettered zeal among researchers is now more guarded than in 1965, as each group devotes half its mental energy to calculating which research strategies and partners are most likely to enable them to start up a biotech corporation based on closely held ideas-as-property for potential profit (which usually does not materialize). Today an observer might write: "Researchers are most extraordinarily ingenious about which strategies will most likely attract venture capitalists and be patentable."

Mario Negri's real utopia of openly collaborative research to figure out how disease mechanisms really work and how to get an effective ingredient to its target may be the exemplar of a new paradigm for much better research at much lower costs. Might restoring patent exemption for medicines and providing greater public funding for independent research end the proliferation of me-too variations created to exploit government-protected high prices?

Nonmaleficence

As the other side of beneficence, the admonition "above all, do no harm" underscores another principle of the Mario Negri Institute. The Institute pioneered techniques for identifying adverse events from medicines[45] and has spoken out against a drug once it finds evidence of harmful side effects. In Chapters 5 and 7, we will describe how this principle opened up new lines of research but also caused the Institute to suffer for carrying out the duty to warn people against drugs being sold and taken by patients for which no good scientific evidence existed that they were beneficial or safe.[46] If the Institute's ethics were emulated more widely, prescription drugs would not be the fourth leading cause of death.[47] Institutional autonomy for research integrity again plays a seminal role as a means to a greater moral end. Garattini told the editors of *Nature*, "This is the value of being an independent institute—you can say what must be said."[48]

To do no harm, leaders at the Mario Negri Institute have advocated much more cautious procedures for launching new medicines. "One cannot do clinical trials that adequately identify harms, and therefore regulators cannot really say new drugs are safe or protect the public from harms or drug disasters," said Garattini based on his seven years of experience at the EMA.

"Safety and efficacy should be based on NNT—the number needed to treat to make one patient better—and NNH—the number needed to harm one patient." Once a drug is approved, there should be "controlled prescribing for the first years, only for the approved indication, and active vigilance by an independent safety board."

By contrast, current practices maximize the number of patients put at risk for harmful side effects before either the safety or effectiveness of new drugs is known—massive launches as soon as regulators approve a new medicine, including surreptitious marketing for unapproved uses through well-paid networks or leading specialists, writers, and journalists.[49] "The bias against scientific evidence of harms is why toxicology is not flourishing," Garattini continued. "Toxicology involves by its nature 'breaking the toys' of the companies. We need *active*, independent pharmacovigilance, not passive reporting."

The normative and practical ethics of the Mario Negri Institute may strike readers as noble but impractical, even as impediments to growth and success. Yet it has grown and won the hearts of millions as a revered, impartial yet caring source of innovative research and scientific advice that has been called upon to serve the nation. In the Institute's twentieth year, the editors of *Nature* titled their assessment, "American Inspiration in Milan: Mario Negri Pharmacology Institute." They reported:

> The Mario Negri Institute for Research in Pharmacology in Milan is tops. It is consistently in the US National Institutes of Health (NIH) list of top ten most-funded foreign institutes (at least twice it has taken top rank) and its director, Professor Silvio Garattini, was one of only four Italian scientists to have reached the Institute of Scientific Information's list of 1,000 most-cited scientists.[50]

In the spring of 2012, we asked Garattini, "Whom would you most like to read this book?" He replied, "Young people. So they will know things don't have to be as they are and they can change them . . . [pause] and administrators and politicians. So they will see how valuable new organizational forms can be."

Part I

Developing a Research Institute for Society

I

Origins and an American Vision for an Ethical, Independent Research Institute

When he was only 33, Silvio Garattini gave up a stellar career at the University of Milan as deputy chair and heir-apparent to the Department of Pharmacology to realize his vision of an independent pharmacological research institute, free of academic fiefdoms, stifling bureaucracies, and political or commercial influence, to develop better drugs for humanity. His strong, independent spirit and drive were developed during a childhood of hard work and self-sufficiency.

Born November 12, 1928, Silvio was the eldest of three sons who grew up in a humble home in Bergamo. Silvio's father had become an orphan at an early age, losing his father to a heart attack and his mother to a broken heart. He had to raise himself, and Silvio said his father raised him and his brothers strictly. Even in elementary school, Silvio's father reviewed his homework, and, if he thought it inadequate, he made Silvio do it again. He became Silvio's most important role model. "He taught me to think critically, and not believe everything you see."[1]

Silvio described his mother as quiet and sweet. She suffered from an early accident with scalding water that contributed to her becoming partly paralyzed and in constant pain. The boys were close and ran much of the household between them. In addition, one of his brothers contracted spondylitis when Silvio was 12 and became disabled. Spondylitis stiffens and inflames the disc spaces between the vertebrae, and his brother had to lie supine on a special bed to keep the vertebrae separate. Health insurance at that time only covered a limited number of visits; so Silvio's father, who had a low-paying job at a bank, did the payroll for a local business in the evening for additional income to pay for the specialty care.

During World War II, Silvio was exempted from the army because his thorax was too thin; but, in 1944, his father was called to the military and asked his 16-year-old son to take over the work. "This gave me an early sense of organization and bookkeeping," he said, the first foundation in a constellation of skills and experience on which he would draw for years to come.

When he turned 15 in 1943, Silvio and his parents talked constantly about which kind of school Silvio should attend next and decided that he should attend an industrial technical high school in Bergamo to acquire practical skills. Silvio took classes in the morning, especially industrial chemistry, and spent all afternoon doing labs, where instructors graded students on the precision of their assays. When he graduated at age 19 in 1947, Silvio received "the most important degree I got in my life." Knowledge of chemistry and refined lab skills added two more foundations on which Garattini built his career. He could not find a job in chemistry, however, and earned his keep as an analyst at a steel factory. In this unwanted job, Silvio envisioned his future—medicine.

During this period, Silvio acquired a strong moral outlook that has shaped the Institute and the rest of his life. His father was anti-Fascist and did not want him to join Giovani Balilla, the Fascist youth movement. He was very thin and did not qualify for the military. When he was 14, Silvio joined the Azione Cattolica, the main Catholic association at the time, where he participated regularly in meetings and social activities in Bergamo. By the time he was 20, he became a regional manager of the student branch of Azione Cattolica and organized conferences, several about religion in contrast to the anticlericalism of Marxist groups, and he overcame his shyness through public speaking.

From these experiences, Silvio concluded that "You shall love your neighbor as yourself" is the most important commandment and the foundation for social ethics. One pillar standing on that foundation is human dignity and respect for each person, regardless of different individual qualities and characteristics. The sanctity of human life is inherent in the moral principle of human dignity. Human dignity calls for absolute honesty and the absence of malice or manipulation. One shall not cheat, manipulate, deceive, or deal falsely.

A second pillar is compassion and charity, especially for the poor, the sick, the suffering, and the dispossessed. One should do all one can to respond to unmet needs and to the calls from those in need, like the Good Samaritan who interrupted his journey to respond to a half-dying man and outcast.

A beam bolted across these two pillars is the principle of solidarity among others in the community and society and the pursuit of common good with them. Our responsibility toward one another is the foundation for human rights. This provides the basis for governments building institutions of common good, such as education and research.

Envisioning a future in medicine motivated Silvio to undertake a feat of will. Silvio's graduation from the working-class industrial technical high school did not qualify him to apply to a university or to medical school, while graduates of Liceo Classico (classical high school where affluent children learned Greek and Latin) or Liceo Scientifico (math, physics, chemistry, and philosophy) could apply directly. To overcome this institutional form of class discrimination, Silvio needed a degree from a Lyceum, a three-year course

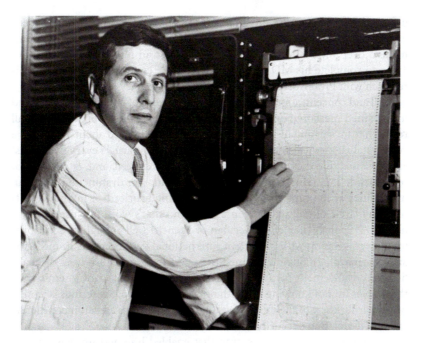

Photo 1.1   Silvio Garattini in Milan, age 35

he could not afford. So three months before the Lyceum exams, he quit his job, crammed in his room day and night, and passed. This collapsing of three years into three months enabled him to apply in 1948 to the medical school at the University of Milan, which accepted him. He found a part-time job as a secretary to cover living expenses while taking first-year classes.

In his third year of medical school, the course in pharmacology appealed as an area that drew on Silvio's training in chemistry and lab work in ways that could enable him to help sick patients. The chairman of the department, Professor Emilio Trabucchi, asked for volunteers to give a lecture, and Silvio prepared one on antihistamines. "I took advantage of my chemical background. I could show different types of structures and demonstrate which groups showed activity. The professor was impressed and said, 'Why don't you come and work here?' "[2] In this moment, Silvio's disadvantage of attending an industrial technical high school turned into an advantage, because none of the more affluent and educated colleagues knew organic chemistry and its techniques for measurement. On several future occasions, Silvio drew on techniques used in industrial chemistry to pioneer their application and methods in medicine and pharmacology. With Professor Trabucchi, he began a research project on the kinetics of procaine or Novocain.

In 1953, Silvio gave a guest lecture at the Lombardy Academy of Science and Letters, where the professor of medicine assumed he was already a doctor. When he learned that Silvio was only a 24-year-old student and one he did not recognize as having taken his course (because he had not), he became irate and refused to grant Silvio access to the examination in clinical medicine. This prejudicial use of academic power and its professorial fiefdoms made a deep impression. Silvio was forced to transfer to the University of Turin to complete his MD degree in 1954, while commuting to continue his research with Professor Trabucchi.

Will and concentration, together with knowledge of organic chemistry and fine-grained measurement of chemical traces led Silvio to organize a small research team starting in 1952. He authored or coauthored about 10 articles a year in Italian medical and scientific journals—a new article every five weeks! He explained that they were short, not seriously refereed, and, of course, not read outside Italy. This led Silvio to recognize another dysfunction of Italian universities at the time: the ritual of producing articles bya marginal, self-referring circle of colleagues who cited each other's work because they did not know English (nor often German or French) well enough to contribute to, or even keep up with important international developments in medicine and pharmacology. Silvio explained to us, "Articles in English were disqualified for advancement because Italian professors did not want to embarrass themselves for not knowing it." With notable exceptions, the serious scientific world hardly knew of their existence. One might call this a guaranteed hierarchy of self-isolating obscurity.

A key feature of Silvio's research that enabled him and his team to win grants and contracts centered on developing pharmacokinetics, based in part on techniques he transposed from organic chemistry. In 1953, he started using colorimetry and then added spectrofluorometry and gas chromatography at the end of the 1950s.

By 1955, Silvio earned a "Libera Docenza" or PhD in chemotherapy, and in 1958 another in pharmacology. He also received the Marzotto Prize in Medicine in 1954 for research on drugs for tuberculosis and the Prix de la Ville from Bergamo in 1955. The following year he received the prize from the Cariplo Bank. He was appointed as an assistant professor in the Department of Pharmacology, and in 1957 Professor Trabucchi de facto appointed him as the deputy chair of the department at age 29. "I worked day and night, and some nights I didn't sleep at all," he said. Meantime, Trabucchi became a Member of Parliament and spent much of his time in Rome, leaving Silvio to informally run the department and cope with the academic bureaucracy first hand.

The Bigger Picture

Why would a brilliant young scientist, chosen by a powerful patron and rapidly promoted to deputy chair and heir-apparent to an academic fiefdom, want to risk all to create a new institute independent of the public university system? The bigger picture was described by the distinguished medical sociologist Renée C. Fox, in a widely read 1962 article that the editors of *Science* took almost unchanged.[3] It provided such a fine-grained analysis of obstacles faced by young scientists in Europe, especially after they had experienced the egalitarian atmosphere in the United States during a visiting fellowship, where what counted was fresh ideas and quality, not hierarchy and connections. Fox's "Medical Scientists in a Château" created an international controversy and a deep rethinking about post–World War II research programs designed to restore Europe's great scientific prowess, because it described how such programs were stymied by a country's own institutional structures, rules, and customs. Fox wrote about medical research in Belgium; but much of it rang true for pharmacological research in Italy and other countries.

Fox began by describing the "sociologically encompassing" list of guests invited to a medical scientific colloquium. "The diversity and importance of extramedical influences on research and research careers is suggested by the presence . . . of political and religious personages, nobles, financiers, and patients and their families." An ancient château was chosen as the site, and the invitation list strained for equality among the classes, factions, academies, societies, government departments, and institutes. Ritualistic attempts to create cross-cutting equality led to projects being "slow-moving, often delay-ridden, and sometimes indefinitely blocked." For example, a major new hospital started 25 years earlier was not yet completed. Blockage or paralysis, in turn, led to finding circumventions, to using or creating *petits chemins*, and to the "complicated, time-consuming, never-ending process of writing eloquent, inquiring, imploring, demanding, grateful letters; of making formal and informal visits to strategic officials; and of sitting on numerous commissions." Parties involved developed elaborate ways to meet competing demands of units or parties equitably, rather than rewarding scientific merit. The principal scientific commissions and councils were made up of senior professors who ruled over their fiefdoms, so that the research applications under review usually came from one of them, a self-perpetuating circle of an aging scientific elite who decided who among them would receive how much.

The château of the academy seemed to have a basement and a top floor, Fox suggested, with the middle floors nearly empty. The professor hires junior researchers to positions with low pay, little security, and basement status— and they are grateful for the patronage. Every decade or so, one of them might be elevated to the top floor. Belgian political parties, an observer wrote, "are equally consecrated to impotence. The necessity to act splinters all their divisions: in the face of this kind of peril [the need to act], without fail they put off until tomorrow what they could not settle today." This influential account of post–World War II science in Belgium resonates with the frustrations of young scientists like Garattini in the 1950s.

Turning more specifically to Italy, the great sociologist of comparative education, Burton Clark, wrote a book that complements Garattini's assessment of a career in academia, *Academic Power in Italy: Bureaucracy and Oligarchy in a National University System*.[4] He traced the Italian universities to their twelfth century guilds and described how over time doctrinal rigidity became an important retarding force. "The Italian university proved especially hostile to science," he wrote in 1977. Historic centralization was reinforced during the Fascist period. Thus "Italian public administration is an extreme case . . . of balkanized bureaucracy." More widely, only 20 percent of young people attended secondary school in 1960, and half did not complete primary school. Only 4 percent of young adults had a university degree, and the median education of adults was fifth grade. In various ways, Clark wrote, "the Italian system has systematically and on a massive scale discouraged students from going on."

The central-agency bureaucrats in effect shielded professors who ran their own local fiefdoms. This created a double balkanization—small pyramids all within one huge national pyramid of centralized bureaucracy, but weak in central power. Although academic positions were centrally determined and appointments reviewed by the Ministry in Rome, the real power lay in the local chairs, like Trabucchi, who were often reelected for years. This was the institutional context in which Garattini and his colleagues found themselves.

An Inspired Trip and Conference

One of Garattini's friends, Alfredo Leonardi, had an American mother who was related to the Pfieffer family who founded a patent-medicine company in the 1880s and was bought by William R. Warner Company in the 1920s. Through acquisitions, it grew to become the Warner-Lambert pharmaceutical company, which was acquired by Pfizer in 2000. As a fellow, frustrated Italian physician and young researcher, Leonardi suggested a trip in the summer of 1957 to "America," as many Europeans like to call the United States, to visit American research institutes. Already by then, Garattini was winning grants from the US National Cancer Institute, which in the spirit of the Marshall Plan was funding projects to build up European research teams. He also had a contract with the US Army to study the safety of contraceptives, because women were being recruited into the ranks.

That spring, Garattini organized an international conference in Milan on psychotropic substances that brought to his door as his guests leading researchers from Oxford, Paris, Geneva, Montreal, Brussels, Berlin, and, especially, United States—from the NIH, Yale, UCLA, Pittsburg, as well as the research centers of major pharmaceutical companies. Professor Trabucchi supported the idea, which was important because Garattini was too young to organize a major international conference without a senior sponsor. He and his colleagues investigated serotonin, found mainly in the gut, and found tiny traces in the brain—the early exploration that led to SSRI drugs for major depression. Ever the master of measurement, Garattini exploited the advance from the spectrophotometer to the spectrofluorimeter to measure these traces in low concentrations. But as an empiricist, he thought the evidence that SSRI drugs helped reduce major depression was mixed, as was evidence for other antidepressants. "There has been no important progress after 1959," he told David Healy in the mid-1990s.[5]

After the conference, Silvio coedited the proceedings in *Psychotropic Drugs*.[6] In part of a historical overview of psychopharmacology, David Healy characterized it as "well the first modern book on psychopharmacology [based on] the very first psychopharmacology meeting."[7] Drawing on his student conference days, Garattini, only 29, organized this internationally seminal meeting. He felt there "was really a new branch of pharmacology." This proved correct, and Garattini's group made important contributions.

The conference led to founding the Collegium International Neuropsychopharmacologium (http://www.cinp.org). "Neuropharmacology, in fact, was born in St. Tropez, during a meeting between Dr. Brodie, Dr. Costa and myself." Brodie and Costa were two giants of the field at the time. Alfredo Leonardi, a young and imaginative scientist who would cofound the Mario Negri Institute with Garattini, organized the meeting in St. Tropez. Most seminal was Brodie, "the man who established the basis for pharmacokinetics, drug metabolism, and the importance of measuring blood levels,"[8] key features of research by Garattini's group and the work they would soon develop at the new Institute.

With these contacts, Garattini corresponded with leading American researchers, such as Bernard Brodie and Julius Axelrod, and arranged appointments to visit various branches of the National Institutes of Health, the Rockefeller Institute, the Gustavus and Lousie Pfeiffer Research Foundation in New York, and several academic (New York University, Sloan-Kettering, Stanford University, MIT, University of Chicago, Galesburg Hospital, NIH) and industrial (Lederle, Wallace, Warner-Lambert) research centers. Although Silvio worked his way through scientific English with a dictionary, he knew little conversational English and studied intensively for two months before departing at the end of July 1957.

The summer visits to the United States opened the eyes of the two young researchers to new possibilities. First, they saw that research could be a full-time profession, as distinct from "a means of collecting credits and publishing papers [in journals few read] to improve one's university career."[9] "In Italy, if you were at the university, you did research and you published, because this was the way to get promoted. If you were in industry, of course you did research the industry required [to increase profits]."[10] But, in an independent research institute, you could devote yourself to the best research as an end in itself.

Second, they realized there could be a variety of institutional arrangements for serious, full-time research—foundations that did intramural research by their own staff as well as foundations that did extramural research by funding others; government research institutes independent of political meddling; and public as well as private universities with research institutes set up within them. Garattini gave lectures about their research wherever he visited, and some invited him to join their research staff. He was particularly impressed by how the Institute of Psychiatry in Gettysburg worked side by side with clinical services, an arrangement he came to emulate years later as part of an ideal research institute that did translational, personalized investigations in order to find out how best to treat a patient's condition, 30 years before "translational" and "personalized" became features of science policy.

After he returned from the United States in September 1957, Garattini decided to tell his research team and young colleagues that either they should all go to one of the American institutes where he had been invited, or set up their own pharmacological research institute in order to avoid the strictures and meddling of Italian universities and public bureaucracies. It could be private yet serve the public and be nonprofit. "I said, 'If we are serious about doing this research, either we go to the US or we do something different here.' And the idea was to do something in our country."[11] The 15–20 researchers around Garattini resolved to seek funding to establish an independent research institute in Italy and began looking for funding. He liked the foundation model because it is more independent of government or academic bureaucracies and yet can be dedicated to serving society on a nonprofit basis. Responses to his talking about this pie-in-the-sky idea varied. "Some people laughed. Some people were not interested. Some said: you are too young, you should stay at the university." In the meantime, Garattini won a grant from Warner Lambert to investigate the biosynthesis of cholesterol, a grant from the National Institutes of Health on antitumor chemotherapy, and a contract with the US Army on the biosynthesis of cholesterol. He organized another international symposium on the metabolism of lipids in 1960 and edited *Drugs Affecting Lipid Metabolism* in 1961.[12]

A Jeweler with a Vision

Mario Negri was a well-known goldsmith and jeweler who owned an elegant shop on the glamorous Via Montenapoleone in Milan. Born in 1891, he became a master jeweler and bought out the shop—a self-made man known for his personal integrity. He then decided to find a way to manufacture attractive pieces rather than make them by hand so that the middle classes could afford fine jewelry. He built an integrated business, owning every phase and the shops in which the pieces were sold. He made millions but did not change his modest lifestyle. Instead, Mr. Negri became fascinated with drugs and research studies in biomedicine. He purchased a small pharmaceutical company, Farmacosmici, a subsidiary of Burroughs-Wellcome, which was then a nonprofit pharmaceutical research enterprise that gave its profits to the Wellcome Trust.

In 1958, Mr. Negri went to Professor Trabucchi to ask about difficulties getting a drug approved, a business man with little formal education at the door of a great professor: "There is a business man who wants to talk to you, Professor. Shall I let him in?"

Being very busy with political affairs, Trabucchi suggested he talk with his able young associate, Silvio Garattini. Mr. Negri found his advice helpful enough that he returned later to ask other questions and to request a collaboration on studying new chemicals. In the following years, the two discussed other pharmacological research questions, as well as the state of pharmacological research and the need for an independent research foundation.

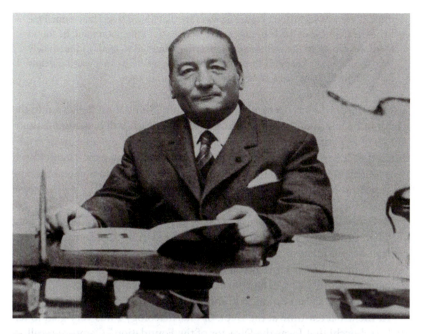

Photo 1.2　Mario Negri: from master jeweler to philanthropist of research

When I asked Mr. Negri, like I asked everyone, "Why don't you help us set up a foundation where we can do independent research?" he responded simply, "Why not?" Then he added, "But you are too young! Let's think about it."[13]

Garattini and Mr. Negri met several times and discussed what kind of research the foundation should do, what kind of rules should guide its operation, and how it could obtain funding. Mr. Negri's wife died and he became more interested in Silvio as a young man with a vision of an independent, first-class research institute. Then cancer struck Mario Negri quickly, and the chances of their plans becoming a reality began to fade. "But then," Garattini recounted, "about a couple of weeks before he passed away, he called me and asked to visit him in the hospital. He told me, 'Don't worry. I have done what we discussed and whatever happens to me, everything will be fine.'"[14] Garattini wrote us:

Mario Negri passed away on April 6, 1960 with our deep sorrow. He had no family except a nephew who was informed about Mario Negri's intention to establish a Foundation. A couple of weeks after his death, the notary sent out a note for the opening of the will. Prof. Trabucchi was invited and when he came back he reported with enthusiasm that Mario Negri left 900 million lira [about $1.5 million at that time] to establish a Foundation that should be located at the University because several professors were members of the Board of Trustees.

One can imagine our desperation. All our hopes and efforts were vanishing. It was a very bad day! A few days afterward, I called the nephew of Mario Negri to get some information and, in particular, to ask why I was not mentioned in the will. He was surprised because he was sure that Mario Negri had named me to be the Director of the Foundation. He went back to the notary and he found there was a note in the will that the notary had omitted to read. I immediately informed Alfredo Leonardi through the window, where he was waiting below for my signal. There was a great enthusiasm in our group.

Mr. Negri's will left his fortune to establish a "foundation dedicated to the health of people and pharmacological research, which will be named Istituto di Ricerche Farmacologiche Mario Negri." Silvio and his colleagues established that it would be a place "where Italian and foreign experts can investigate medicines capable of curing diseases" in three areas: chemotherapy for cancer, medicines affecting the metabolism of lipids, and psychotropic medications.

He established a board of trustees that included the rector of the University of Milan, the dean of the medical school, the head of the Institute of Pharmacology, the president of the Policlinico, his nephew, and three "professional people," but no one from regional or national government. Mr. Negri envisioned the Institute as a center for international research that would set up exchanges with "savant estrangers" and host international symposia.

"At the usual tea-time at the Dept. of Pharmacology I was very glad to tell Prof. Trabucchi that I was the Director of the Foundation," Garattini recalled. "At that point, since all the members of the Board were named ex-officio, I was the only person that was authorized to make all the necessary steps to establish the Foundation. However, Prof. Trabucchi and the Dean of the University started a lot of pressure to avoid the detachment of the Foundation from the University. Since I was very close to getting a chair, they wanted to convince me to accept the chair; but I was determined to carry out the will of Mario

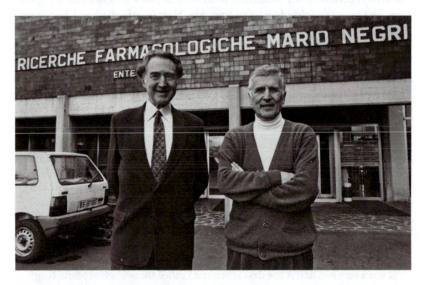

Photo 1.3 The Institute's co-founders, Alfredo Leonardi and Silvio Garattini

Negri to establish a Foundation independent from academia, industry and government. It was not easy."

Trabucchi urged Garattini to accept a professorship as well as direct the new Institute so that it would be part of the Department of Pharmacology. But Garattini said this was not possible, because having the Institute independent of any university or other institution was critical to Mr. Negri. Garattini said, "His great entrepreneurial merit was that of always looking forward and never stopping. He was speaking about innovation and research sixty years ago, when these words were practically unknown."[15]

The endowment consisted of 250 million lire in cash and an estimated 650 million in stock of Farmacosmici. Although the stock seemed bound to rise, Garattini persuaded the finance committee of the Institute to sell it. This established a strong precedent of independence from corporate as well as government ties that was to shape other critical decisions in the coming years, even if the revenues of Farmacosmici could have been very important for the survival of the Institute. He did not want the Institute to develop or make decisions dependent on how it might affect possible profits or relations with another institution.

Establishing Institutional Independence

Garattini set about establishing the Mario Negri Institute for Pharmacological Research with both the Italian and American governments. In the United States, the Treasury Department recognized it as a nonprofit organization in 1961—a vital status for grants, contracts, and donations from American organizations, foundations, and the NIH. In Italy, it had be recognized by Presidential Decree, yet another example of how political rules, regulations, and influence create obstacles that can compromise clear scientific priorities and projects. Garattini drew on all the leading politicians and ministers with whom he had worked as deputy chair of the department to ask for help. It took one year; but a Presidential Decree was signed in 1961. With a touch of irony, Garattini said, "First we were recognized by the American government and then later by the Italian government."[16] *Chemical and Engineering News* hailed it as "another milestone on Italy's road toward more scientific and industrial sophistication," set up "outside the traditional educational, industrial, and governmental channels."[17]

Even more vital was to gain recognition and credibility with first-rate researchers and their technical staff. Garattini already had his own team of 31 at the University of Milan and invited colleagues whose work he liked to leave and come with him. In effect, he was asking them to leave their university posts and cast their lot with a kind of research institute that had never existed in the country before—in fact existed only on paper and in his imagination—and that threatened existing institutions embedded in the power structure of the state by implying that first-class research was difficult to achieve in them. Not all agreed to come across, but Garattini persuaded 21 of his team to join him.[18]

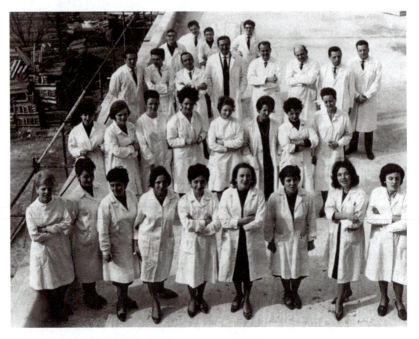

Names of people in the photo of 1963:

First line, from left to right: Consolo Silvana, Dal Bo Maria Lida, Krassich, Perdomini, thesist, Jori Armanda, Veneroni Erminia, Marcucci Franca, Airoldi Luisa

Second line, from left to right: Bonaccorsi Aurora, Kruger, Bernardi Daniela, Mapelli Rosanna, Albricci Annisa, Bizzi Adalgisa, Codegoni Annamaria, Guaitani Amalia

Third line, from left to right: Mussini Emilio, Garattini Silvio, Valzelli Luigi, Leonardi Alfredo, Morasca Luciano, Palma Valentino, Giachetti Antonio, Nanni E.

Fourth line, from left to right: technicians in training: Marchesini Massimo, thesist, Guadagni Luigi, thesist.

Photo 1.4 The founding pioneers of the Institute

Professor Garattini (as nearly everyone came to address him) had to decide whether the new Institute should operate on the interest from the endowment or try to use the entire endowment to build an institute and grow from there by competing for grants or contracts. He sought the advice of the president of the bank in Lombardi from which he had once won a prize, Cassa di Risparmio delle Provincie Lombarde (CARIPLO). He advised Garattini to use the endowment to grow and offered a low-interest 25-year loan of 130 million lire, which with inflation would in fact cost the new Institute very little.

Garattini then looked for a site and realized that one of his board members was the president of Milan's largest hospital, which owned large tracts of land. One tract in Via Eritrea was available for a low price in a low-income area on the outskirts of the city, and Garattini bought it, eager to start building. A local carrot farmer, however, said they would have to wait for him to harvest his crop before breaking ground. Garattini bought out his crop on the spot: "Never has so much been paid for a field of carrots!"

Meantime, the pioneers had to continue working at the university department in close proximity to Professor Trabucchi and the staff who were staying in place. One of these was Rosanna Mapelli, who became Garattini's secretary for the next 49 years. On June 29, 2012, we drove with the Institute's English editor, Judith Baggott, out to Ms. Mapelli's classic, lovely home with a pretty garden, to find her walking toward us, 82 but eager to greet us. She first met Professor Garattini (as she called him) in 1954, she recalled, at the Department of Pharmacology, where she also met her husband, a pharmacologist. She had left a job at a pharmaceutical company to become Professor Trabucchi's personal assistant, and he promised her a contract but never drew one up; so she worked for him without pay. When we asked about this, she told us she did not object or inquire and lived with her parents.

She recalled that after his summer trip to America, Garattini was convinced his team needed an independent research institute, even though Trabucchi held Garattini in high esteem. When Mr. Negri left his fortune to endow the Institute and selected Garattini as its Director, we asked her why so many were willing to leave their posts and join him? "They knew him well, and they had worked together for years," she replied. "They wanted to do their own work, set their own course, and pursue the research they thought was most promising." She said that right away, with Leonardi in charge of public affairs, Garattini started giving public talks, going on early television, and writing columns in popular newspapers and magazines.

We also asked her why so many of the pioneers were women? She replied that Garattini was very open about gender and also the kind of degree one had, so long as one was talented and did good work. Working at the Institute, with its informal atmosphere, led to many marriages.

Plans for an independent research institute drew fire from universities and senior faculty, who discouraged their advanced students from going there. But the new institute drew international attention and also support within Italy as a catalyst for strengthening Italy's presence in the field of science.

From the beginning, Garattini persuaded his group to join him in embracing new principles that promoted independence and the opportunity to do outstanding research. First, the founding members agreed to publish only in English scientific journals and to turn the university rule on its head: Only articles in English would count as serious contributions. Second, they agreed that all research findings should be available to any serious party who wanted to see them, including failures and negative results. Open science and sharing both methods as well as results accelerates scientific progress. Third, they agreed to break with the long academic tradition of snubbing or not talking with the media and public about the complexities of high science by doing the opposite—speaking and explaining what they were doing and why to the

(a)

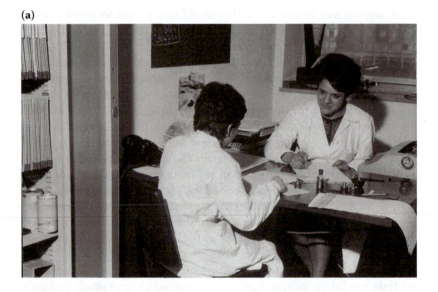

(b)

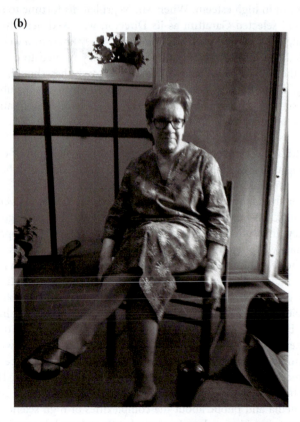

Photo 1.5 Silvio Garattini's long-time secretary, Rosanna Mapelli, (a) 1964 and (b) 2012

media and lay audiences. Fourth, Garattini led the pioneers to agree to an informal, flat organizational structure, no more than 2–3 layers of hierarchy and an open-door form of leadership at each lab and for the Institute as a whole. In addition, the difference between the highest and lowest salary was less than fourfold as it continues to be.

2

The Formative Years— Leadership, Culture, and Organization

In a classic on organizational culture and leadership, the distinguished professor of business management, Edgar Schein holds that "the only thing of real importance that leaders do is to create and manage culture . . . the source of the beliefs and values that get a group moving in dealing with its internal and external problems."[1]

In the years before the Mario Negri Institute opened its doors in 1963, Silvio Garattini formed an organizational culture as he brought colleagues together to research projects of shared interest and to win grants. Garattini did two other things of real importance: He provided original ideas and unique methods that enabled the teams in his group to win grants or contracts, and he taught them how to write first-class grant applications and scientific articles. As young researchers, they worked in teams and shared their research findings and developed an egalitarian peer culture. In contrast to the hierarchical university culture around them, where one never challenged what "the professor" said, they critiqued each other's methods and findings in the spirit of open science observed in leading American and British laboratories. Thus much of what Edgar Schein describes about how organizational culture begins was already taking place as this renegade band of talented researchers carried on with their research at the university during the day and met after hours to plan and develop a strong collective identity around shared values and goals.

Schein defines organizational culture as a pattern of basic values, norms, practices, and habits of thinking that a group develops as it solves problems of external adaptation and internal integration.[2] In this case, the young researchers found common ground in their discontents with the university fiefdoms and culture, described in Chapter 1, that stifled the new kinds of research, methods, and practices they valued. The first steps that Schein identified include: obtaining a shared understanding of one's core *mission* and strategy; developing consensus on *goals* based on that mission; developing consensus on the *means* to achieve those goals; and agreeing on *how to measure* progress toward those goals.

Garattini set as the mission of the new Institute to do research of international quality to improve people's health, based on independent, transparent science, and openly used to educate doctors and patients about how best to address their health needs. Over many conversations, the original pioneers developed a consensus and commitment to this mission. Besides keeping control of their data and findings, they also kept control of their research and methods by not accepting funds for research on subjects outside their expertise. These are familiar values and practices of classic science dating back to the founding of the Royal Society in 1660, but not so easy to achieve when companies offer substantial funds to investigate different topics of commercial interest to them. Seeking patents can have the same distorting effects as researchers shape their research to maximize chances of attracting venture capital. As we shall see, this led Garattini and the Institute to decide not to patent any of their discoveries.

The pioneers of the Mario Negri Institute were determined to minimize how the preferences of major funders might compromise their independence by distorting the direction or the quality of research, because this creates what is called "institutional corruption" or the corrupting of an institution's societal mission.[3] In pharmacological research, the young pioneers had seen how corporate funders influence and often compromise what drugs are developed, how research is done, and how the findings are published or suppressed. These problems have continued to bias research on medicines right into the twenty-first century, misleading decades of physicians and their patients, and producing scores of drugs with few benefits to offset their risks of harm.[4] The Mario Negri pioneers had the rash conviction that if they kept control of the research design and methods for addressing a problem, and if they did really superior research based on the classic ethics of rigorous science, with methods, data, and outcomes open to outside review, then corporations, governments, and others would fund their work. In 1980, Leonardi and colleagues summarized the nature of research at the Mario Negri as "investigating the innermost mechanisms of living organisms, by discovering why certain diseases occur, and by learning what happens in the body when a 'foreign' substance, such as a drug or medicine, enters it. The Institute's research path starts at the molecular level and extends to studies involving the whole body."[5] A 1990 report of the Institute summarized its culture this way:

> a moral institute completely independent of industry, the state, and universities, working with maximum freedom, without bureaucratic interference, without political pressures, with the efficiency of a private organization but working for the public. All results are never protected by patents and are available unconditionally to everyone.

A second goal was to establish experiences for advanced training for younger and more established researchers in how Mario Negri research teams did their work. Together with active participation in international networks and organizing symposia, these activities quickly connected the new Institute to an international community of first-class researchers, especially concerning their initial research work.

A third early goal was to reach out and connect to people from all walks of life, to manifest what Erik Olin Wright calls a "real utopia"[6] of an independent, nonprofit research institute dedicated to finding better medicines and sharing the best of medical research in a demystified, transparent way that addressed the concerns and needs of individuals. This idea flaunted the customs of scientists and professors then, who did not deign to talk with the public about the complexities of their research. Garattini and Leonardi turned these customs on their head by reaching out to lay audiences about their work and relevant issues of concern on television and the radio, in newspapers and magazines, and in public lectures.

Pharmaceutical companies, of course, have extensive public relations operations, but with the goal of expanding markets and increasing profits, especially with patent-protected products, by creating or increasing awareness of disorders for which they have drugs to sell. Examples include "educating" women about menopause as a "deficiency disease" in the 1980s that could be "treated" by taking hormone replacement therapy, or fostering a fear of high cholesterol as a serious health risk, or creating "osteopenia" as the commercialized diluted form of osteoporosis to get millions to take drugs with little benefit to offset their risks of harm.[7] By contrast, as a community of independent scientists, the Mario Negri Institute provided lay audiences with something they had never experienced: the best scientists in the country giving them straight talk about their concerns and about health risks, including ineffective and dangerous drugs described in Chapters 7 and 8. Led by the warm, exuberant Leonardi, who seemed to know everybody in Italian society, and by the soft-spoken Garattini, who routinely wrote columns in national periodicals and appeared on talk shows, everyone soon came to know about the new Institute. Garattini has continued these activities throughout his long career and they are described in Chapter 4.[8]

Institutionally, this goal or vision of a private research institute dedicated to the needs of people shaped the Institute's role in helping to determine the risks to residents when the nation's worst chemical explosion occurred in 1978 (Chapter 5), in telling people about dangerous drugs their doctors were prescribing during the 1970s and 1990s (Chapter 7), or in founding a center where people with rare diseases could get expert assessment and advice in the 1980s (Chapter 3).

Over time, the Institute became a beacon of scientific integrity on which society and governments came to rely. From this goal they built up a broad following of people eager to learn more about how research is done, about their health problems, and about how to avoid harmful or doubtful interventions. For example, Garattini's skepticism about herbal remedies rested on how poor the scientific evidence was about which active ingredient was doing what in which organs. His critique of homeopathic products rested on evidence that the active ingredients are too diluted to have any effect at all. In time, as explained in Chapter 6, the Institute research staff also helped

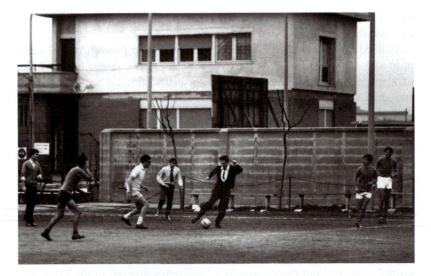

Photo 2.1   Last photo of Silvio Garattini with a tie

assemble national networks of specialists across the country in order to design and run large-scale clinical trials on important questions to help sick patients and to upgrade services on a national scale.

Finally, Garattini led the Pioneers to agree to an informal, flat organizational structure, with no more than two or three layers of hierarchy and an open-door form of leadership at each lab and for the Institute as a whole. To symbolize this principle, Garattini stopped wearing a tie after he returned from his visit to the United States. He did not wear a tie even when meeting the president of Italy or receiving the Legion d'Honneur from the French government in 1984. There was Garattini in his white turtleneck, surrounded by dignitaries in black tie and tails. The last photo found of him wearing a tie was taken in 1965.

Organization

Initially, research at the Institute clustered around three areas: psychopharmacology, where Garattini had already achieved international prominence, cardiovascular disease, and cancer—a new field of little interest in pharmacology at the time. A defining skill and characteristic of the research was the ability to measure small quantities of an active ingredient and trace its effects in various organs, the blood, or the brain. Measurement broadened out to early mastery of clinical epidemiology as a new field and to what today is called "personalized medicine." When a film crew came to shoot a segment about pharmocogenetics and "personalized medicine" in 2012, Claudio Pantarotto, the head of the external relations office, remarked, "We did that in 1968." Professor Garattini explained that a lot of early work centered on pharmacokinetics—how a drug is absorbed, distributed, metabolized, and excreted. It formed the heart of quantitative pharmacology. Measuring drug concentrations with sensitivity and specificity is difficult because there are so many other elements and factors affecting a given intervention. These measurements became ever more fine-grained as instrumentation advanced from colorimetry in the 1950s to gas chromatography and then liquid chromatography and mass spectrometry in the 1960s. A much more complicated picture resulted than companies presented when they developed and promoted new compounds.

First, drugs are metabolized into a large number of metabolites that exceed the quantity of the drug administered. Metabolites may be pharmacologically active, in some cases in the same direction of the drug administered, but in other cases antagonistic to it. Some metabolites may be inactive from a pharmacological point of view but toxic to some tissues or organs. Second, drug concentrations vary by person for genetic reasons, because enzymes that metabolize drugs are coded by DNA, and also by "environmental" factors such as smoking or use of other drugs at the same time. Third, drugs must interact with given receptors, but the expression of those receptors varies and also depends on genetic factors. Thus depending on all these determinants of drug action, the same drug administered for the same disease may be more or less effective or toxic in different patients. If "personalized medicine" refers to a detailed assessment of how a given patient's body and genetic makeup absorb and respond to given drugs, the results may show greater benefits, or great toxicity.

This kind of research, as one comparative sociologist of science, Karin Knorr Cetina, has noted, is organized into small teams in small labs doing experiments, where change is relatively rapid as researchers act on and measure closely what happens after each experiment.[9] She contrasts this with plasma physics, where large teams use huge equipment and work on one project for a long time. In biological research, a team brings a part of the world into the lab. At the other extreme, like astronomy, one cannot possibly bring one's subject in and experiment on it. Thus, work at the Institute was organized by research units, which in turn were clustered into laboratories. Only years later, when units and labs became too numerous, was a third organizational tier of departments created. These small-scale characteristics of the research also affected the organization of space and thus the design of the Institute's first building and its second, state-of-the-art, building in 2007.

At the time, the trend at universities was to have very large laboratories hosting many units and people. Laboratories were often impersonal clusters of equipment and supplies. But the technical and organizational nature of pharmacological research led the Mario Negri leaders working at the University of Milan in 1961 to design a new kind of building with labs that fit the characteristics of the work and team size. Silvio Garattini, Luigi Valzelli, Emilio Mussini, and Alfredo Leonardi developed the idea of designing small laboratories and offices so that each researcher could have a personal space that they could set up to suit their research needs and style. Each lab team has its own way of doing its work. "Certainly the visits to the UK and the States were inspiring," Garattini wrote us, "and represented a model for the Mario Negri building." Near each suite of offices was space for shared equipment and services.

The animal lab received special attention. Instead of one large animal room or warehouse, the senior group designed several smaller rooms for the mice and rats, with controls for temperature, humidity, and a 24-hour light-cycle of 12 hours of light and 12 of darkness—ideal for regular sleep. Compared to most labs then, where rats and mice sweated out the summer months in close quarters and huddled together in the winter, one researcher described the first animal facilities as "fantastic." As explained in Chapter 4, Garattini played a key role in designing more humanitarian cages that became the new international standard for humane homes.

The Mario Negri senior group, consisting of Alfredo Leonardi, Emilio Mussini, Luigi Valzelli, and Garattini, designed a building four times larger than the pioneers needed. "We wanted a fairly large building since we anticipated that the Mario Negri, should grow," Garattini explained. They kept the building and labs simple, functional, and easy to clean. In order to complete the building quickly so the researchers could get out of the university and into their own space, the architect and builder first constructed the exterior shell for just the labs and offices. Construction began in October 1961 and was completed in just 18 months. It took another eight months more for the staff to complete the interior to their needs and taste. Ample, free parking was part of the design and took advantage of the large, 12,000 square-meter property that Garattini had bought at the edge of the city. The cafeteria, library, and lecture room took eight more months to build. The lecture room held 220 people and had facilities for simultaneous interpretation for hosting international meetings, a critical part of the Institute's strategy to leapfrog over Italian practices and researchers to create strong networks with the world's leading scientists. The lists of speakers and attendees vindicated this bold strategy as did the annual volumes with contributions from these speakers in what became known as the *Mario Negri Monograph Series in Pharmacological Research*.

The Institute opened its doors on February 1, 1963. "When we moved in, it was far from complete—just a building," Professor Jori told us 49 years later on July 9, 2012. "We had a grand opening and invited many prominent people to come, only to have a black-out! So we rushed out to buy candles. There were only two stores in the neighborhood with candles, so we bought all they had. Then we lit and placed a candle on each step—it was so romantic!" Improvising is a key skill of all good scientists, even at a grand opening gone black.

In order to foster the mission and organizational culture of the Institute, the senior team also created common spaces and functions near the small personal labs to bring staff together. They designed a central place where staff ran into one another to get their mail and a common cafeteria where staff could meet and exchange ideas during lunch or coffee breaks. There was no executive dining hall, and no one punched in or out of a time clock until changes in the law required it decades later. In fact, never checking on people's working time was one of "three simple rules" Garattini used to operate the Institute.

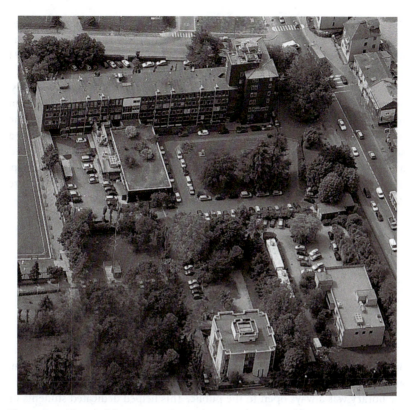

Photo 2.2   Home of the Institute for 44 years

The other two were do not spend money you do not have, and do not to accept any contract or grant that is more than ten percent of the total budget.[10] "Self-motivation is key," said Garattini. People stayed on into the night or came back after dinner, as impassioned researchers have been doing for decades. The senior scientists arranged regular meetings three times a week where researchers presented their work or shared problems and exchanged information and ideas. "We foster a culture of collaboration with constructive criticism," Garattini explained.

The Research Library

The Gustavus A. Pfeiffer Memorial Library for research was designed from the start to be large and the intellectual crucible of the new Institute. With generous help from the Pfeiffer Foundation, who funded it, and also a professionally trained research science librarian, the library at the Mario Negri Institute became a center for training other research librarians throughout the country and elevating national science. Although the library was legally private, it later became accepted as part of a consortium of public libraries for the Lombardy Region. Since the Lombardy Region paid for a large number of scientific and medical journals, it saved the Institute money. In time, the library became part of the Cochrane Collaboration, founded in Italy in 1994 by Garattini and Alessandro Liberati and described in Chapter 7.

Nearly all books and journals were in English, a remarkable feature in Italy, even to this day, that encouraged all staff to read English, still an exception more than 50 years later. Even more than eating together in the cafeteria, the new science library became the center of intellectual life. Staff competed for a seat. When important journals published their latest issue, researchers signed a queue card to read it. A system of circulating the latest issue was set up, but access to articles outside the library's collection was more difficult. Ettore Zuccato, Head of the Laboratory of Food Toxicology, recalled:

> Every week we would all look at a weekly list of new scientific and medical articles to see what we might like to read. The Library had a reasonable number of journals, but many articles were in other journals. We would then go to the University of Milan Index, find the journal, and complete a pre-filled postcard to the University, asking for a copy of each article. It worked, sort of, and about half the time you would get an article in a week or two. If the article came from the United States, it would take more than a month.

Everyone met in the Library to talk over the latest articles. Unlike public and university libraries at the time, the Institute library opened by 8:30 a.m. and stayed open until 10 p.m. Staff had keys to use it even after it "closed," and the library was always open to the public. This helped dedicated students or others who were willing to make the trip.

The founding research librarian, Vanna Pistotti, organized the nation's first research library as part of the Pfeiffer endowment. "I came here in January 1967, on the tenth," she told us, and explained how different research librarians are. Regular librarians catalogue, lend, and keep track of books and such—a circulation librarian. They may not know much about what is in the books at all. Reference librarians know a lot about content and what can be found where so that they can refer patrons to the appropriate works or locations. By contrast, while research librarians also know a lot about a given subject, they teach patrons how to research their own questions to find what they are looking for. They are really information science librarians, she explained. "I was very curious so I liked this American way a lot."

Vanna Pistotti went to many courses on scientific libraries and professional librarianship. In 1972–73, Garattini sent her to an important course in Paris to learn about Medline and electronic search methods. "I was a pioneer in Italy and taught other Italian librarians how to be an information science librarian. I taught courses for doctors on how to do searches on the web."

"In the 1970s, everyone came to the library, and it was open to the public as well," Pistotti recalled. But everyone had to make their own copies of articles and return journals to the right place. The library was open all the time. "People came in at night, all days, except Sundays. You could come at night and see the lights on." Decades later, this continues to be an exceptional level of access.

(a)

(b)

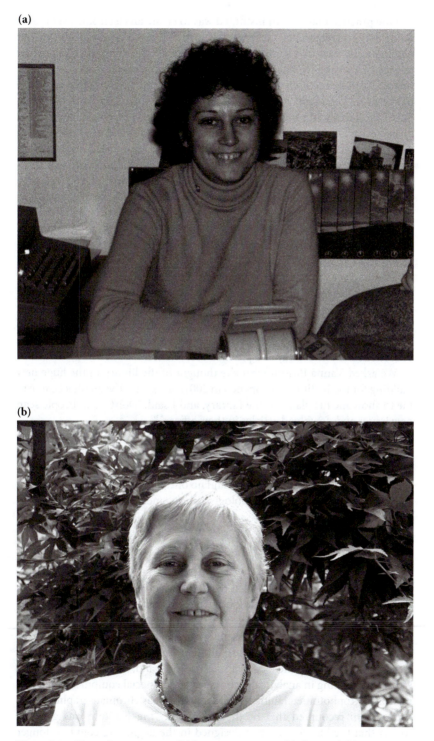

Photo 2.3   Vanna Pistotti, research librarian since 1967, (a) then and (b) now

One practice that Pistotti instituted was to create an electronic list of journals that each researcher most wanted to track. It would go to him or her automatically each week, with links to any new issues. Another important service that Pistotti instituted was for the Library to check all the references that an Institute researcher used in any paper about to be submitted to a journal because "researchers are not so careful about referencing," she observed. This significantly improved acceptance rates, because reviewers and editors dislike errors in the references. "As we taught them how to use EndNote [an electronic software for managing references] and get or check references on major electronic indexing, we got them to where they did this themselves."

Pistotti also organized the practice that every paper written by a member of the staff was circulated to everyone via a download click, so that colleagues could know about it and read it if they wanted. Also, all articles published by Institute staff went into a database that is searchable by title, author, keywords, journal, impact factor, and department. The library collects all articles in a year into an annual volume.

The Institute's researchers get about 300 articles a year accepted into refereed, scientific journals. All totaled, they have published over 12,000 articles since 1963, and Institute staff have published around 5,000 articles for the public in the lay press. They have edited or authored about 1,675 books, though over time doing edited books of conference proceedings and other collections has fallen away as a practice everywhere.

We asked Vanna Pistotti what she thought of the library in the huge new building for the Institute that opened in 2007. She said, "The architect came to me to show me his plans for the Library, and I said, 'Don't do it. People scan new issues and download articles in their offices.'"

We mused, "I guess he didn't listen to you." She replied, "Before, it was to be much bigger than it is now." Today, some senior researchers refer to the new large, luxurious library as The Mausoleum, or Jurassic Park, where extinct species (called books) sit on shelves, and no one comes to look at them, except for the occasional visitor or sociologist who comes in searching for arcane knowledge.

Early Expansion

By 1968, there was a staff of 71 led by 29 researchers with advanced degrees and organized into eight laboratories: two for research into anticancer drugs, one in vitro and the other in vivo; a psychopharmacology lab and another for research on the autonomic nervous system; a laboratory for clinical pharmacology (a new, developing field); another on drug metabolism; a lab for general pharmacology (headed by Professor Jori); and, finally, an eighth laboratory specializing in analytical techniques using special equipment such as a microspectrophotometer, ultracentrifuges, and a gas chromatographer.

Garattini recounted that by the late-1960s: "the Institute was growing so fast that the building we had designed in the beginning could no longer

accommodate all our researchers." A third floor was added to the main building in 1971, and thanks to Leonardi's family connections and excitement about
the new international model for independent pharmacological research, the
Pfeiffer family generously donated funds for a residence of guest accommodations. The George W. Pfeiffer Memorial Residence provided 24 apartments for
international and national visiting researchers, common rooms, and a conference room for 100 people.

In 1983, a six-story "tower" was added, the gift of the Angelo and Angela
Valenti Foundation, as well as gifts from the Italian Association for Cancer
Research, the Pfeiffer Foundation, and other major donors. In 1987, another
building was completed. Named after Catullo and Daniela Borgomainerio,
it provided space for epidemiology and molecular biology, "two areas of
research we became interested in."[11]

Space for a guesthouse for international visitors and fellows was part of the
original Mario Negri design. Together with the large conference hall for international conferences, foreign fellowships, and other programs, these features
indicate that from the start, Garattini and the senior group envisioned "the
Mario Negri" as a center for international research and training.

The number of researchers with advanced degrees rose steadily, from 29
in 1968, to about double or 62 in 1974, as they won more grants and contracts. Research staff doubled again to 135 in 1980 and again to 270 by 1990.
About two-thirds were women. Technical and support staff rose more slowly
in tandem so that the total technical staff reached 119 in 1974, 213 in 1980,
and 402 in 1990. Another substantial group consisted of advanced "postdoc"
students, students learning to become lab technicians described in Chapter 3,
or foreign visiting researchers: 85 in 1974, 107 in 1980, and 225 in 1990. The
number of research units within each lab increased, and the building became
crowded in a way fondly remembered by those interviewed, everybody working close together, helping, joking, forming friendships and collaborations,
falling in (and out) of love, and getting married.

In 2013, we interviewed Dr. Silvia Marsoni, who spent many years at the
Mario Negri and codirected trials on cancer drugs but has gone on to be the
scientific director at the Istituto di Candiolo in Turin. We asked what she had
learned after she began at the Mario Negri in 1976, and she said, "Mario Negri
taught us three things: to be skeptical, to be critical of one's own data, and
never to compromise—you know when you do."

The Paradox of Independent Interdependencies

In their classic book on organizations and environment, *The External Control of Organizations: A Resource Dependence Perspective*, Jeffrey Pfeffer and
Gerald Salancik write, "Organizations are inescapably bound up with the conditions of their environment."[12] To many, it must have seemed sheer organizational folly for a group of researchers to declare the independence of their new
Institute from government, corporations, and the national university system

where nearly all research took place. From Pfeffer and Salancik's perspective, the resource dependencies of any research institute—even one with a generous endowment—are obvious and deep. And indeed, senior university faculty and deans scoffed at Garattini's radical new institute and took steps to discourage or prohibit young researchers from joining it. When Garattini wrote to the National Research Institute, the main funder of research in Italy, they did not even reply.

Garattini realized, however, that what constituted the new Institute's organizational environment were the rapidly growing international constellation of research funders and the international networks of leading researchers who are the gatekeepers for major funding as well as journal article selection. Italy was not funding much scientific research anyway, and national networks controlling local grants and journals in Italian sat on the periphery of the main environment for first-class research. The new Institute's interdependencies on funders of grants or contracts, and on getting published in world-class journals, were clear; but, paradoxically, developing and building those interdependencies depended on being intellectually independent from national institutions to do first-class research.

Aided by his friend and colleague, Alfredo Leonardi, Garattini organized with other senior researchers one international meeting after another that brought the key nodes of international research networks together with the new Institute's researchers. Charmed by Italy and its pleasures, even when they paid their own way, participants established lasting relationships with the young teams. Garattini made sure a new book resulted from each conference that contained the contributions of the speakers, both great and aspiring, bound between two covers to go on the shelf as a Mario Negri Monograph and reference, or to show off to colleagues.

From the day the Institute opened, Garattini and his colleagues also encouraged and hosted international researchers, even from Japan, Australia, and China, for both short-term and long-term stays. Leonardi would find them suitable accommodations and squire them to the most interesting intellectual seminars, clubs, and cultural events, including performances at La Scala. The Institute leapfrogged most university departments, which were still publishing only in Italian. By degrees it brought national medical and pharmacological research up to international standards. The practice of sending promising researchers abroad for a year at a world-class research center, often arranged using networks of colleagues in the United States, the UK, the Netherlands, Germany, and France, reciprocated this cross-fertilization of skills and ideas, mostly developed by one of the leading researcher's close ties with senior colleagues abroad.

Another dynamic of "independent interdependencies" lies in being well connected in and across several interdependencies so that paradoxically, the more interdependent you become, the more independently you can act. Pfeffer and Salancik may have underestimated the importance of network connections so vividly described in the new classic by Christakis and Fowler, *Connected*.[13] No one seems to have made and kept up with more lifelong friendships than Garattini, unless it was Leonardi. For example, Garattini kept leaders at Burroughs-Wellcome informed about his research plans, which led to an interview with the chairman of the Wellcome Trust, Sir Henry Dale, corecipient of the Nobel Prize in 1936 for pioneering work in the physiology of medicine.

Sir Henry was so impressed by Garattini's research productivity and plans that he arranged to equip the new Institute building with first-class scientific instruments at no charge. Thus by the end of its second year the Institute had first-class laboratories four times the size it needed, mostly financed by low-interest loans and gifts. In 1964, a minister paid an official visit to the Institute, a remarkable symbol of acceptance and respect by the government after the first year of this radical institutional challenge to the status quo.

Garattini's rules for independence, such as controlling the research design and execution of a project, or no more than ten percent of turnover from any one source, or control of publication, were also ways to control the new Institute's interdependencies in order to manage their possible distortions or biases early in discussion about a project.

Garattini established a cultural, organizational, and financial pattern that would characterize the Institute for years: a frugal, self-effacing culture of scientific inquiry inside the Institute, connected to a wide, diverse network of distinguished scientists and supporters outside it. Garattini taught his teams how to win grants, and, initially, grant applications or contracts went out under the collective name, Istituto di Ricerche Farmacologiche "Mario Negri," not under the names of the principal investigators. After a few years, Garattini made the important leadership decision to stop doing his own, internationally renowned research in order to provide unbiased support to all the research teams at the Institute and to make unbiased decisions for the Institute as a whole. This reinforced a growing and central strength of the Institute: having top people from all the key specialties collaborating under one roof, working and commenting on each other's work every week. For many, this is a researcher's heaven, and today the same vertically integrated, multispecialty team structure can be found in the highly innovative Cancer Therapy Evaluation Program and the Vaccine Research Center, both part of the US National Institutes of Health and described further in Chapter 9.

Governance worked largely by consensus among the senior research staff and officers. Decisions on requests from laboratories were taken every day and decided case by case. There was almost no hierarchy. For over 50 years, Garattini kept his door open and anyone could pop in. Pfeffer and Salancik define organizations as "collections of individual efforts that come together to achieve something which might not otherwise be accomplished through individual action,"[14] a telling focus on individuals by famous experts on organizations and their environment. The Mario Negri Institute came together in exactly this way. Pfeffer and Salancik add that loose coupling is an important safety device for organizational survival in an environment. Everyone agreed that some money should be set aside for hard times and that there should be a common pot: One year a lab is rich but the next it may need help covering expenses. These practices continue to the present, as does the need for them. Alfredo Leonardi offered an insightful perspective on the organizational culture of the Institute. He wrote that the ethos of frugality and low salaries bound community members together in a shared mission and passion, "the conviction of doing something useful for society and the enthusiasm for scientific endeavor."[15]

Finances

Based on current research when the Institute opened its doors in 1963, funding came from a range of national and international sources.[16] According to the 1963–68 report and other documents from the basement archives, 43 percent of funding came from international sources (largely the United States) in 1963 and rose steadily to 56 percent by 1968. Judith Baggott, the Institute's editor, commented that "Mario Negri was famous for doing top-flight work at lower cost, because our salaries [and overheads] were lower." National sources declined from 57 to 44 percent. Two-thirds of all funds in 1963 came from private sources, mainly research contracts with pharmaceutical companies to do basic research and American foundations like the Pfeiffer Foundation's generous donation for a professionally staffed research library, declining to 60 percent by 1968 and 55 percent by 1983.[17] The largest contract came from the Ministry of Education (for training described below and in Chapter 4), and large research contracts came from the US Army and Department of Agriculture, as well as from the National Institutes of Health (NIH) and two international atomic commissions.

One other advantage that the Mario Negri Institute had was lower budgets and overhead. This meant more good science and product per research dollar. According to Benedetto Saraceno, a former WHO's Director of the Department of Mental Health and Substance Abuse who started his career as a researcher at the Mario Negri, the Institute paid "very modest salaries, and it still does. We used to joke that to be here you either have to be rich or crazy. Many lived frugally. Nevertheless, people stayed because of the excitement of the work, a somehow heroic atmosphere, being at the leading edge of science." While supportive, encouraging, and synergistic, Garattini kept a close eye on expenses. He personally reviewed each request to attend a conference or seminar and all the details. "He would not allow us to make color slides—only black and white," one researcher recalled. Frugality together with synergy worked. By 1968, the Institute was the largest recipient of NIH grants in Europe. "We will always and forever be grateful to Americans for their decisive, early support," Garattini told us in May 2012.

Since 1975, finances have been overseen by Maria Pezzoni, the director of accounts. Born in 1935, she exudes serious intent and high energy, complemented by her kindness and sense of humor. "In 1971, the accountant here asked me to come. I had worked as the bookkeeper and financial administrator for a company, but it closed and I got a job at a new company where the

(a)

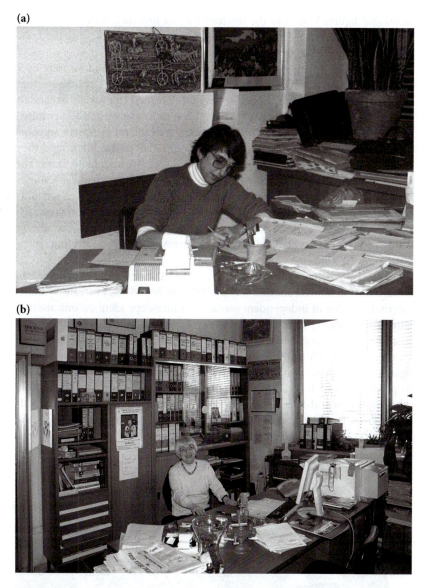

(b)

Photo 2.4   Maria Pezzoni, director of accounts since 1975

boss was harsh; so I was eager to find a new position. Here, I met Professor Garattini, and he was very friendly, as was Leonardi. Professor Leonardi became a real friend. But I was paid much less than before. I lived in Brescia and did not have a car; so I stayed at the Institute all week and went home only on the weekends."

Pezzoni found that all accounting was done by hand, and it took three people to do it. (She dug out of the basement for us the original books of the Institute from the 1960s, each with page after large page of fine, handwritten notes and figures.) She had the Institute buy its first mechanical accounting system, and, in 1975, Garattini made her director of accounts. Since then, she has signed everything for the Institute.

Ms. Pezzoni dug up the financial records back to 1961, and we went over some figures. We learned one category of personnel is Life Contracts. Other categories were multiyear, renewable Service Contracts (for people like Judith Baggott), Fixed Term Contracts for one, three, or five years, and Fellowships.

Pezzoni kept updating equipment, notably a new kind of American computer called a Mac. "We bought our first computers in the 1980s, and they were all Macs.[18] The sales rep gave us ten, and soon we bought 40 more. The staff were delighted—they were so much easier and faster than the complicated PCs." Accounting migrated over to Macs, and, by 1994, all accounting was done on them, she said. The Macs also transformed writing research papers. "It was amazing," said Judith Baggott. "Researchers who had always written papers by hand and said, 'I *never* type my papers,' soon starting typing them on their Macs."

Besides the demanding rule that no more than one-tenth of income can come from one source, another way the Institute coped was to create a parallel internal paradox of independent researchers interdependent on one another through a shared reserve and governance. Led by Garattini, the Mario Negri Institute quickly established itself as a whole that was greater than the sum of its parts, a research institute in a country where rules and customs worked against good science, which used its independence to negotiate with funders to produce research equal to the best in the world. As Benedetto Saraceno, who became world-famous for his work at WHO on behalf of people suffering from psychiatric problems, recalled in 2013 of his early days at the

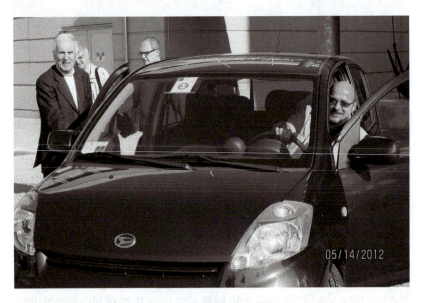

Photo 2.5   The director's driver and "limo" (a 2007 Daihatsu Sirion)

Institute, "When I travelled abroad, I was treated and recognized as someone coming from a prestigious research institution."

While low salaries and tight budgeting gave the Institute a financial edge in competing for grants and contracts, competing university research institutes do not have to budget for their buildings and salaries, paid for by the government. Overhead costs at the Institute were kept low—about 20 percent at the time, rising slowly to 35 percent today. University groups could apply for only direct research costs. The rule against contracts or grants exceeding 10 percent of total revenues meant that research units and labs had to seek and win more funds from more sources—a difficult and never-ending task. But if a company pulled out its projects after the Institute told the public about harmful side effects from a drug or a cluster of drugs, as did happen, the Institute was able to carry on and seek alternate sources of funding.

Commercial-Free Science without Patenting

Patents are an Italian invention. The first was granted in Italy in 1421 for a period of three years to the Florentine architect Filippo Brunelleschi, for a barge with hoisting gear that was used to transport marble along the Arno River. As they developed, patents were not applied to medicines, because they were regarded in many countries as social goods to be made available to anyone who needed them, not to those who could afford patent-protected prices. Society, that is, public funding, as well as charitable contributions funded most basic research to find better medicines, and this is still the case, even though companies fund the final testing and thus control the process of defining uses, testing for approval, and promoting to doctors.[19]

Doctors, medical researchers, and scientists constantly experiment to find out how a disease works and what might prevent or relieve it. Although economic competition has long been credited as the engine for innovation, curiosity and a desire to solve puzzles and help those suffering are strong motives, too. Patenting commercializes research and scientific thinking, and many profitable products, like most new drugs, do not substantially help patients get better. It can also impede innovation by creating barriers or thickets to everyone else trying to innovate.[20]

When Italy decided in 1978 to remove the exemption of medicines from patent law, Garattini and the Mario Negri Institute decided they would not finance part of their research through patenting new discoveries or developments. They gave moral and scientific reasons for this decision. Morally, they are paid to invent and discover for patients and society, so their inventions should be available to all, like Jonas Salk when he refused to patent his vaccine against polio. Practically, both the prospect of patents and the patenting process can seriously compromise a team or lab's research away from investigating the more important scientific or clinical questions that are commercially unpromising.

The no-patent rule also means that companies can share their proprietary secrets with Mario Negri scientists without fear of their being stolen
or surreptitiously patented. The rule fosters collaboration and trust. Some
staff disagree about this rule and advocate middle ways to enable income
from inventions to fund the Institute's work while minimizing distortion of
research. For example, patents could be held by the Institute and revenues
from royalties could go to the common pot. To date, however, these have not
been developed. The no-patent rule contributes to the Institute's reputation
for moral integrity and dedication to the public's welfare.

The challenge of maintaining the Institute's ethics and getting funds for
research today, during a protracted recession, was candidly described by
Ariela Benigni, an internationally known researcher who heads the Department of Molecular Medicine at Negri-Bergamo and played a key role in kidney
regeneration described in Chapter 3. We asked about the terms of commercial
contracts, and she replied, "We propose the research design to carry out what
the company requests, and we control the data and its analysis. We don't do
trials that companies want us to do . . . We are completely autonomous in all
we do . . . We don't screen compounds, for example, unless they are relevant
to the pathophysiology of the disease [we are investigating] . . . One should
always compare a new drug with an older drug in use, even if it is a "new class"
that uses a new pathway, because it is meant to benefit the patient, and one
wants to see if it is of greater or lesser benefit."

These policies create difficulties, she continued. They mean her team has
to write and submit a new proposal for a grant or contract every ten days. We
turn down companies who want screening studies to choose the best products
to market. Sometimes we propose to a company a promising compound to
test, but they are not always interested. We ask companies to compare a new
with an older drug, and they don't want to, because the older drug may prove
superior to the new one.

Today, the Institute faces greater challenges than it did as a fledging organization trying to deal with its own paradox of declaring institutional independence
from government, industry, and universities in order to achieve a real utopia of
independent control over the design, data, and publication of its research, while
being utterly dependent on external organizations for its funding.[21]

First, Lasting Impressions

When we arrived at his office, Mario Salmona was waiting for us with a sheet
of paper. "I thought I would dig out my original application in 1971 to show
you," he said. "I applied for a job, and the response was astounding—I received
a reply within 48 hours! The letter asked me to tell them when I wanted to take
an exam for the position. I took it and receive an acceptance, accompanied by
an enclosed a three-page outline of rules and procedures within three days! I
was hired . . . fantastic!!" He then earned a master's degree while working—
very hard to do. "As Silvio did?" we asked; he nodded. By the time he was 30,
he became the youngest head of a laboratory at the Institute.

Gianni Tognoni, one of the great innovators in modern pharmacology and an impassioned advocate for global health justice, left the priesthood to attend medical school and pursue his interest in psychotropic drugs. He visited the Mario Negri Institute in 1970 and met Garattini. "He said, 'We're establishing a lab in clinical pharmacology. Would you like to join us?' This was before I had completed my medical school exams! I talked with him on September 8th and came to work on September 9th."

"What was it like, working at the Institute, then?" we asked. "Very simple, very participatory. Small groups. We practically lived together, and it was easy to work nights and weekends. Everyone was so young, so open, so easy to contact and talk with. We worked and planned projects together. We talked freely. Silvio Garattini and the others were very open, adventuresome. He was always very curious."

Claudio Antonio Pantarotto, who started as a very productive researcher and ended up as head of external relations, had a unique experience:

> I was looking for work (in 1968) and applied to the Mario Negri Institute. I got a reply the next day to come in for an interview and testing. There were 15 or 16 candidates, all with university degrees except for two of us. I didn't know what "research" was or what it meant. A key exam question was, "If city water is flowing through a pipe and up a smokestack, what level will it reach?" Another applicant said, "People with a university degree think about problems. People with high-school diplomas solve them." One after another struggled with it. I replied that city water is under 2 atmospheres of pressure, and water rises 10 meters per atmosphere, so the answer is 20 meters. That was correct, and I was hired.

Benedetto Saraceno, who became a unit and then lab head at Mario Negri before he was tapped by the WHO for a series of senior posts directing international mental health policy, first heard about the Mario Negri during the revolution of 1968 when he was juggling medical studies with demonstrating in the streets. We asked what he heard about it then and he replied, "I knew it as a strange institution that did top research and had a different culture—knowing English well, reading the international research literature, and being much more rigorous than research at Italian universities. My two brightest friends in 1968 worked there."

We asked him for his impressions in the first few weeks after he came to work at the Institute. He said, "My impression was enormous—a complete absence of any bureaucratic attitude among the leaders and a focus on outcomes, not how you achieved them. I was impressed by the extreme intellectual openness of the Institute . . . Every day was an enormous learning experience, and a great contrast with the poor knowledge and research in Italian medical schools."

International Contributions

As described in Chapter 1, the Mario Negri pioneers started making international contributions as they came together before the Institute began—the

1957 conference, the pioneering volume that resulted, the founding of the International College of Neuropsychopharmacology (CINP), and their own research. It was only in the 1960s that the concept of measuring concentrations of drugs in patients' blood and their effects became well known. Institute researchers, especially Garattini, learned how to measure their duration, decline, and disappearance as well. This raised the exciting prospect of measuring beneficial and toxic effects in a single patient so that one could modify the dose. However, complications dealing with the penetration of drugs in tissue and with the expression of the target posed major challenges.

Unlike some other laboratories, the Institute's researchers could measure the actions of drugs in terms of physiological, biochemical, and behavioral parameters. The researchers also investigated how the mode of transportation in the body and the formation of metabolites affected some drugs' benefits or toxicity. These studies were particularly important when measuring tiny concentrations and effects of drugs in the brain, and thus their mechanism of action. Researchers also learned to measure the distribution of a drug in a tissue, which is today possible at the microscopic level with the use of mass spectrometry. Such studies are still being done, especially in clinical trials.

Once the new Institute opened, Garattini and the pioneers organized an international course on spectrophotofluorimetric techniques in biology that was attended by 120 researchers and supported by the NATO Institute for Advanced Study.[22] In 1964, they organized an international symposium on nonsteroidal anti-inflammatory drugs, with 220 attendees and supported by the European Society of Pharmacology and Biochemistry. In 1965, another 220 researchers came to the Institute's new building for an international catecholamine symposium, supported by the US National Institutes of Health (NIH) and the American Society for Pharmacology and Experimental Therapeutics. This occurred because the Organizing Committee for the NIH trusted Garattini and the Institute as a prime European site. These and other conferences put the Mario Negri Institute for Pharmacological Research on the international map. As Garattini wrote in a report, the Institute was born in Italy, but research has no boundaries.[23]

The staff, led by Garattini, also edited one—and sometimes two—volumes a year of new scientific papers in English, published by a prominent scientific press. By 1990, in its first 27 years, the Institute had organized 70 international congresses attended by 8,780 researchers, 112 national congresses, and 544 seminars or conferences. It established a series, *Monographs of the Mario Negri Institute for Pharmacological Research*, edited by Garattini, with Raven Press in New York.

In addition, the Institute research staff organized about two courses or symposia a year for the national community of pharmacological researchers, each attended by 120–170 scientists, and some supported by the national government. This level of activity had not been seen before at any other research institute. Publications in international scientific journals, usually in English, grew from just 3 in 1963 to 25 in 1968, plus another 38 in press, as the staff learned the difficult skills of writing first-class articles in English.[24] Scientific publications grew to 170 in 1983 with 34 in press.[25] By 1990, Negri staff had published 3,478 scientific articles.[26]

Cancer research was a main focus of Mario Negri work. By 1980, the Institute had contributed considerably to the development of 30 drugs useful in treatment.[27] Investigations were linked to and supported by the US National Cancer Institute. Garattini also played a formative role in developing EORTC, the European Organization for Research and Treatment of Cancer. He served as president from 1965 to 1968, when the current EORTC became the major independent body for coordinating investigator driven clinical trials of anticancer drugs, as it continues to be today (www.eortc.org).

International Networking and Training

The international scope was reinforced by two practices of the Mario Negri Institute, which have continued to this day. First, the Institute quickly became a postdoc training center for reciprocal visits and stays by both young and established researchers from abroad. Combined with the international symposia organized every year, and facilitated by the international residence for visitors, a rich, cosmopolitan culture of first-class open science developed, with everyone contributing their best ideas for solving problems posed by diseases or specific drug-candidates. Visitors came from universities and research centers in California, Massachusetts, Illinois, New York, and Pennsylvania, as well as The Netherlands, Britain, Denmark, Spain, Poland, Mexico, Czechoslovakia, Japan, Hungary, and Finland. By 1990, 342 international researchers from 44 nations had worked in residence an average of 11 months each.[28] The Johananoff fellowships helped bring over senior scientists each year to the Institute.

Second, many young staff researchers with promise at the Institute were sent abroad to a major research lab for a year or more for additional training and to learn new advanced techniques, usually in the United States or Britain, but sometimes elsewhere like The Netherlands, Sweden, or Germany. The Wellcome Trust fellowships helped in arranging short visits abroad. Garattini, Leonardi, and others drew on their extensive knowledge of international fellowships, visiting postdoc appointments, and networks of personal relations with leading scientists to find suitable arrangements. Several of these resulted in young researchers returning with new, leading-edge skills or even a new area of research.

Enrico Garattini, Silvio's eldest son and head of the Laboratory in Molecular Biology explained how his trip abroad changed his scientific career. In 1983, after four years working as a student of medicine in the laboratory of enzymology at Mario Negri, he was sent to the Roche Institute of Molecular Biology in Nutley, NJ. Molecular biology was just coming of age, and it looked as if it would be important. The Roche Institute was the best place to go; it was set up by Sidney Udenfriend, a giant in the field, as a showcase for Roche. It did only basic, pure science, and Roche left it alone, until ten years later it closed the

Institute down. This is the danger of basic research funded by pharmaceutical companies. It may not fit the next administration's corporate vision.

Enrico ended up staying there four years, and when he returned in 1987, his group was among the first to apply molecular biology to pharmacological problems. Computer science was also booming, and Silvio bought 50 Macintosh computers: "They were all over the place in 1987." This was a radical and prescient choice. "They were *such fun* to work with."

In describing his fellowship abroad, Maurizio D'Incalci, now the head of the Department of Oncology, portrays sociological aspects of career development for a young researcher at the Institute:

> In 1974 I was a first-year medical student at the University of Milan and visited the Mario Negri Institute. There, I discovered that what we were learning in class from texts had huge gaps, and that there was a fascinating world of the unknown . . . I could see this was a way to combine research with clinical medicine to make it better. I kept coming over from classes to the Institute, and in 1977, Professor Garattini asked me to stay.
>
> Mario Negri was very different from Italian universities. Leaders did not stand on ceremony and protect their fiefdoms. In the second year, while participating in ovarian cancer experiments, one of the Mario Negri scientists mentioned there was a summer research internship in London at the Imperial Cancer Research Fund, and would I like to go? I jumped at the chance to improve my broken English and do research in London.
>
> When I returned from London, I had a research idea and talked it over with Garattini—a 21-year-old medical student talking with the Director! He said something I have always remembered: "I don't think it will work, but why don't you try it." In subsequent years, I have done the same thing when I thought an earnest young researcher had a reasonable idea: "I don't think it will work, but why don't you try it." By the way, Silvio was right—it didn't work; but I learned a lot trying.
>
> Military service in Italy was mandatory for one year, but I did not want to miss a year at the Mario Negri; so I applied as a conscientious objector so I could do two years of alternative service at the Institute. Alfredo Leonardi knew people high up in every part of government, including generals, and he had already arranged for Mario Negri to be a site for alternative service. The whole process was awkward and embarrassing; but it enabled me to continue my research at the Mario Negri Institute. Leonardi was wonderful. He loved people, knew everyone.

Recognizing talent early and nurturing it is a vital part of Mario Negri's organizational culture: It grows its own leaders. It could never afford to buy in international leaders anyway; but the deeper advantages lie in leaders acculturating into a relatively self-effacing community of research scientists who are all committed to better care for patients, especially the poor. Mario Salmona, head of Molecular Biology, put it this way:

> Something you may have missed is that all the heads of departments grew up here. We grow our scientific leaders. We never import them, like many places.

They internalize our values and culture—and we couldn't afford to import stars anyway. So we've been planning succession for a long time, by hiring very talented 35-year-olds and letting them grow up here. The human capital here is very important—a great asset. It took 50 years to develop.

A prime example is Roberto Fanelli, a central figure in Chapter 5. Hired out of high school in 1965, he applied his skills in analytical chemistry for the next eight years as he also worked through an entire university education to a doctorate in biological sciences in 1973. Then Garattini arranged for him to spend a year abroad at the Institute for Lipid Research at Baylor University, the leading edge of new analytical techniques in pharmacology. "It was fantastic, aside from the weather! I learned a lot. I have been adding different kinds of spectrometric machines ever since." A year later, his highly refined skills served the nation after the tragic Seveso explosion described in Chapter 5. Fanelli kept expanding applications in environmental epidemiology, and in 1997 he was made head of the Department of Environmental Health Sciences, which he has been leading ever since.

Leonardi's early arrangements for the Mario Negri Institute to be designated for alternative service for conscientious objectors helped recruit several young men who became international researchers. Also helpful were part-time work-study programs that allowed aspiring researchers to take university courses while paying the rent as lab technicians at the Mario Negri. Ettore Zuccato, for example, now the lab head for environmental sciences, arrived in 1972 and started medical school part-time "It was very demanding, but I had no choice," he said. It took him 14 years, but he got 110 out of 110 on his exams (summa cum laude) and honors for his thesis. During that time, Mario Negri arranged for his getting advanced training at the University of Maastricht, all paid. "Now they no longer allow work-study programs, only full time. It's a pity because it excludes bright, ambitious kids who don't have money," he said. He thought about taking residency training in pediatrics; but one has to wait three years or more for an opening, while working nearby with your potential sponsor for no pay—simply impossible unless your family is affluent. In 1988–89, a much more supportive Mario Negri arranged a second fellowship at King's College, London for Zuccato, with pay.

Remembering the Institute as a Real Utopia

As lifelong partners through medical school and PhDs at the University of Leuven, Maria Benedetta Donati and Giovanni de Gaetano did groundbreaking research on the effective treatment of heart disease, ten years before it was tested in the first GISSI trial described in Chapter 5. Silvio Garattini spotted them and invited them to join the Mario Negri family. Donati became the scientific director of Mario Negri Sud (Chapter 4), and her husband the director of a lab. Recently, they wrote a retrospective about their experience:[29]

Italian universities were still under the influence of the so-called "baroni," old professors who had long managed to change everything so that nothing changed. At that time, a faithful and servile attitude towards one of them rather than being competent and independent was often more useful to obtain an academic position.

The Mario Negri Institute was a remarkable exception not because English was actively used there, but mainly because instead of offering an academic career, it offered the pleasure to fellows and research personnel of challenging themselves to explore the intimate mechanisms of the brain or the heart and to find out new remedies for old or novel diseases.

During our first years in Milan [1973–78], it became more and more clear to us that the main object of our research activity was to produce reliable results to answer clinically relevant questions . . . We adopted to research for our young coworkers a famous statement of Immanuel Kant: research should always be viewed as an end and never as simply a means (to progress in your career or to get money or power). We would have considered a different attitude a betrayal of their persons on their part.

At Mario Negri Institute, nobody could apply for a patent, as Silvio Garattini, both founder and Director of the Institute, was strongly convinced that it should be a non-profit institution offering health benefit to the population, rather than economically exploiting the scientific results obtained. Instead of being kept secret and unpublished for a patent, data should be rapidly published and largely diffused, from publications in peer-reviewed international journals up to meetings with medical doctors, students, laymen, mass-media. At that time participating in a radio or a TV programme was considered inappropriate for a scientist who should only address himself to his peers in scientific contexts. At Mario Negri Institute, science communication was instead developed as an ethical aspect of research itself. '*Data are not data if they are not communicated,*' was one of the statements that both of us accepted with enthusiasm.

What Do You Do with a Bright, Irrepressible Daughter?

On July 9, 2012, we entered the office of Armanda Jori, one of the last surviving members of the pioneers. She rose quickly for a woman of 79, sharply dressed with color and style, energetically smiling. She immediately started talking . . .

"I was born in 1933 and grew up in Milan. My father was a tax accountant and also a local minister in the Socialist Party for 25 years . . . I attended the classical high school, Parini, and graduated in 1952."[30] She explained that her father expected her to marry, but she had other plans.

"I started at the University of Pavia—it's very old and had a good course in pharmacy—and got my degree in 1956—very fast, with a summa. My degree was in Chemistry and Pharmaceutical Technology [*Chimica e Tecnologia Farmaceutica*]."

After graduation my cousin was sick and her parents called on Professor Trabucchi, because he was the head of Pharmacological Research at the University of Milan; so I met him there. He asked what I was doing. Then he invited me to work for him. Garattini was there as an assistant, and I started working on his investigations.

We asked, "Then the next year Garattini went to the US. What was that like?"

"Oh, he was very excited, and when he came back he talked with us a lot about needing to have our own institute. He became very discouraged about the way things were at Italian universities.

"Then Mario Negri came in 1959 with some questions to talk with Professor Trabucchi. But he was a member of Parliament and very busy; so he recommended that Mario Negri talk with his talented young colleague, Silvio Garattini. As a result, he and Garattini got to know each other."

We asked about the decision of the original 21 pioneers to cast their lot with Garattini. "Several felt conflicted," she said, "bothered about setting up a separate institute. And some of them decided not to come, while others did in the end. Professor Paoletti, for example, worked for Garattini on his projects and was part of his team. But he had tenure and could not bring himself to leave the University."

"Garattini had a charismatic personality and was very persuasive," she continued. "Mario Negri designated him as Director for Life; so the die was cast. Professor Trabucchi tried to get me to stay. He even offered me a salary! But I decided to go with Garattini."

We asked, who was on salary then? "Leonardi, Palma, Valzelli, Mussini, Morasca—that's all. The three secretaries might have been paid . . . no I guess not." [Mapelli told us she received no pay at the University.] At the Mario Negri, all staff received a modest salary.

We asked, so for most, they were leaving unpaid jobs? "Yes. I got my first check in 1963, when we began in the new Institute building."

We asked, what about the period between 1961 and 1963 when you all had to continue to work in the Department at the University while the lab was being built? It must have been quite awkward.

"Yes, very old friends split apart. Those who stayed could not believe the others were leaving. They were shocked that Garattini was taking away so many people from the Department. The Union (as she called this dedicated group who had decided to leave) could not meet in the Department and had to meet at my house."

"We had to see Trabucchi every day, to tell him how many animals we would be using. He was concerned, not for the animals but for the cost. We would tell him, say, 25, and he would reply: 'Twenty-five?! Do you really need 25? I think you can get by with 20.' It was impossible."[31]

"I obtained my Libera Docenza in 1967," Professor Jori continued. She reached again into her bookcase and took out her thesis volume, a collection of early articles and papers—the way a thesis is done now at Utrecht and other prominent European universities. We noticed that her earliest published article in English was dated 1959! We asked, how did you do that? Had you done English in school?

"No, I just picked it up. Scientific English isn't that hard," she said, at least for her.

We asked, when did you get your first grant? "I can't remember . . . Garattini would send applications out from the Institute [as a collective principal investigator] and the budget would be allocated, this much for one lab and that much for another." Judith Baggott added that she remembered grants were done this way.

"American funding came very early," Dr. Jori added, "and from the UK too."

We asked about the early organization of the institute. Dr. Jori replied by writing on a sheet: S, S, S, L, L, L as she explained there were 3 Sections and 3 Labs. "But really, they were not very different."

We asked about life after 1963 and she said there was much more autonomy than at the University. It was a good atmosphere, and the average age was 28. She became the head of a lab.

We asked, were women paid less than men? She said she didn't think so and said she earned the same as Valzelli (a professor)! "That was something." All the salaries, however, were very low compared to industry.

"I was Head of the Lab for 25 years . . . up to 1978. And then because of family needs I went half time and started doing public relations, corresponding and contacting donors, acknowledging every gift, even 5 euros. We treat all gifts the same. We write up the progress in the areas of interest to different donors and how their gift is being put to good use."

3

Expansions to New Campuses and Integrated Research

Starting in the late 1970s, the Mario Negri Institute began to expand into three new campuses and into new fields. Coordinated by Professor Garattini and a core senior group, all reflected the ethos of the Institute's social ethic to use first-class independent research to improve the health of patients and the public. This social ethic was strongly reinforced when the nation decided in 1978 to move from insurance-based universal health-care system based on the workplace to a single payer system regardless of workplace.[1] Garattini, Tognoni, and other leaders realized this turned health services into a unified whole that could serve as a laboratory for applied research to improve patient care.

The advantages of a national health service for translational and clinical research are often not mentioned in debates about whether it would be more cost-effective for a nation to have national health insurance or a service. During the same period, the movement against asylums, or large state hospitals for the mentally ill serving as virtual warehouses, led to their being emptied

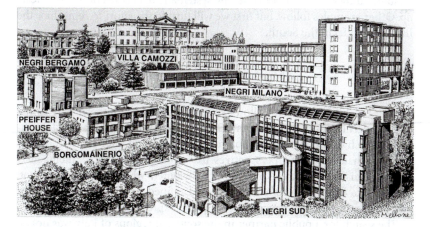

Photo 3.1 The Mario Negri labs on four sites by mid-1980s

and replaced by networks of service providers. National associations of doctors, especially general practitioners, collaborated on developing therapeutic formularies. In these ways, a national groundwork was laid for developing new ways to join research with patient care.

In 1982, work started on an expansion of the Institute's headquarters in Milan, funded by many donations large and small from thousands of citizens and some institutions. The Institute has never had a department for fundraising or gifts and annuities. Yet giving to this research institute evolved as numerous talks, columns, and other activities by its leaders to communicate with the public what good science had to say about a range of issues led to trust, respect, and gifts (see Chapter 4). Work also began on extending the Mario Negri model to a large site in Southern Italy for research and training, based on funding from the Cassa del Mezzogiorno and a ministerial committee for developing areas in Southern Italy. Renovations began on converting an eighteenth century convent into a new research center in Bergamo that would permit close integration of lab research with bedside clinical care of patients. A second, large center—actually a converted 100-room mansion from the early 1800s overlooking its own park—integrated basic research with help for patients with rare diseases and developed into a model for national and European networks of centers for rare diseases.

Linking and integrating pharmacological research with patient care was an old dream of the Institute's founders and achieved in other ways. For example, Maurizio Bonati, currently the head of the department of public health at the Mario Negri, began to develop a unit on perinatal clinical pharmacology by organizing a network of neonatal centers in 1985. Neonatologists, obstetricians, and researchers came together to address the complex challenges of better care for babies with serious respiratory problems. This enabled Dr. Bonati and Institute staff to monitor high-risk babies before, during, and after birth and to help integrate primary, secondary, and tertiary levels of care. The network allowed new drugs to be tried for babies who did not respond well to established therapies, accompanied by systematic data collection and follow-up. Other examples follow, but first we will turn to the effort to reproduce the Institute model in the South.

Negri-SUD

During the 1970s, research fellows kept coming from Southern Italy to the Mario Negri Institute in Milan, and Garattini generated the idea of establishing a branch of the Institute in Southern Italy. It could offer unusual opportunities, challenges, and perspectives to young people there. Intelligence, as Garattini used to say, is randomly distributed while resources are not. Researchers from the South joined in and refined how the Institute might give others there a real chance to develop and express their talents.

The search for a public partner in the southern regions of Italy was not an easy undertaking: On one side the regions of Campania and Calabria could not offer conditions suitable for independence, a core principle of the Institute. However, a partnership was formed with the Puglia Region; but it collapsed after the assassination in 1978 of the regional and national political leader Aldo Moro and a subsequent change in the regional government.

Finally, in 1980, the provincial government of Chieti in Abruzzo, and the Cassa del Mezzogiorno approached Garattini to express interest in establishing a branch of the Mario Negri Institute with the help of development funds from the EU for strengthening the economies of lower-income areas. There was a large site available that had been slated for a new psychiatric hospital but had been stopped by the 1978 law that mandated the dehospitalization of mental health patients. Nearby was the young University of Chieti, focused on training programs, and a potential partner for training researchers. Having a plot of land, a building, and funding to remodel it into labs provided by the province were deciding factors.

The vision was to develop an industrial park for high-tech bioscience companies by having the Mario Negri Research Institute, a branch of the National Research Council (CNR), a Sports Medicine Institute of the nearby Chieti University, and the branch of at least one pharmaceutical company as anchors for the park. As plans progressed, the CNR and Chieti University dropped out, and the pharmaceutical company preferred to build a facility closer to Rome. However, Garattini and the Institute decided to go ahead, with the assurance of EU development funds for projects in an economically deprived area, and the financial support of the Cassa for the first three years. Garattini's idea was an organizationally innovative progenitor of what later became known as Public-Private Partnerships. On December 5, 1980, the Consortium Mario Negri SUD was set up with the provincial government of Chieti, outside the village of Santa Maria Imbaro. It was also supported by the Special Project for Applied Scientific Research in Southern Italy initiated by the National Research Council.[2]

In 1982, the Mario Negri Institute in Milan started advertising for applicants from the South to come for three years' training in order to take jobs at the new Negri-SUD institute. Garattini, together with Giovanni de Gaetano, de Gaetano's wife, Maria Benedetta Donati, and other leaders began planning how they would staff and organize the new institute. As a native of Southern Italy, de Gaetano felt a strong commitment toward young people there and did not hesitate when Garattini invited him and his wife to head up Negri-SUD. A first decision from both researchers was that everyone working at the new Institute should reside in the area. In order to avoid the negative experience of small peripheral universities, where professors spend only one or two days a week there and do not establish any firm link with colleagues, students, and the local environment, no commuting would be allowed. Ground was broken to build a major new edifice, with 14,000 square meters (150,640 sq. ft.) of research space on the 42,000 square meter site, and other buildings were renovated for different functions. A second Pfeiffer Library was built, along with labs, a cafeteria, and residential apartments for up to 40 young researchers to come for a 2–3 year research fellowship. Total cost was about 40 billion lire, or 20 million euros. The careful planning, training, and preparations took five years.

Negri-SUD began its activities on September 1, 1987. A few months later, on February 1, 1988, the twenty-fifth anniversary of when the original Institute had opened its doors, scientific research officially started. About 20 research staff came from the Milan Institute and 20 were young fellows from the region. Total staff built up to about 260 by the end of 1997. The founding director, Giovanni de Gaetano and his wife, Dr. Donati, the scientific secretary, organized research and training programs, conferences, and other scientific events to put Negri-SUD on the map and connect its researchers with networks of leading researchers around the world. In the first decade, they held 20 international and 45 national research congresses, one every 2–3 months. The scientific results obtained in the Negri-SUD laboratories were

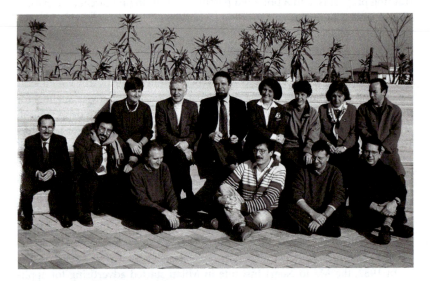

Photo 3.2a   Key staff at Mario Negri-Sud

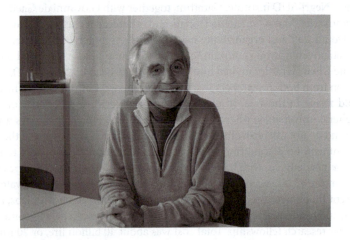

Photo 3.2b   Gianni Tognoni

published in many top international scientific journals, such as *Nature, Cell, New England Journal of Medicine, PNAS, The Lancet, Blood*.

After the fall of the Berlin Wall in 1989, special training grants became available for young researchers, and 75 came from 25 countries, mostly from Eastern Europe, India, and China. At the same time, 25 Negri-SUD researchers and fellows had spent at least one year working abroad in scientific institutions. Altogether, Negri-SUD awarded 410 research training fellowships during its first ten years, funded largely from a combination of the National Research Council, the Mario Negri Institute, and European funds aimed at developing science and technology in lower-income regions.

Because these funds were not for specific research projects, they provided general research training support. Researcher fellows could be assigned where it best suited them and the senior research staff. The Mario Negri style of hands-on, apprenticeship-type training on the job made graduates very attractive, and many went on to top research programs. Since Italy did not have a PhD degree until the end of the 1980s, Negri-SUD started a PhD program in conjunction with the Open University in the UK that was later extended to the home Institute in Milan.

Negri-SUD and the Surrounding Area

From the beginning, researchers at Negri-Sud set up programs to address the cultural heritage and industrial realities of the area. Collaborative programs were established with many secondary schools not only from nearby Lanciano but also from the entire Abruzzo and surrounding regions. A "Summer Student" program was organized during the months of June and July that hosted about 50 students each year to spend one full-time month in the different Institute laboratories. The original "Negri-link" program was the first in the country to allow secondary schools to be connected to a novel Internet system. Students in a Lanciano school used it to develop the first Italian electronic school journal. Each year, "Science Week" brought dozens of scientists, clinicians, journalists, and sportsmen to meet students in the morning and deliver lectures to the general public in the afternoon. A pioneering video-conferencing system was used to allow local students sitting in the auditorium of a local bank to interview the Nobel Prize winner Renato Dulbecco in Milan.

Negri-SUD researchers established relations with local producers of wine or olive oil, and a number of research projects were devoted to the possible influence of dietary habits on human health. The first EU-funded project on wine and health (EU FAIR Program, 1997) was headed by Negri-SUD researchers. The regional Ministry of Agriculture publicly declared that Negri-SUD had significantly contributed to the international image and commercial success of the typical local wine, Montepulciano d'Abruzzo. De Gaetano recalls the great development of the wine industry in the 1990s went in parallel with the Negri-SUD collaboration with local wine producers and regional agricultural authorities. "I personally accompanied Abruzzo wine producers to Stockholm, Brussels, London . . . In each place, they were presenting their bottles to marketing people while I was presenting our research data to doctors, science journalists and so on."

In recognition of Negri-SUD's increasing role as "the new name of the regional development," business and government leaders established one of the EU-promoted "Territory Pacts" in Abruzzo, which had its legal seat at the Negri-SUD headquarters. This pact brought together key actors with special skills and resources to develop economic activity, networks, and markets for economic growth. Later, the Italian Government singled it out for an official visit by the minister of the treasury, Carlo Azeglio Ciampi, who soon after was elected president of the Italian Republic. Negri-SUD also gained sufficient prestige and inspiration to once again overcome the tradition of not giving to research institutes but rather museums, the Church, and charities, as the Institute in Milan had done 20 years earlier. Besides many small donations, two large ones included a valuable painting and a gift to establish the Environmental Laboratory.

International Contributions

Research programs at Negri-SUD, de Gaetano and Donati felt, should not exclusively cover the personal expertise of their team in thrombosis, atherosclerosis, and related vascular fields. Thus, other research leaders from Mario Negri-Milan joined Negri-SUD, providing high-level complementary skills in cell and molecular biology, neurodegenerative diseases, computer science, and clinical epidemiology.

By the end of the 1990s, Negri-SUD had an impressive range of departments and laboratories. Daniela Corda and Alberto Luini headed up the Department of Cell Biology and Oncology that included laboratories of cellular and molecular endocrinology, experimental oncology, molecular neurobiology, the molecular pharmacology of tumor cells, intracellular transport, and signal transduction. The morphology unit run by Dr. Alexander Mironov, a Russian investigator, kept expanding. Maria Benedetta Donati directed the Department of Vascular Medicine and Pharmacology, which included labs investigating genetic and environmental risk factors for thrombotic disease (headed by Licia Iacoviello), blood platelets and leukocytes (Chiara Cerletti), tumor cell biology (Andreina Poggi), and the relationships between thrombosis, atherosclerosis, and cancer (Roberto Lorenzet). Gianni Tognoni chaired the Department of Clinical and Epidemiological Research and worked with Roberto Marchioli (lab of epidemiology of cardiovascular diseases), Antonio Nicolucci (with projects in oncology and diabetes and a Center of the Cochrane Collaboration), and Marilena Romero, who headed the Laboratory of Pharmacoepidemiology and went on to become the head of the research center at the Italian Association of Clinical Pharmacy. A school of scientific journalism was set up to which editors from *The Lancet* and *Nature* and many other distinguished journals came to give seminars. In collaboration with the province of Chieti, a Department of Environmental Studies was also established and chaired by Domenico Rotilio to monitor water, air, and soil contamination. They also developed strategies aiming at providing models of safer planning of industrial and agricultural projects and activities.

The most important characteristic of the research conducted during the first decade of Negri-SUD was its multidisciplinarity. Luini and Corda's group devoted much effort to examining the sophisticated information systems (called signal transduction) within a cell and the mechanisms of secretion of active substances from the cell. The role of the intracellular Golgi apparatus in protein trafficking and in the passage of information inside/outside the cell enabled these researchers to identify several biochemical intermediaries that were relevant to rare neurological disorders such as Lowe's syndrome. This area of study also involved the effects of oncogenes on cell communication and the possible existence of biomarkers in the tissue of growing tumors. Beta-adrenergic cell receptors and dopaminergic neurons were the object of important observations by Antonio De Blasi and Ennio Esposito's group, respectively. A cell and molecular biology approach was also followed by Chiara Cerletti and Virgilio Evangelista, who developed a widely accepted scheme of interactions between blood platelets and leukocytes, through a series of widely cited papers published in *Blood*, the journal of the American Society of Hematology.

A pioneering epidemiologic research led by Donati and Licia Iacoviello drew on the data from the 12,000 acute myocardial infarction patients enrolled in the nationwide GISSI 2 trial (see Chapter 6) to identify those suffering from a familial form of the disease. Blood samples were then collected from these selected patients in almost all Italian regions and delivered by special courier, under liquid nitrogen, to Santa Maria Imbaro. Genetic polymorphisms of the blood coagulation Factor VII were identified and correlated with the risk of this form of disease. It was the first approach of this kind and the results were published in the *New England Journal of Medicine*.[3]

Diabetes Research at Negri-SUD

Research on diabetes at Negri-SUD has changed national and international practice because it was so well tied into clinical care. Antonio Nicolucci established the first Mario Negri laboratory on diabetes, and it has grown steadily, despite earthquakes and the recession. Using the GISSI model of doing trials by organizing and involving clinicians (explained in Chapter 6), Nicolucci worked to sign up 325 diabetic clinics that treat about 500,000 patients, nearly half the national total. He says that drug companies are making this kind of independent, clinician-based research increasingly difficult, because what specialists did free as part of good clinical care in a national health service is now handsomely rewarded by companies—about 1,000–3,000 euros per "subject" recruited. In a way that Michael Sandel describes when moral motives such as compassion, duty, and altruism are commercialized, Nico-lucci reports that commercially paid specialists compromise quality.[4] They apply the research criteria more loosely, because it's not their study and they earn more with each patient they recruit.

Further, companies fund thousands of trials not needed for regulatory approval in order to get large numbers of specialists involved, almost as members of the marketing team. Participating in trials has become a significant new source of income for many specialists, further corrupting the ethos of a national health service, or health care as a social good provided on a nonprofit basis.

Despite these institutionally corrupting practices,[5] Nicolucci's Negri-SUD researchers work together with the network of diabetes clinics to investigate important questions on a voluntary basis, like the once-standard guideline that diabetic patients should take aspirin because it will reduce the serious risk of cardiovascular events.

Initially, the Negri-SUD team found that clinics differed considerably in how they treated patients with diabetes. But by developing a specialized soft-ware package, integrated data collection across medical record systems, and an index of process and outcome measures of quality, the project has been able to improve quality of care toward agreed standards.[6] On the basis of nationally analyzed, anonymous data, centers can continuously compare their performance with the top-performing centers (an achievable goal) and "gold standards" of care.[7] The authors' names fill two columns of small type. One might call this a "continuous quality improvement (CQI) observational trial with feedback." American consultants and policy leaders love to talk about CQI but refuse to acknowledge that it cannot happen in a free market where every provider is free to practice how, with whom, where, and on what. CQI requires developing together and sharing goals, measures, data, and practices within a common financial and institutional framework focused on systemic quality, not revenues, profits, or market share. Years of research have found that high-quality health care in a so-called free market is an oxymoron, except for the handful of winners at the top. And even their patients lose from lack of integrated care once they're discharged.

An important research contribution has been provided on the role of aspi-rin in diabetes. In a meta-analysis of randomized clinical trials, researchers at Mario Negri-SUD found that taking aspirin does not reduce the already-high risk of cardiovascular disease among patients with diabetes. As primary pre-vention, however, aspirin significantly reduced risk in men but not women.[8] In a large, observational trial, the Negri-SUD team compared 186,425 patients with or without diabetes who took low-dose aspirin with 186,425 patients who did not, over 5.7 years, for 1.6 million person-years of observation.[9] The team found that patients who took aspirin had a 55 percent greater chance for hospitalization from major bleeding, but aspirin did not increase the risk for patients with diabetes beyond their high risk from diabetes itself. Guidelines have changed throughout the world.

This and other studies have been possible on a voluntary basis, without financial incentives for the clinicians who participate, and they are promoted by a scientific society (Associazione Medici Diabetologi). Clinicians perceive the initiative as a powerful instrument to monitor and improve their practice: In six years the number of diabetes clinics joining the project has grown from 80 to over 300. This is tangible proof that it is still possible to do practice based research, independent from the market-oriented approach of pharmaceutical companies.

A study of international importance in the 1990s tested the belief—largely from America—that taking more aspirin would reduce the chances of a heart attack even more: that more of a good thing would be even better. The results of a landmark trial testing the efficacy-safety profile of low-dose aspirin contributed to a radical change in the therapeutic strategy for this disease.[10] A later trial, also published in the *New England Journal of Medicine*, produced for the first time evidence on what should be the preferred level of hematocrit to be adopted in patients with polycythemia vera (a disorder of the bone marrow) to ensure the most favorable outcomes in terms of cardiovascular events.[11] At present, the Mario Negri-SUD group is the coordinator for Italy of trials promoted by the US National Cancer Institute in the area of myeloproliferative diseases.

With the development of a strong department of informatics, the area of pharmacoepidemiology, run by Dr. Marilena Romero, Vito Lepore, and Antonio D'Ettorre, became an internationally recognized leader in the analysis of large administrative databases that are recognized as a uniquely powerful tool in outcome effectiveness research, a central pillar in the planning and evaluation of public health–oriented epidemiology.

External Challenges to Mario Negri-SUD

The well-known unfavorable events marking the political and economic development of Italy in the first decade of this century have had a profound impact in the southern regions. The cuts in public funding, and the progressive decrease of research funds of the pharmaceutical firms active in Italy, have led some groups working in basic science to seek more favorable working conditions elsewhere, and have greatly affected the overall sustainability of the Institute. The Abruzzo Region with its unstable political governments has failed to maintain its commitment to provide support for at least general operating expenses. The lack of any tradition of private donations (which have been and are so critical for the development and sustainability of the Mario Negri Institute in Milano and Bergamo) does not compensate for the failure of the public partners. While the scientific production of the groups active in the field of clinical epidemiology keeps up its pace of excellent publications (with a mean yearly impact factor of 7–8, even in the difficult, recent years), the Negri-SUD, 25 years after its opening, faced the challenges of an uncertain future.

At the end of the 1990s, larger forces began to undermine the foundation of Negri-SUD. First, the regional government did not pick up on or leverage the advantages and strengths of the Institute as a catalyst for building a science-based economy, as the choice and backing for Negri-SUD would have initially suggested. A regional law to support general operating expenses and selected projects of regional interest of the four main research centers in Abruzzo, including Negri-SUD, was proposed several times by de Gaetano but never approved. Giovanni Tognoni, who has been director since 2001, says there is a "political class" in the South that is not interested in what is best for its own people. Officials are forced to resign because of corruption charges. The public schools are academically inferior. There seems to be no political leadership or will to create and sustain enlightened biomedical research (an old theme noted by Burton Clark decades ago in Chapter 1). This has had an ironic knock-on effect on the students being trained in the South—a key part of the mission and vision for creating the Institute. Research jobs have been scarce; so graduates have gone north to find them, thus reproducing the old pattern of the south-to-north brain drain. Negri-SUD did its job by providing first-class training for talented students from the south, but the government did not complement this effort with biomedical industrial development. Government officials seem to regard Negri-SUD as a costly orchid rather than as a center of research and training that can spur economic growth.

Second, the economy of Abruzzo improved just enough to rise above the criteria for receiving the large, vital EU funds as an economically deprived area. The economy has grown steadily and faster than other parts of Southern Italy, but largely around traditional economic sectors such as automobile manufacturing and wine production. Average income has risen from 53 percent of average in Northern Italy to 76 percent.

Third, Negri-SUD had to fend for itself when the CNR and Chieti University should have brought additional research and training resources. This made the weight of uncovered general expenses heavy for a single institution. Moreover, the free buildings and land meant Negri-SUD had no collateral for securing general loans from banks and had to rely solely on unpredictable research grants or contracts for revenue.

Fourth, the economic recession starting in 2008—the worst since the Great Depression—meant the Ministry of Research and the Ministry for the Environment never paid the Negri-SUD staff two million euros for work completed, even though the Ministry received the money for it from the EU. Apparently, they regarded paying bills from Negri-SUD as less pressing than other financial obligations. The entire budget for Negri-SUD was only seven million euros; so workers had to take a 20 percent cut in their pay to keep their jobs, and morale plummeted.

Finally, in the city of L'Aquila a severe earthquake occurred in the spring of 2009 that damaged thousands of buildings in the capital of the Abruzzo region.[12] About 300 died and 40,000 people became homeless and went to tent camps. The earthquake damaged many businesses and the economy. Food prices shot up and rents tripled. While Negri-SUD was not affected directly, dealing with these problems, in addition to the recession, drew the attention of government officials away from the Institute's plight.

In response to unpaid bills, large debts, and the impact of the recession on research funding, some legal and structural measures have been taken. About 50 of the staff have been reclassified so that a special legal provision enables the state to pay their salaries. The institute was reconstituted as Fondazione Negri-Sud, a more flexible legal form. The region became an equal, one-third partner with the Mario Negri Institute as well as the Province of Chieti. As part of this change, the debts of Negri-SUD were paid off by the three partners, in proportion to their previous involvement. This meant that the Institute in Milan had to pay 75 percent, while dealing with its own problems from a general reduction in grants, contracts, and donations. The situation became very difficult because there were too many people compared to the limited budget resources. Negri-SUD continued its scientific activity with a smaller number of scientists, mostly devoted to epidemiological research and clinical trials, until the economic crises and withdrawal of state support forced it to close in spring 2015.

Replicating the Mario Negri Model Again?

These five larger forces illustrate Pfeffer and Salancik's case for the "external control of organizations" through resource dependency. But the success of replicating the Mario Negri model, until the state withdrew its support, shows that the Mario Negri Institute is not a unique model but rather a coherent, tough set of institutional practices and ethics that has survived serious environmental challenges and can be reproduced in a region or a nation that wants to supplant costly, inefficient, and wasteful commercial pharmaceutical research that largely develops minor innovations with high risks of serious toxic side effects, by sponsoring pharmacological research with open, public participation to develop better medicines and practices for longer, healthier lives. In fact, a team of about 20 headed by de Gaetano and Donati, was invited by the Catholic University of Rome to reproduce the Mario Negri model of institutional integrity in the hills of Campobasso.

"Once again, we opened new laboratories, selected new young people from the region, started *ex novo* new research programmes."[13] With collaboration from local GPs, the regional health authorities, the priests in charge of different parishes, elderly cultural circles, the lay press, television networks, and the public schools, the new Center drew random cluster samples from township registries and started going from house to house to participate in a sophisticated, multifaceted, longitudinal epidemiologic study to find out what contributes to cardiovascular risk and/or cancer and how to reduce it (the MOLI-SANI project). The story underscores the importance of becoming culturally and institutionally integrated into an area and generating a shared vision for a "real utopia" of biomedical research. Using far fewer exclusion criteria than companies do made the sample as representative as possible of the real patient population; so that the results would reflect real practice. Using carefully defined, standardized recruitment protocols, together with structured, digitalized questionnaires about personal and clinical information, the team signed up a total of 24,318 residents. The Pfizer Foundation and the Ministry of Research (MIUR) jointly funded the start of the project (i.e., the enrollment of the participants) with unrestricted grants. The study—still ongoing in its follow-up phase, has generated a series of findings and major articles between 2010 and 2012. One finding we like is that regular consumption of dark chocolate keeps the Grim Reaper at bay.

A principal alternative to taking drugs *after* people acquire risks of serious disease is good diet and exercise to prevent or reduce those risks. The "Mediterranean diet" holds a mythic status as the secret to lower risk among Italians, French, or Greeks compared to the Americans or Brits. Is there any truth to its magical claims? Or is it the wine they imbibe along with the salads, fruits, or vegetables? Researchers at Campobasso have carried out rigorous trials and found that a diet centered on legumes, cereals, fruits, vegetables, and moderate consumption of red wine, rather than processed meat, refined grains, animal fat, and sugar reduces obesity, diabetes, cardiovascular disease, some types of cancer, and all-cause mortality.[14]

Operating independently within the rules, customs, and finances of a university meant that 3–5 year contracts were needed so that the team could operate under its own rules and procedures of independence. In time, however, university officials regarded the center as a foreign object and used its immunological defenses to cancel the contracts in December 2012. This experience reflects Garattini's intuition in 1961 to not set up the Institute as part of the University of Milan and its Department of Pharmacology.

Negri-Bergamo

In this beautiful hillside city, with its ancient upper squares of fine art and dining and lower boulevards for strolling and more fine dining, Garattini had been a favorite son and trustee of the 1200-bed Bergamo Hospital (*Ospedali Riuniti di Bergamo*) since he was 33 in 1961. Born in Bergamo, he wanted to establish the first laboratory of biomedical research and consummate an earlier mission to integrate basic research at the bench with clinical care at the bedside, a mission not possible at the Milano site where there are only laboratories. The obvious partner was the rising star at Bergamo Hospital, Giuseppe Remuzzi, a physician-researcher.

Remuzzi had begun several years earlier as a medical student at Bergamo Hospital. His organizational skills and leadership soon became clear. The hospital, he found, was an excellent place for clinical work, but weak in the areas of research and training. He persuaded the chief of Medicine, Francesco Vaccari, to allow him to organize learning groups of staff and residents who would read, present, and discuss topics or readings in selected specialty areas. No one chose blood coagulation; so the young Remuzzi took it and became interested in platelet dysfunctions in pregnant women. In 1975, at age 26, he was hired at Bergamo Hospital in the nephrology division, while continuing to cultivate his interest in hematology.

Remuzzi became interested in renal dialysis and transplantation. A wealthy man was admitted with severe renal failure caused by a rare kidney disease. He was successfully treated and was grateful to the nephrology staff, then led by Dr. Giuliano Mecca. He was particularly struck by the enthusiasm and dedication that Remuzzi and his young colleagues showed to patient care and research. Remuzzi asked him to sponsor fellowships to leading medical centers abroad for members of his little clinical research team at Bergamo so that they could get first-class, hands-on training. He did, and, in the following years, one went to Strasbourg, another to Leuven, a third to Cambridge, and a fourth to London.

In the meantime, Remuzzi established a connection with the Mario Negri Institute in Milan through Professor Emilio Mussini, a long-time friend of Professor Vaccari. Mussini was a leading figure at the Mario Negri Institute in Milan but his interests differed from Remuzzi's; so he introduced Remuzzi to a couple of young investigators, Giovanni de Gaetano and Maria Benedetta Donati. After their MD degree at the Catholic University in Rome, they had just arrived at Mario Negri from Leuven, where they had been working for the last five years in the field of platelet and coagulation physiology and pharmacology and discussed their PhD thesis in that ancient Belgian University. The connection proved very convenient for both parties, and a collaboration was then started, soon reinforced by the inclusion in Negri staff of a brilliant, beautiful young scientist of Remuzzi's group, Dr. Manuela Livio, whom he married.

Things progressed quickly, and by 1977 this home-grown cub team in their 20s had their first research article published in *The Lancet*.[15] It concerned the nature of bleeding in patients with renal failure and was a harbinger of research-based medical breakthroughs yet to come. Remuzzi and his colleagues at the Mario Negri also organized their dream international conference where they invited international leaders from the fields of kidney disease and the field of hemostasis. They hoped to get people from apparently distant areas of research to talk together and exchange data and formulate hypotheses on the role of hemostasis in the pathogenesis of conditions such as glomerular diseases, hemolytic uremic syndrome, and uremic bleeding. Each speaker had to write a paper, and these became a book.[16]

Meanwhile, after many years of laboratory research with some interactions with clinical work, many senior staff at Negri-Milan had become convinced that a closer relationship with a hospital would enable them to extrapolate data from the lab to the clinic and also to have feedback and ideas from the clinic to the lab (what is now called translational research).

Soon after Remuzzi started his collaboration with de Gaetano and Donati, they introduced him to Garattini, who promptly realized his great capacity for integrating laboratory and clinical research. Given numerous and continuing ties with the Negri-Milano, they invited Garattini to see the integration of advanced clinical care for seriously ill patients they had achieved with basic research on the mechanisms and dynamics of diseases. Together, they began to think about establishing some joint activity in Bergamo that would also fulfill Garattini's ambition to do something for Bergamo as his birthplace. Remuzzi, de Gaetano, and Donati still remember a discussion with Garattini during which 1.5 billion lire was considered the minimum amount of money needed to start a new laboratory in Bergamo.

Another problem was to find a suitable building and site. Remuzzi's uncle, the engineer Camillo Remuzzi, suggested an old convent almost in ruins. Garattini recalled, "I thought that putting together the recuperation of an old building, property of the Casa del Giovane, a non-profit organization to help young people, with the possibility of setting up in Bergamo for the first time a biomedical research laboratory, could be regarded as a good cause for the townspeople and help find the money."

The project required 1.5 billion lire. Since Garattini knew the presidents of three Bergamo banks, the Banca Popolare di Bergamo, the Credito Bergamasco, and the Banca Provinciale Lombarda, he decided to ask them to help and at the same time contribute equal shares of the new laboratory as a gift to science, to the city, and its future. The banks agreed to fund the remodeling of the convent under an agreement with the Casa del Giovane. De Gaetano remembers the three presidents of the Bergamo banks arriving at Mario Negri with their checks. "They looked like the three Kings, arriving at Jesus's cradle."

Other donors followed the announcement of the new initiative. Garattini wrote us:

> I recall an old rich lady whom I visited a couple of times because her husband I knew was affected with Alzheimer. The third time I visited her, she said she wanted to help the new laboratories and she gave me an envelope. When I opened it, I almost had a heart attack: it contained an anonymous savings-book for one billion lira! Very useful money to provide furniture and equipment for the Bergamo site, now called Negri Bergamo to distinguish it from Negri Milano.

By 1984, Negri-Bergamo was completed, with full ties to a major regional hospital. Staff loved the modern labs in the beautiful sixteenth century building on a lovely site. Negri Bergamo started by concentrating on nephrology and organ transplantation, in close collaboration with the Bergamo Hospital, where Remuzzi became responsible for the Department of Nephrology. The lab was open to the doctors of the Bergamo Hospital, and the hospital became open to researchers from the Institute—the first public-private medical department in the country.

Remuzzi kept searching for ways to slow down kidney failure. Joined by then-junior colleagues, Ariela Benigni, Carla Zoja, and Marina Morigi, they recalled in a July 2012 interview how their initial pay as young researchers was so low that two of them had to teach high school to make ends meet. They wondered if they could ever make a living doing research. Now they are known to nephrologists throughout the world for research that has transformed clinical practice and the lives of patients whose kidneys are failing.

INTEGRATED TRANSLATIONAL RESEARCH

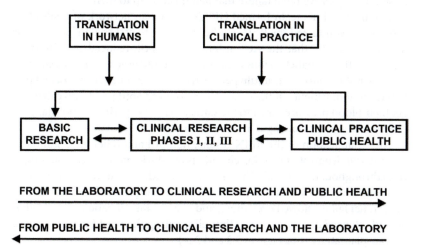

Figure 3.1   Integrated, translational research by 1984

In 1982, Remuzzi and Donati's teams jointly discovered that a single injection of adriamycin, an anticancer drug, caused a nephrotic syndrome in rats.[17] In plain English, they had an easy-to-produce animal model for creating kidney disease and therefore could examine closely the mechanisms of renal disease progression and how it might be slowed down or stopped. In that period other studies contributed to understanding the pathogenesis of preeclampsia by examining prostaglandin metabolism and indicated low-dose aspirin as preventive treatment for pregnant women at high risk of developing it.[18]

In the meantime, Negri-Bergamo scientists devoted themselves to trying to reproduce kidney disease experimentally in rats or mice, in order to find out what could slow down its progress. Remuzzi's team at Negri-Bergamo made significant contributions throughout the 1980s, showing the role of proteinuria, the leakage of proteins through the filters of damaged kidneys. Then they discovered that ACE inhibitors, normally used for reducing blood pressure, also reduced the leakage of proteins. This dual effect significantly slowed the loss of renal function in a few laboratory animals with kidney disease and nicely predicted what is now the treatment of choice for patients with chronic renal disease. Thanks to the translational nature of the Negri-Bergamo integrated research, the results obtained in animals led straight to a human clinical trial, named REIN (Ramipril Efficacy in Nephropathy).

Much of this research was inspired by original observations of Professor Barry Brenner and his coworkers at Harvard University. Brenner's group had previously shown that elevated blood pressure in the capillaries of the element that filters the blood in the kidney and forms urine was responsible for the relentless deterioration of renal function observed in most kidney diseases.

The implications of this research were far-reaching—a new therapeutic tool to arrest progressive renal failure that had no cure up to then.

Remuzzi and his team formed GISEN, an Italian network of nephrology centers that conducted the REIN study. This was the first trial in humans that found in 1995–97 that the ACE inhibitor, ramipril, reduced proteinuria in patients with nondiabetic kidney disease and *slowed progression of renal insufficiency*, not because of its antihypertensive effect but because it blocked protein excretion. Patients in the control arm received antihypertensive drugs to get their blood pressure down to the same level but experienced no change in proteinuria and no slowing of renal deterioration.

After publication of the REIN results, ramipril and other ACE inhibitors became the drugs of choice for chronic proteinuric, nondiabetic nephropathies throughout the world.[19] The patients in the REIN trial were then enrolled in a follow-up study that continued the treatment protocol with ramipril.[20] Their renal failure slowed even more, and in a number of patients *renal failure actually stopped or even reversed,* thus eliminating the need for renal dialysis or transplantation. (See Figures 3.2 and 3.3.)

These studies have provided the foundation for further research that has led to formulating a global approach to halt the progression of kidney disease at what is called the Remission Clinic. The nephrology team has used a combination of drugs and lifestyle changes on hundreds of patients to stop or reverse renal failure. This multimodal strategy targets urinary proteins with combination therapies, intensified blood pressure control, stop-smoking regimens, and infusion of healthy lifestyle practices in outpatients that "normalize urinary proteins and prevent renal function loss in patients otherwise predicted to rapidly progress to ESRD (end-stage renal disease)." "This approach . . . stabilized kidney function in most cases and almost fully prevented progression to ESRD."[21] It thus prevents the need for dialysis or transplantation.

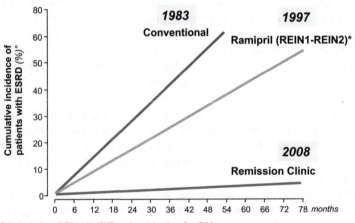

* Patients from REIN with CKD and proteinuria ≥ 3 g /24 h
° Percentage of patients with ESRD means actually percentage of patients that need dialysis

Figure 3.2   Stopping renal failure

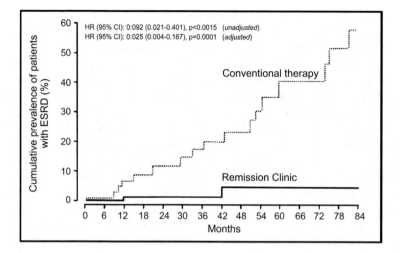

Figure 3.3 Preventing renal failure

Next, the team at Negri-Bergamo turned to diabetic nephropathy, an ominous complication of diabetes and the leading cause of end-stage renal disease in most countries. Half the patients undergoing dialysis in the United States, for example, have diabetic nephropathy, and by 2020, approximately 785,000 will need dialysis or transplantation. In the early 2000s, several large, international clinical trials showed that angiotensin receptor blockers (ARBs) could slow the progression of renal failure in both type 1 and type 2 diabetics with established nephropathy. A few trials have shown a benefit from ACE inhibitors as well. However, those with advanced kidney disease progressed to end-stage renal failure, though more slowly.

Prevention and early intervention work much better than later intervention. This was the reason for designing studies in which treatment with ACE inhibitors was initiated before the earliest sign of diabetic nephropathy, when only microalbuminuria (tiny amounts of albumin in the urine) could be detected. Mario Negri-Bergamo then designed the BENEDICT trial, which showed that the ACE inhibitor trandolapril, given to diabetic patients with hypertension but without signs of nephropathy, could prevent the onset of microalbuminuria, while other blood pressure drugs did not.[22]

Increasing the Supply of Kidneys

Negri-Bergamo's contributions to arresting renal failure have been complemented by another new strategy, increasing the supply and use of kidneys for transplantation, because available kidneys are only one-third the number of people waiting for them. Besides reducing the number of people who need a transplant by arresting kidney failure and thus reducing "demand," might there be a way of increasing the number of kidneys available? Remuzzi's team began doing biopsies of people over 60, the source of half all kidneys donated.[23] They found that a significant proportion of older people's kidneys still worked well, others adequately, and still others poorly.

Dr. Barry Brenner, the distinguished professor of nephrology at Harvard University, had suggested that transplanting two adequately functioning kidneys might restore sufficient kidney function, thus opening up a new way to do transplantations on significantly more people with kidney failure. Brenner did not pursue the idea, but Remuzzi's team at Negri-Bergamo did. In their best mouse model that approximates human kidney functioning, the researchers found that transplanting two adequately functioning kidneys worked well.[24] In theory, then, one could not only save the lives of two people if someone died with two healthy kidneys but one could even use adequately functioning kidneys in pairs. Supply could be increased significantly. In fact, this work by Remuzzi and Mario Negri staff is saving lives by accepting kidneys from old donors and doing dual transplantations of adequate kidneys.[25] Five-year survival rates and other outcome measures are nearly as high.[26] In the United States, half the kidney transplantation centers now have no age limit for donors, and scores of Americans who would have died on the waiting list in years past now have new kidneys, thanks to the pioneering work at the Mario Negri Institute.

Under Remuzzi, the Mario Negri team is working on two other strategies. Progenitor stem cells have been identified in the kidney. They normally are devoted to renal repair, but during a disease they cortically proliferate and migrate, contributing to kidney injury. Scientists at Negri-Bergamo have found the way to reduce this abnormal behavior by restoring the renal architecture.[27]

Finally, strategies to regenerate the whole kidney are being pursued, because drugs with renoprotective properties are not enough when the lesion is too severe. One involves reconstructing nephrons, the filtering unit of the kidney, starting from embryonic tissue that can be integrated into a living animal to carry out kidney functions including blood filtering and molecule reabsorption.[28] Scientists at Negri-Bergamo are also working on re-creating a new organ in the laboratory, starting from a kidney decellularized and subsequently recellularized with embryonic stem (ES) cells or induced pluripotent stem (IPS) cells. In these ways, Mario Negri-Bergamo continues to be a world leader in preventing renal failure, restoring renal function, and transplanting more kidneys to more patients on the waiting lists.

Worldwide, Remuzzi, Benigni, and others are leading campaigns to address kidney failure in Africa and other developing regions.[29] In the last of a six-part series about global kidney disease, the authors point to the prevalence of kidney disease, the need to gather accurate information about how many suffer at stages 1–4 (11.6 percent of the US population), and the potential for affordable treatments. As president of the International Society of Nephrology, Remuzzi is promoting campaigns such as the Global Alliance for Transplantation and Saving Young Lives, which focus on inexpensive but effective ways to minimize kidney failure.

The Center for Research on Rare Diseases

In 1977, a patient from Southern Italy came to the attention of the Milano team: She was a young lady affected by Glanzmann's thrombasthenia, a congenital rare bleeding disorder. The team discovered that the defect was not restricted to platelets but also affected skin fibroblasts, thus explaining a concomitant defective tissue repair in this patient.[30] Garattini was impressed by this case report and by the fact that other diseases studied by Remuzzi and de Gaetano's group, such as hemolytic uremic syndrome or thrombotic thrombocytopenic purpura, were rare, still obscure clinical entities. He became increasingly interested in other cases of children with rare, mysterious conditions and their parents' lonely pilgrimages to medical centers in Italy and abroad to get help, usually at great expense and with few results.

Garattini proposed that the Italian CNR form a working group on "Rare and genetic diseases" that included de Gaetano among its members. In the meantime, he developed the idea of founding a center for such patients, usually very young and bearing genetic mutations. During a meeting in Brussels, Garattini discussed this idea with an officer of the European Union and together they wrote a concept paper on the need to consider rare diseases as a priority because nobody was willing to develop therapeutic strategies for them.

Meantime, the idea evolved that Mario Negri should establish some clinical facilities for these patients. Garattini, Remuzzi, and Leonardi together set out to sensitize the public and the health authorities to the need for a program for rare diseases and orphan drugs like the Rare Disease Act of 1987 in the United States. They soon realized that research on rare diseases must first clarify the criteria for diagnosis, gather firsthand information from patients and their families to clarify the disease's etiology, and bring together enough cases for clinical research to begin. These steps coincide with what patients and their doctors want, too:

- Gather information about their condition and build up a body of knowledge through registries and a data base;
- Give patients this information so they can rapidly reach the best Italian or foreign center dealing with their disease;
- Educate practitioners to recognize rare diseases and to ask for help; and
- Have some beds available, in order to do clinical research on rare diseases, combining in this way the efforts performed in the laboratory with the opportunity to have patients for research—not for care because they would create competition with the NHS hospitals.

During the twenty-fifth anniversary of the Mario Negri Institute in 1988, a lawyer contacted Garattini and told him that a person wanted to donate one billion lire (about US$ 770,000) to the Mario Negri Institute on two conditions: that she remain anonymous and that the donation be made public in hopes that it would inspire others.

Garattini, Remuzzi, and Leonardi looked around in Bergamo for a suitable place and found a great mansion with 365 rooms and hand-painted ceilings and moldings, built in early nineteenth century on the outskirts of Bergamo, in Ranica.[31] It had about 9,000 square meters of space (97,000 sq. ft.), plus outbuildings that overlooked the countryside from the top of a large, sloping park. It had been built by the parents of Count Gabriele Camozzi, who helped Giuseppe Garibaldi establish the unity and independence of Italy. Gabriele Camozzi also served as captain of the National Guard during the uprisings of 1866. In time, the property was given to an order of nuns and became the place where Pope John XXIII went for his "spiritual exercises."

Then an entrepreneur bought it and applied to convert it to condominiums. The Italian Art Authority, however, rejected his plan and said this historic mansion should be devoted only to activities of public interest. This depressed the high price of the property to "only" 1.5 billion lire, a great deal of money for the Institute. Garattini asked the advice of his good friend, Senator Enzo Berlanda, who arranged an introduction to the head of the Compagnia di San Paolo bank from Turin, Dr. Zandano. He expressed interest but was concerned that millions more would be needed to restore the mansion. Garattini replied by promising to invite him to the dedication of a fully restored building, without asking for any additional money. With this assurance, Zandano gave the 1.5 billion lire.

Once the building was purchased, Garattini turned to financing its renovation and conversion into a center for medical research and education. The lady who gave the anonymous billion agreed to disclose her identity as Cele Daccò and invited him to meet at her home in Lugano, in Switzerland. She very much liked the idea of a clinical center for rare diseases and asked how much it would cost to do the renovations. Garattini gave his estimate of 12 billion lire, and she agreed to support it entirely. Renovations took six years, and in 1992 the building was dedicated as the *Centro di Ricerche Cliniche per le Malattie Rare Aldo e Cele Daccò*. Garattini took pleasure in inviting the bank president, Dr. Zandano, along with Luigi Granelli, Minister of Research to the dedication. He had kept his promise.

The Daccò Center is designed as a complex for implementing clinical research. It includes the Rare Diseases Information Center, a fully equipped hospital section for research, ISN-GO or the Commission on Global Advancement of Nephrology, the International Society of Nephrology program for preventing and treating progressive renal diseases in emerging countries. Two other key groups are the Angelo and Angela Valenti Health Economics Center (CESAV) and GiViTI, the Gruppo Italiano Valutazione Interventi Terapia Intensiva for reducing deaths from desperately sick patients in intensive care units across the entire country. Eight years later, an additional outbuilding was renovated in 2002 for animal organ transplantation with the help of the Associazione per la Ricerca sui Trapianti (ART).

The Daccò Center has well-equipped laboratories to analyze genetic mutations in patients with rare diseases—about 80 percent of all rare diseases. It also has a day hospital with ample space for patients and scientists, rooms for

(a)

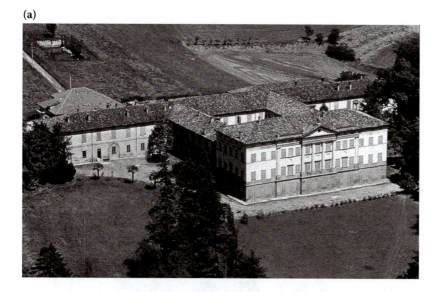

(b)

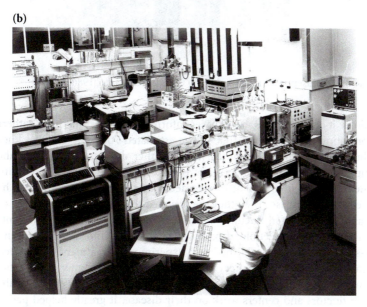

Photo 3.3 (a) The Daccò Center and estate, and (b) a lab inside

the many research courses held throughout the year for nurses, doctors, statisticians, and others, a chapel, and a large conference room. The staff is composed of doctors from several medical specialties and basic sciences, research nurses, biostatisticians, laboratory technicians, and young trainees. An automated data system coordinates input from patients, clinical information, and lab results from different people simultaneously from different locations. It can generate analyses in research and for trials in real time.

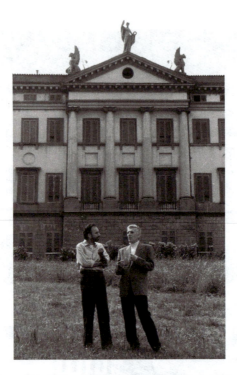

Photo 3.4   Giuseppe Remuzzi and Silvio Garattini at Daccò, 1986

Since it opened, the Rare Diseases Information Center has been gathering information on more than 1000 of the estimated 7000 rare diseases known to humankind. Specially trained nurses gather detailed information about symptoms, experiences, and course of illness from patients who call in or come in with their clinical history, to determine whether or not they do have a specific rare disease. Then they are assigned to a team of nurses at the center and to one of ten doctors (and a network of consultants). The center's information includes etiology, pathogenesis, genetic information, preventive measures, registries, established and experimental treatments, and referral research and treatment centers. For the most part, the center helps patients learn about their disease, about rare-disease networks if they exist, and about which doctors and centers work on their disease. It greatly helped patients, some of whom had been wandering the world, searching for someone to tell them why they have the conditions or behaviors they do, and telling them they are crazy, cursed, or "bad seed." Years later, two surveys of patients with rare diseases found that 25 percent reported waiting 5–30 years for a diagnosis, and 41 percent reported being misdiagnosed initially, resulting in inappropriate interventions and great distress.

The center has inspired the creation of rare disease centers in every region, a national law that passed in 2001, and a national registry. It also contributed to the European Union passing an orphan drug act in 1999. The *Centro di Ricerche Cliniche per le Malattie Rare Aldo e Cele Daccò* was selected to coordinate the rare disease network of the Lombardy Region. Because of its depth and experience, it helped several other regions set up similar centers. It receives about 200,000 euros a year to do this work. The overall program is run by the Italian Health Research Institute. The program helps family doctors and specialists, who may see one case in their lifetime, confirm or disconfirm their suspicions that a patient has a rare disease and provides information about how best to care for their patients. It also trains doctors and nurses about the rare diseases in which it specializes.

This center collects data on all rare diseases it sees but specializes in a few. Specific research projects have been developed for some rare conditions such as atypical hemolytic uremic syndrome (HUS) and thrombotic thrombocytopenic purpura (TTP), Fabry disease, Alport syndrome, Takayasu arteritis, and steroid-resistant nephrotic syndrome. The work of the center can also turn round the traditional progression of research, from bench to translational research to patient care. Remuzzi and Schieppati write, "rare diseases often need the opposite path: we observe rare patients in the clinical practice, then we find out that they have a genetic defect, and finally we reproduce the defect in an animal model to extend the observation further beyond the clinic."

ARMR—A Research Foundation for Rare Diseases

During a Christmas party in 1993 for women leaders, Garattini arrived unexpectedly and Garattini told the gathering that they were restructuring Villa Camozzi into a center for rare diseases. After showing them around the villa, Garattini asked if they would raise funds for the furniture.

"We had to bring the city [of Bergamo] to Villa Camozzi," recounted Daniela Guadalupi, a nonstop entrepreneur, with her husband. "I called all the presidents of the twenty-eight community service clubs and convinced them to pay for dinner for any of their members, no matter how many accepted. One thousand came and the best restaurants of Bergamo offered to prepare the dinner. We raised enough in that night to furnish all the rooms."

After this success, Garattini asked Signora Guadalupi to create an association for rare diseases. She got all 28 presidents to become cofounders of ARMR, the Foundation for Help for Research on Rare Diseases. Located at the Mario Negri Center for Rare Disease, they have raised funds and awareness: "You know, behind a rare disease there is loneliness," she mused. ARMR has won two gold medals from the president of the Italian Republic. "We are pure volunteers," she explained. "None of us has relatives with a rare disease— I think that is a good sign."

ARMR has also raised funds for research fellowships, and one went to Cinzia Rota, a young researcher working at the Mario Negri Center. In 2010, while on her honeymoon before starting a new life, she learned she had won an international prize for young investigators. She flew to Seoul, Korea, to receive the prize and then handed it over to the Mario Negri Institute.

Saving Lives from a Deadly Disease

Atypical HUS is one of nine rare diseases that are researched at the Daccò Center. Prevalence is 1–2 per 100,000 population, and about 50 percent of patients die. At the Camozzi center, Marina Noris is responsible for genetic aspects of rare diseases and a key member of Remuzzi's team. Together with Erica Daina and Elena Bresin, the team has been able to reduce mortality to just 2 percent. Because the disease is genetic, patients are not cured. They have to take the drug for life; but they are healthy and avoid both renal failure and dialysis.

The key discovery came when Remuzzi, Noris, and the team conducted early tests of the drug, eculizumab (Soliris), in humans. A very sick patient came in, and Remuzzi wanted to try it in the first human use—there seemed little to lose and much to gain. Eculizumab was the sole product of Alexion, then a small pharmaceutical company that charged $300,000 for a year's supply then and has raised its price yearly to $569,000 by 2014. Patients must take it for life. Remuzzi contacted executives at Alexion and asked for a free sample to try their drug for a new use, based on successful outcomes with mice. Alexion refused, reportedly saying that the patient was too sick and if he died, it would damage the reputation and future sales of their precious drug. Remuzzi was furious, and the patient died. Subsequently, Remuzzi's team proved that it was very effective in humans.[32]

The Mario Negri team has organized the International Registry of HUS/ TTP and collected biological samples and clinical data that have clarified that the disease is caused by the impaired regulation of the complement protein system due to genetic abnormalities. Such knowledge provides the basis for the use of eculizumab and is the result of a collective effort at the Institute. The team has kept 30–35 patients from dying and returned them to normal life. The Italian NHS pays for it, and it is free to the patients. This contrasts with the United States, where companies are free to set their prices and then insurance companies "contain costs" by obliging subscribers to pay 20 percent of the cost, in this case, about $104,000 cash to stay alive each year, substantially more than the average American family income for a year.

The fully integrated bench-to-bedside research of the Mario Negri Institute since the 1980s, done through collaborative research with no pursuit of profits or patents, enables its teams to seek answers at the genetic, molecular, and cellular levels based solely on what research strategies will most likely help patients with life-threatening or debilitating disorders.

The Expansion of Mario Negri in Milan

In 2007, the Institute staff packed up everything in the original, much-beloved laboratories and moved to a magnificent new building, located within walking distance of the train line from the center of Milan to Malpensa Airport. A large, 48,000 square-meter industrial site had been found next to the Bovisa polytechnic university, on which the Institute's architect, Giovanni Remuzzi, designed an elegant set of labs, fitted with the latest equipment, two conference halls, six meeting rooms, a multimedia hall, a large cafeteria and café, a computerized library, an animal lab, and administrative offices. Across from this four-story, 290,000 square foot building are 33 apartments for foreign and Italian researchers. The Mario Negri teams have about three times more space than before, with room to spare for new research labs, and it took some time for people to get acclimated to so much space. "Crikey!" exclaimed an awed senior research on a recent visit, "We don't build labs like this in England."

As the construction crew put up the building, Fabio Brighenti, head of technical services and responsible for furnishing the laboratories, recalls visiting dignitaries being shown around by Garattini. He would take them up several flights of stairs over here, then down another set over there, then around and up back there, "and we'd take bets on which one was most out of breath and would drop out in the next five minutes . . . they couldn't keep up with him!" He had building instructions printed in Arabic, Italian, Spanish, and Romanian. "And then there were crew who spoke a Bergamo dialect," he added. The building features an advanced cogeneration energy system by Siemens that minimizes energy used to heat and cool all the equipment as well as different parts of the building.

Then the 2008 recession hit, much deeper and longer lasting than anything the Institute had experienced. We asked Garattini about the 1973 oil-crisis recession and he replied, "Then, I could see across to recovery and people knew there would be jobs again. But this time, young people see no sign of real economic recovery, and research funding has become difficult." Late last year, science news from *Nature Neuroscience*, reported that national funding for Italian research institutes would be cut for the third year in a row, by ten percent.[33] On another occasion, Garattini said, "The future is not bright because the government regards funding research as an expense rather than as an investment. And students take science courses but do not learn the principles of science and how scientific thinking changes your view of the world. The concept of probability and risk, and the difficulties in establishing causality lead to understanding why science is so important." Nevertheless, the books for the Institute show little change. One would not know from them that a recession had happened at all. Total research funds increased 2.5 percent in 2008 and have fluctuated by less than 1 percent a year since then, a remarkable achievement.

By 2009, the leaders of the Mario Negri Institute made a fundamental decision to seek qualification as one of the 45 Italian Scientific Institutes for Recovery and Treatment (IRCCS) that qualifies for earmarked national funds. This would be the first time that the Institute would depend on regular, though competitive, government funding, though only through submitting qualifying research projects and requests for upgraded equipment. Qualification required a change in the law, from stipulating that an institute had inpatients to including extra-bedded patients. Considerable resistance from current members had to be overcome, because the Institute would be a strong competitor for IRCCS funds.

Being an IRCCS member will provide opportunities for good collaboration with other members in the region, because IRCCS is the research arm of the NHS, and regions run health services. Basic funding depends on points earned from the number, quality, and impact of scientific publications. The Institute will score well and also qualify for a second fund for scientific equipment. Collaborative projects can win funds for projects restricted to IRCCS members. Overall, IRCCS should provide 3–5 percent of the Institute's funding or perhaps more. But the Institute also needs endowments to provide basic support that undergird research grants and contracts in a given disease area every year.

Today, the Institute has 10 departments in which 51 more specific laboratories and 55 specialized research units are located. (http://www.marionegri.it/mn/en/sezioni/dipartimenti/) Numbers keep changing but there are about 190 research staff in Milan and another 78 in Bergamo and Ranica, 110 support staff, and about 120 postdocs, as well as visitors and scientists funded by external sources, who bring in so many new perspectives and ideas to the permanent staff. The new labs are equipped for pharmacogenomic research, which will be intensified with the aim of finding ways to personalize therapies with psychotropic, cardiovascular, and antitumor drugs. New biotechnologies will be applied, particularly new gene therapy vectors and stem cells to treat heart failure. New models will be developed for the study of neurodegenerative diseases like Alzheimer's, Parkinsons, Amyotrophic Lateral Sclerosis, and epilepsy. The Institute will also continue research in its traditional areas of interest, including angiogenesis, metastasis chemotherapy, mother-infant diseases, pathologies of the elderly, tumor epidemiology, cardiovascular pharmacology, and environmental pollution.

International Outreach

From its early years, certain senior researchers, such as Gianni Tognoni, Maurizio Bonati, and Giuseppe Remuzzi have volunteered to address forms of global injustice and inequality. They have also developed projects in lower-income countries to help by providing their skills in epidemiology, or public health, or in specific disease areas to improve access and treatment. For example, as a young researcher with Tognoni, Benedetto Saraceno undertook outreach projects in Central and Latin America that spanned the 1980s and "the training of mental health personnel, the promotion of an epidemiological approach to mental health care, and the assistance to the local health authorities in the field of mental health policy."[34] Garattini provided critical support from general funds, and the work spanned more than a decade in collaboration with several countries' departments of health as well as with the WHO regional office. This work became the basis for WHO selecting Saraceno to direct programs in global mental health policy through the 1990s and 2000s. He describes first arriving at the Mario Negri in Chapter 2. International outreach reflects the moral principles of dignity and solidarity with those suffering through compassion as described in Chapter 1.

There are more, sustained, often barely funded, projects like this than we can describe that certain members of the staff have undertaken because of their sense of mission toward the underserved and oppressed. They involved studies and training there and bringing back professionals for training here. For example, over several years, the Laboratory for Mother and Child Health under Maurizio Bonati has trained five physicians from Ghana, Egypt, Tanzania, and the Sudan, seven pharmacists from Zimbabwe, Egypt, Ghana, Burkina, and Eritrea, paying for all expenses and sometimes receiving funds from international agencies or associations. After one to two years' training, they have returned to their homeland and often developed or directed national programs. For example, Ossy Kasilo was sponsored in Tanzania by an Italian Catholic missionary to learn pharmacy at Pavia University before she came to the Mario Negri to learn how to organize drug information centers. She returned to help develop several centers, evidence-based formularies (pioneered at Mario Negri—see Chapter 7), and independent review bodies in Zimbabwe and the Congo with distance mentoring from Mario Negri staff. This has proven to be an effective way to make a difference based on Mario Negri research staff providing intensive training for a year or two, followed by sustained support and advising at a distance.

In Latin America, published contributions to the medical literature reflect sustained projects concerning pediatric leukemia in Nicaragua over nearly 30 years, pediatrics in Colombia, cardiovascular prevention in Ecuador, nephrology in Bolivia, and others. Since 1998, the Mario Negri Institute has supported the Colsubsidio Prize for best research in pediatrics in the Americas, which was designed to create a network and forum for exchanging knowledge and best ideas about child health. Bonati's lab has developed international courses on drug evaluation for safety and efficacy, methods, and related topics that can be adopted to different national environments. Other projects have concerned reducing infant deaths through vitamin and nutritional supplements in Ecuador, decreasing high maternal mortality in Bolivia, and improving pediatric care in the Sudan, Egypt, and Nepal. Certain Mario Negri leaders, most notably Gianni Tognoni, have devoted countless hours to campaigns concerning international injustices, violation of human rights, and health inequality. The Institute itself has sometimes devoted funds from its own pooled reserves to support projects as part of its social mission and belief in clinical epidemiology as a service to society and humanity (see Chapters 6 and 7).

From One Student to a National Network

International outreach also occurs through advanced students who come from many developing countries and return to assume roles of leadership and develop new programs, often with expert back up and support from their Mario Negri mentors. Such is the case of a young Bolivian physician, Raul Plata-Cornejo, who came to Negri-Bergamo for a three-year training program in nephrology, funded by the International Society of Nephrology (ISN).

On returning to Bolivia, he founded the Instituto de Nefrologia in La Paz, a unique small clinic for specialty treatment of patients with kidney diseases. Then, with guidance from faculty at Negri-Bergamo he started a screening program for kidney disease, diabetes, and hypertension among poor communities in remote areas of Bolivia.[35]

Dr. Plata also created small health-care units (Unidad de Salud) throughout the Andean region of Bolivia to help poor people at risk for renal failure. At least ten other doctors and technicians followed after him to train at the Mario Negri-Bergamo, all with ISN scholarship and a commitment to return home. Some have joined Dr. Plata at the Instituto. He became one of the most prominent nephrologists in Bolivia and was also elected as president of the Bolivian Society of Nephrology.

More recently the engineering team from Negri-Bergamo has designed and is helping to set up a tele-health system so that nephrology patients in rural areas of Bolivia can receive better follow-up care. (No patents, of course.) Nephrologists at the Instituto de Nefrologia will now be able to provide remote, long-term kidney care to patients at peripheral centers across the country. This will be life-changing: Patients can get specialty care without having to leave family and work to reach an urban specialty center. The project will enable nonspecialist physicians to carry out follow-up care using instructions they receive from nephrologists at the Instituto in La Paz. They will also perform patient evaluation and data collection for quality assessment at the Instituto. Under the guidance of the Negri-Bergamo team, clinicians treating patients across the network collect data using an electronic health record system that is available in real time to nephrologists at the Instituto. These innovations in delivery can be replicated in any country, from the vast rural stretches of the United States to rural China, and anywhere else in between.

From National to Global: "Zero by 2025"

Drawing on the work he has been doing with Plata in Bolivia, Professor Giuseppe Remuzzi became the chair of a new Research and Prevention Committee at the ISN, where he developed a program called Detection and Management of Chronic Kidney Disease, Hypertension, Diabetes, and Cardiovascular Disease (KHDC). This program screens high-risk individuals in rural communities so they can be treated for chronic kidney disease and its risk factors. With support from ISN, Remuzzi also organized the team of bioengineers and experts in informatics at the Daccò Center to create a Kidney Disease Data Center (KDDC). Through the Web, it collects patient data from the prevention programs awarded by ISN in emerging countries. So far, data from more than 100,000 people from Latin America, Africa, Eastern Europe, and Asia have been collected and results published periodically in international journals.[36] The KDDC has also been central to the ISN carrying out its responsibilities as the only officially recognized partner of the WHO in renal disease.

When Remuzzi was elected president of the ISN in 2013, he launched a new initiative, "0 by 25": Zero people should die of untreated acute kidney failure (AKF) in the poorest parts of Africa, Asia, and Latin America by 2025. It has a Mario Negri ethos and a moral mandate: the need to address AKF, often in young patients, in countries lacking good nephrology, using preventive and compassionate low-budget strategies. Treatment of AKF should be as much a human right as treatment of HIV-AIDS. Remuzzi and nephrologists around the world have developed globally applicable strategies that permit a timely diagnosis of acute kidney injury or failure and provide access to renal replacement therapy for patients with potentially reversible diseases in resource-poor countries. They use low-cost intervention centers to screen for factors that put patients at risk for renal failure, carry out early interventions, and use peritoneal dialysis. "0 by 25" builds on and complements the Saving Young Lives project, a constellation of ISN capacity-building programs, and hundreds of volunteers from around the world.[37] The "0 by 2025" project is the latest and largest example of ways in which researchers at the Mario Negri have a multiplier effect on international efforts to reduce global health inequalities.

4

Educating the Public and Future Researchers

From the earliest years, as we mentioned in Chapter 2, one of the main goals of the original group of young, talented researchers as they founded the Mario Negri Institute for Pharmacological Research was to share their model of research integrity with the public, as well as with doctors and their patients. The Institute's three pillars were research, training, and communication. Their sense of research with a social mission led them to breakout practices like speaking against unhealthy dependencies on dangerous drugs like cigarettes, or treatments without evidence, or pseudoscientific fads by doctors like useless cures for cancer. Mario Negri leaders became public intellectuals who also weighed in on a number of other issues.

The first half of this chapter describes some of these outreach efforts. They include several issues that Garattini and others opposed or advocated, and we will go into a couple of them in more detail to convey the nature of the controversies. Mario Negri leaders have not shied away from controversy and have staked evidence-based positions against popular sentiments. In some cases they have prevailed and in others not; but the public came to admire them for their honesty without political prevarications, a refreshing contrast to many other leaders in society. Around one issue we will discuss, Garattini received death threats.

In the second half of the chapter, we move on to how the same core of advanced, independent research served as the basis for training graduate students in advanced research methods, specialized subfields, how to write scientific reports and papers in English, and how to apply for grants. The Institute senior staff organized for researchers from dozens of countries to come and work on research projects. Some programs, like the school for training laboratory technicians or the Institute's summer school for high school pupils, served as bridges over which some students in entry-level programs cross to more advanced training for research careers.

The People's Pharmacologist: Educating Local and National Publics

Perhaps as a response to experiencing the closed, secretive hierarchy of university professors who held themselves above accountability in their self-perpetuating academic fiefdoms, Garattini and Alfredo Leonardi, the Institute's scientific secretary and later secretary general, determined that not only would the Institute's research be transparent and accountable, but they would inform the public, patients, and doctors about it, as well as about what makes good science. In public talks they would explain what a randomized control trial is, and why is it critical to go to all that trouble to have one. Or what does "significantly better" mean, and why is a placebo often not a helpful benchmark for gauging the benefits and harms of a drug? They also spoke out against biased or pseudoscientific research and its unproven products so heavily marketed for profit. The Mario Negri campaigns against "bad science" and "bad pharma," as Ben Goldacre puts it, were so large that they take up all of Chapters 7 and 8.

No senior scientist had come down from his ivory tower before to describe research and answer questions from lay audiences. Garattini, Leonardi, and others got invited by clubs, associations, and other groups. Moreover, Garattini had earned an early reputation as a young star who won awards, and as a bold (also striking-looking!) innovator who was staking a large endowment from Mr. Negri on the bet that a research institute independent of government, universities, and industry could attract steady streams of funding for research. Garattini, the warmly enthusiastic Alfredo Leonardi, and later Giuseppe Remuzzi, and other scientists from the new Institute were invited to talk to audiences on the radio and television. Soon they were speaking almost twice a week—about a hundred times a year. Garattini still keeps up this pace in his 80s. He started writing regular and guest columns in national newspapers and magazines, and he served as a regular guest on national talk shows. An unwavering focus on good scientific evidence has enabled him and colleagues to weigh in on controversial issues in a balanced, fearless way by simply stating what the evidence shows.

Garattini and other Mario Negri scientists also explained to audiences why clinical trials may invalidate even the most experienced expert's recommendations—evidence-based medicine instead of eminence-based medicine. They explained how statistics can show that a drug may have a "significant effect" that is clinically trivial. The question to ask is whether a statistically significant difference makes a clinical difference for patients; often with new drugs the answer is no. Likewise, new drugs significantly better than a placebo may in fact be no better—or even worse—than current drugs in use. They explained why it is important to publish all research results, especially failures and toxic side effects. Yet usually the public hears and reads only about the successes and benefits, largely because a large network of science writers and journalists on retainers with companies write most of the stories.

Soon, people learned about this unique institute of dedicated, underpaid scientists doing things no doctor could do, investigating at the frontiers of pharmacological knowledge for ways to treat patients more effectively. We gave examples in Chapter 3 and will give more in the concluding chapter.

Responding to Community Needs

Soon after the pioneers began working in their new laboratories, people from the area phoned in or arrived at the door to ask about the drugs they were taking. Mario Negri staff did not respond by saying, "Sorry, you've come to the wrong place. Try the local hospital." The researchers understood what numerous sociological studies show in deprived neighborhoods like Quarto Oggiaro, that low levels of education and poor wages make access to health care difficult.[1] Instead, no call or visitor was turned away, and they would find someone in the building (often a research-physician) who could help. No one had ever experienced something like this: an open-door research institute that did not screen out ordinary people but said someone would be right out to help them. The Institute staff then decided they needed to go out and speak at local churches, or clubs, or high schools, to increase what sociologists call "health literacy," a repertoire of understanding, vocabulary, and practical knowledge about a problem and what to do about it.[2]

Working on the outskirts of Milan in the largely blue-collar community, which had still not recovered from the war and the depression before that, the Institute staff watched teenage boys join gangs, commit crimes, and ruin their lives going to jail—some of them quite clever, only doing the wrong thing. Most did not stay in school beyond sixth grade and had no sense of a future. In the mid-1960s, Mario Negri staff decided to organize a small school at the Institute to train teenagers how to become lab technicians, and we shall discuss this more fully in the later section on training. In 1973, Gianni Tognoni and Maurizio Bonati (who grew up as the son of a maintenance man at the Institute) set up evening courses for people in Quarto Oggiaro to help them complete their eight years of schooling after work and receive a diploma so they could get better jobs. Some researchers lived in the area and contributed to the local economy. In time, many residents in Quarto Oggiaro started to make donations to the Mario Negri Institute, small but numerous. When some taxi drivers learned they were taking their passenger to the Mario Negri Institute, they refused to take a fare for the ride.

With time, research leaders decided that a more systematic approach to dispensing evidence-based pharmaceutical advice was needed. In 1975, Gianni Tognoni persuaded the Lombardy Region to sponsor the Regional Center for Information on Pharmaceuticals (CRIF) as an organized way to provide reliable information to pharmacists, doctors, and patients. Their most frequent concern was the use of drugs during pregnancy.

In 1995, Dr. Maurizio Bonati became responsible for CRIF and set up a free telephone number for inquiries. The staff grew to four; but in 2000 the Lombardy Region cut the funding. In response, Mario Negri researchers began to search for new sponsors and were able to arrange for the Bergamo Hospital to continue the CRIF to this day—dispensing almost 40 years of science-based information about medicines to citizens, doctors, and pharmacists. For a few hours a day, someone answers people's questions. Sometimes, to the callers' surprise, Silvio Garattini himself answers the phone and addresses their concerns. They have learned to put information in writing, because oral answers get misunderstood.

Out of CRIF, Bonati, who now directs the Mario Negri Laboratory for Maternal and Infancy Health in the Department of Public Health, developed in collaboration with the union of pharmacies, a pediatric association and the Department of Public Health the broadsheet, *Lo sai mamma?* ("Do you know, Mama?"). Every two months, the laboratory issues another fact sheet for parents about a topic relating to maternal and infant health in simple language anyone can understand. These broadsheets are circulated in pharmacies and widely read. *Lo sai mamma?* is also published, as a column in the Institute's journal for physicians, *Ricerca & Pratica*.

Besides the Regional Center for Information on Pharmaceuticals, the Institute established a second center for drug information, the major Center for Rare Diseases Aldo e Cele Daccò described in Chapter 3, where trained staff respond, largely by email, to hundreds of inquiries from patients, families, and physicians about conditions suspected of coming from a rare disease. It also serves major referral and networking functions. Garattini explains that he and his colleagues have a moral obligation to engage with the public as part of receiving public funds from their taxes, and a duty in gratitude for people participating in clinical trials, as a way to learn from the public their

MARIO NEGRI RESEARCH-BASED OUTREACH ACTIVITIES

MEDICAL COMMUNITY	PUBLIC
• RICERCA&PRATICA (Research & Practice)	• NEGRI NEWS
• NEWSLETTER	• MONTHLY NEWSLETTER
• ARTICLES IN ITALIAN MEDICAL JOURNALS	• THE PRESS, RADIO, TELEVISION
• COURSES IN STATISTICS	• CONFERENCES
• COCHRANE COURSES	• WWW.MARIONEGRI.IT
• COURSES ON RETRIEVING SCIENTIFIC INFORMATION	• WWW.PARTECIPASALUTE.IT
	• MEETINGS WITH PATIENTS

• DRUG INFORMATION CENTER

• CENTER FOR INFORMATION ON RARE DISEASES

Figure 4.1   Outreach activities

concerns or questions, and as a way to counter medicine as a business. The highest compliment Garattini says he has received is being called "the people's pharmacologist."

Reaching Clinicians and Expert Patients

Besides engaging the public through a number of media, Mario Negri researchers have undertaken activities to communicate research findings with clinicians and to engage knowledgeable patients involved in patient groups. Here are two of them.

Dr. Maurizio Bonati is the editor-in-chief of *Ricerca & Pratica* (Research & Practice) a scientific journal started at the Institute in 1985 and still being published (http://www.ricercaepratica.it). The Editorial Board includes Silvio Garattini and Gianni Tognoni. Articles address clinical and practical issues. For example, the March/April 2014 issue included a research report on prescription drugs prescribed to immigrants, an assessment of where we are regarding transparency policy, an analysis of dangers posed by unreliable and often tainted information on Internet sites about medicines, a proposal from the National Institutes of Health for clinical research about off-label uses of drugs, and a column from *Lo sai mamma?* on pain in children. The publisher, *Il Pensiero Scientifico Editore,* has an excellent reputation, and the journal is also affiliated with the *International Society of Drug Bulletins.* The journal also provides on its website several illustrations that can be used in PowerPoint presentations by clinicians—another example of the Mario Negri emphasis on practical knowledge.

Professor Costantino Cipolla, a sociologist at Bologna, wrote that the fourth phase of research, after data collection, elaboration and analysis, and interpretation is communication and practical use.[3] *Ricerca & Pratica* exemplifies how research at the Mario Negri is not a closed activity but an open one that includes dissemination. From the start, it has insisted that researchers publish in English and thus can communicate with a large international audience. The *Mario Negri News* is also written by researchers at the Institute and goes out to 35,000 people interested in the work of the Institute and about the problems regarding research in the National Health Service and work at the Institute.

In 2005, Paola Mosconi founded the Laboratory of Medical Research Patient Empowerment at the Mario Negri Institute, to reflect its "increasing interest in boosting citizens' and patients' involvement in health care."[4] Patients' preferences and their quality-of-life assessment became a focus of research at the Mario Negri at the end of the 1980s, and some Institute projects were conducted in collaboration with patients' associations. Other Italian, English, and American developments occurred in parallel. One particular initiative that Alessandro Liberati actively pursued was *PartecipaSalute* (see Chapter 7).

PartecipaSalute is an interdisciplinary project developed by patient associations and citizens, members of the scientific and medical community, researchers, and experts in scientific communication. It is coordinated by the Institute in collaboration with the Italian Cochrane Center and the scientific journalism agency called Zadig. Initially, it was supported by the *Compagnia di San Paolo* (a large nonprofit foundation in Turin) and has a multidisciplinary scientific board. It has developed several training programs in 2-day modules to train and educate patient association activists. Course topics include the ABCs of clinical research regarding the causes of diseases, the ABCs on how to evaluate the efficacy of an intervention, uncertainty in medicine, conflicts of interest, ethics committees, and strategies of health-care information.[5] Patient activists scored these modules as significantly increasing their knowledge. They have been taught for several years.

PartecipaSalute means "participatory health." As its leaders have written, it "aimed at creating a partnership among lay people, patients' associations and the scientific/medical community . . . [because that community] still fails to see patients and consumer groups as partners with 'equal rights and weight.'"[6] Associations of expert patients (patients with an ongoing condition that has made them experts) have grown rapidly. Chronic diseases and degenerative conditions need the cooperation of the so-called 'expert patient.' Expert caregivers are needed as well—often family members—to integrate hospital and home care. Indeed, self-care and home care are fast becoming the fulcrum of health-care delivery. It is democracy in health care. Participation enables individuals to obtain information about health-care organizations and the possibilities offered by medicine. This is the basis on which people can exercise their rights to access to care.[7]

As a Mario Negri Institute project, *PartecipaSalute* takes into account the epidemiological changes from the classic binary situation in medicine where one was either sick or not to more prevalent kinds of conditions where one can be a patient for years. Often, we are not 'pure' patients, but a presick or a potential-patient, or a semipatient, or somewhere in between. Some patients require periods of treatment involving a high level of technology and intrusiveness (like chemotherapy)—alternating with periods with no medical intervention. As a *BMJ* editorial put it, "Far more than clinicians, patients understand the realities of their condition, the impact of disease and its treatment on their lives, and how services could be better designed to help them."[8] The international movement includes the James Lind Alliance in the UK, the Patient-Centered Outcomes Research Institute in the United States, and Choosing Wisely, as a collaborative effort by several specialty societies to reduce unnecessary tests or procedures and undertake a range of Internet activities.

PartecipaSalute fosters the development of a scientific attitude among expert patients and empowerment through partnerships, using skills of critical assessment, and drawing on reliable expert information. Since 2003, *PartecipaSalute* has developed an impressive number of initiatives to educate and empower patients to mount health campaigns. In the past ten years, thousands of citizens have participated.

The *PartecipaSalute* project contributes to the movement in health care toward partnership models of managing patients with serious chronic diseases and models of participatory governance.[9] Participation of individuals in health-care choices is not only an ethical requirement, it is also a cognitive and organizational one.[10] Health-care institutions cannot on their own recognize and understand the complex health needs of individual patients without taking into account the circles and networks of significant others, neighborhood, work, and community context. Around the patient, there are relatives, associations, and networks.[11]

To make health-care systems more understandable to patients, *PartecipaSalute* has developed tools such as *misuraAssociazioni* (measure associations). Participants are encouraged to analyze the methods of Italian ethics committees and citizens' juries. *PartecipaSalute* provides patients and friends with other tools for empowerment, Web-based resources for every kind of medical condition, and an expanding list of analytic resources like the famous British periodical, *Bandolier. PartecipaSalute* informs expert patients about new tools and studies like the Multidimensional Geriatric Assessment, which the Negri Laboratory on the Evaluation of the Quality of Care and Services for the Elderly is assessing in a clinical study due out in July 2015. Its annual conferences are dedicated to a major theme such as the 2014 theme of investigating why so much good research is underused by patients and what to do about it.

One notable activity organized by *PartecipaSalute* is citizens' juries on controversial medical issues. People gather and deliberate on delicate health issues through structured discussions. Citizens' juries have been promoted by the Mario Negri Institute, the Italian Cochrane Center, Zadig publisher, and the Italian Agency for the Regional Health Care Centers. Recent topics include cystic fibrosis and screening for prostate cancer. Results are publicly disseminated.

The Mario Negri Institute also sponsors a monthly newsletter on attention deficit and hyperactivity disorder (ADHD), a highly controversial sickness.[12] The "epidemic" of ADHD in US schools is a dramatic phenomenon: millions of children are treated with pharmaceuticals that can have dangerous side effects. ADHD appears more like a sign of problems getting integrated into the class than a brain disease. At the same time, American university students make strategic use of getting an ADHD diagnosis so they can use psychostimulants to boost their academic performance. This reflects the shifting, fuzzy borders and constructions of medicalized disorders in the United States,[13] while Italy and several other European countries have developed clear criteria for diagnosing ADHD that limits it use. The Mario Negri Institute has long been wary of medicalizing behaviors or symptoms and cautions against using drugs unless necessary.[14]

The ADHD Newsletter provides up-to-date lists of scientific publications and is a pilot initiative that will be shaped by the suggestions of expert citizens involved. This is part of a project promoted by the Italian Medicines Agency (AIFA) together with the Istituto Superiore di Sanità (National Institute of

Health) entitled "Long-term safety of medicines used for the treatment of schoolchildren with ADHD and epidemiology of ADHD in the Italian population." The Institute also maintains an ADHD Web center that provides materials and info on this topic, financed by the Lombardy Region as part of a project on developed shared diagnostic-therapeutic pathways for ADHD.

Campaigns for Better Health and Research

As public intellectuals, Garattini, Bertele, Remuzzi, and others from the Mario Negri Institute devoted particular attention to certain policies, prejudices, habits, or actions they thought posed a danger to good pharmacological research or to people's health. Often, they weighed in on the unpopular side of a debate or taken-for-granted way of behaving or thinking. Paradoxically, this seemed to increase people's respect for them and the Institute, for taking positions based on evidence and their best judgment, regardless of how contrary to public opinion. Topics included animal testing, genetically modified organisms (GMO), experiments on human embryos, the shutdown of small hospitals in the countryside, increasing the number of incinerators, herbal medicines, and homeopathic medicine. Garattini's case against herbal medicines, as we explained in the Introduction, is simple: People do not know what active ingredients they are swallowing or which ingredients are affecting which part of the body. The case against homeopathic medicines is also simple: They are so diluted that even their advocates cannot tell the difference between them and water in a blind test. Yet at issue is cost to a precious public good, the NHS. Should the NHS provide what patients demand, regardless of evidence of efficacy? Why should the NHS not dole out amulets since there are many people who rely on them as good luck charms.[15]

The Antismoking Campaigns

Finally, Professor Garattini has campaigned against cigarette smoking as the inhaling of a very dangerous "drug" with scores of carcinogens. In 1965, nearly one-third of adults smoked, an average made up of 60 percent among adult men and 7.7 percent among women. Part of increasing gender equality, it seems, has been women becoming more like men in puffing addictive carcinogens, because women more than tripled their rate of smoking to 26 percent by 1990, while men's rate declined to under 40 percent.[16] Since then both have been converging and declining to about one-fifth of adults. Contributing to the decline of the most dangerous drug in society has been the Mario Negri Institute in its rigorous ways. Effective policy has depended on the Institute's Department of Epidemiology, under Carlo La Vecchia, determining the impact of different measures, monitoring patterns of smoking nationally and comparatively for Europe, and measuring the impact of smoking on several chronic conditions.[17]

In the 1960s, Garattini, Leonardi, and other Institute speakers warned audiences about the many contaminants in the smoke and the risks of cancer, even as film directors made sure their female leads smoked to look more alluring as females and made sure their male stars smoked to look more manly! Garattini and his fellow scientists pointed out that the pharmacological mechanisms behind tobacco addiction are similar to those of heroin and cocaine. Having prominent scientists speak out medically and scientifically against one of the nation's most popular habits was certainly surprising, especially since doctors usually said nothing. A minute of concern and advice from one's personal physician has been shown to be quite cost-effective.

Over 40 years, Mario Negri researchers have penned hundreds of essays published in the popular press and scientific journals, conducted interviews and given lectures, and raised people's concerns for the risks of smoking. They also underlined the paradox of a state concentrated on earning money from high taxes on cigarettes while ignoring the huge public health expenditures for lung cancer and other smoking-related diseases. Garattini explained in *Negri News* (XVI/7, pp. 1–2): "The Mario Negri Institute, an independent organization that is concerned and devoted practically to the defense of human health, considers its central duty to express its opinion about smoking." The state did nothing specific about it until the late 1980s.

Garattini's and Leonardi's battle against smoking was unpopular and yet contributed to the wider campaign to limit or prohibit smoking. The first law, passed in 1975, No. 584/1975, banned smoking in some public places like hospitals and public transport but lacked serious enforcement, except in primary schools. Fines for smokers were the exception. Antonio Maturo remembers in 1980 his teacher smoking in his sixth grade classroom in Northern Italy. In trains, the law established nonsmoking wagons, but if there were no signs, people assumed they could smoke. The strong prosmoking culture of the South contrasted with a somewhat more cautious, evidence-based attitude in the North. In 1986, the Minister of Health proposed a comprehensive ban on smoking that Garattini strongly supported, and Mario Negri studies showed public support was quite strong.[18] But then the minister was transferred, and it took another 19 years before a comprehensive ban passed.

By 1991, warnings appeared on packs, saying "Smoking is harmful." In 1994, Garattini took on a very popular TV anchorman, Gianfranco Funari, who had millions of fans. The professor said he was rude to smoke where others gathered, and he set a bad example for young people. Funari countered that Garattini was inelegant in his polo shirts. Some years later, however, Funari contracted lung cancer, changed his mind, and said that Garattini had been right. In 2005, he publicly made an appeal: "Youngsters, I beg you not to smoke. I have had to have five by-passes because of smoking. Smoking has destroyed my life."

In 2005, Italy passed a landmark law prohibiting smoking nearly everywhere except in open air, the strongest law in Europe. Once smoke-free policies where put in place, public support *increased*.[19] Tobacco bans are almost universally accepted. Yet, vending machines still lead to minors smoking.

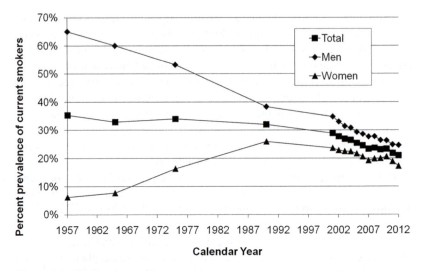

Figure 4.2   Decline in smoking

More recently, the Institute has promoted the idea of raising the price of cigarettes to support biomedical research. Each 20 cents of research tax per pack produces about one billion euro, and can pay the salaries of 6,000 researchers and to grant 12,000 fellowships. Since a package of 20 cigarettes costs on average €4.5 in Italy compared to €6–8 in other European countries, there is plenty of room to raise billions for biomedical research. As higher prices reduce the number of smokers, one could raise the tariff, thus taxing smokers in proportion to their refusal to quit.

Quack Cures

Quack cures, like the Di Bella cure for cancer or the Stamina therapy for neurodegenerative diseases are another matter, more powerful and possibly dangerous. Luigi Di Bella was mild-mannered, cultivated specialist on the faculty of the University of Modena who developed during the 1960s a personalized brew from somatostatin and bromocriptine, as well as vitamins, melatonin, and sometimes low doses of chemotherapy drugs or other substances combined in varying amounts that either shrunk tumors or cured cancer. Both he and his therapy became so popular that according to a survey in the mid-1990s, 42 percent of citizens believed it worked and 53 percent were unsure, while only 1 percent thought it was a sham.[20] When Professor Garattini was asked by a scandal-ridden government to oversee the removal of useless or dangerous drugs from reimbursement by the NHS (described in Chapter 7), some drugs of the Di Bella cocktail was among them. He became the target of attacks and talked widely on why no scientific evidence supported the therapy by the beloved Dr. Di Bella. Then the Ministry of Health supported the assessment by Garattini's team by stating that the Di Bella method was "not scientifically reliable." Because Di Bella's method was popular and losing NHS coverage for the drugs made them expensive, patients mounted protests.

The public became distraught from the strength and desperation of patients and their relatives battling on behalf of Professor Di Bella's therapy. Front-page stories filled the press and the most popular TV talk shows featured the quiet, cool, and ever-popular Di Bella explaining that Garattini and the NHS were depriving cancer patients of his proven therapy. A judge in the South of Italy ordered the health authorities to treat people with the Di Bella therapy for free. Stories of cancer patients taking the therapy brought tears to the eyes of viewers. People rallied in streets for the right to choose how to be treated. Patients as consumers were pitted against medicine as a science. The ex-Fascist party *Alleanza Nazionale* became the political supporter for Di Bella's therapy, and members of Parliament launched initiatives to legally support it. Garattini spoke widely against both Di Bella and the judge's decision. He called Di Bella a charlatan.

In this classic case of evidence-based medicine versus consumer-based and eminence-based medicine (Di Bella, a senior, respected expert, was convinced that his therapy worked), the Ministry of Health ordered a clinical trial. The results showed Di Bella's therapy did not shrink tumors or cure cancer.[21] The National Oncological Committee also insisted on the inefficacy of Di Bella therapy. A later study of cancer patients treated by Di Bella from 1971 to 1997 found his treatment did not improve survival compared to standard treatment.[22] Garattini and his evidence-based decision to forbid NHS coverage prevailed against widespread public support, and the Mario Negri Institute dedicated its thirty-fifth anniversary in 1998 to its role in contesting Di Bella therapy. To this day, however, many patients ask for the Di Bella therapy and some physicians are willing to offer it, for cash.

A much more recent case has occurred around the Stamina therapy that its creator, Davide Vannoni, who established a company and foundation for its promotion, claims to cure a number of neurodegenerative diseases using stem cells. Although medically more complicated, many features of the Di Bella case are present: great pressure for it from the media; broadcasts of convincing video tapes; claims of high success rates on hundreds of cases; street demonstrations; payments of 20,000–50,000 euros per treatment; yet no scientific evidence that it works. Garattini was one of the first Italian scientists to take a strong stand against Stamina therapy, even when a young girl seemed to have benefited:

> We are faced with a situation that is understandable. On one side, a desperate family is witnessing the dramatic sickness of their child and wants to do anything possible to treat her. Therefore the family is in a very vulnerable condition. On the other side, there is a group of people who work without any authorization for the creation and the utilization of stem cells—a highly abnormal situation.[23]

By 2013, several investigations found too few stem cells in Vannoni's cocktail to be effective, traces of dangerous pollutants, and violations of safety and hygiene regulations. There have been charges of fraud, lawsuits from patients, and finally the editors of *Nature* concluding that Stamina therapy is based on false data from a "psychologist transformed into a businessman doctor." The Department of Health subsequently judged the therapy as "dangerous for the health of patients."

Campaigning for Animal Research

In the efforts by Mario Negri researchers, nothing is so valuable as doing research on their rats and mice. In Chapter 3, for example, every step in the research to find out how to arrest renal failure depended on trying out alternatives on certain strains of rats, bred to most approximate the kidney functions of humans. Careful observation and measurement enabled Remuzzi's team to learn from each effort, discard less successful ones, and move on with better ones. What would be the alternative, to induce renal failure or another disease condition in humans and measures their responses?

That said, great efforts have been made since the Mario Negri opened to improve the lives of rats and mice, and to reduce the number needed. In 1962, Garattini designed a much more comfortable home to replace the steel-and-wood cages by using new, transparent thermoplastics and working with Carlo Bernardini at Tecniplast. This cage set a new international standard, and as it became adopted throughout the world, they have together been improving the design and related animal equipment ever since. New technologies for measurement have greatly reduced the number of animals needed, and all staff working with animals must go through special training.

Recently, we ran into Professor Garattini who told us about his weekend. On Saturday, he attended a small, closed gathering of publishers in a region; yet soon after he arrived, professional demonstrators appeared who shouted from behind their placards: "MURDERER!" "ANIMAL TORTURER!" On Sunday he traveled far to speak at a public event in a different region and there they were again, apparently paid to track him wherever he goes. Animal rights advocates target Garattini because he has spoken out for the importance of using animals in pharmacological research with unwavering vigor for 50 years, as convinced of the just use of animals for research as his opponents are convinced that no such use can ever be just. He has admonished research colleagues who cave into militant opposition against using animals to develop better medicines for seriously ill patients. Still worse are research leaders who declare they don't experiment on animals but then surreptitiously do. Declared as heroes who have joined the cause, they betray it on the sly.

PETA or People for the Ethical Treatment of Animals, is the world's largest animal rights organization in the world, with headquarters in the United States, UK, Germany, The Netherlands, France, India, Australia, and elsewhere (http://www.peta.org/). At least in 2013 it featured a video, "Who cares about mice and rats?" Who cares that they feel pain or care for their young or are resourceful—they're just rats and mice. On this point Garattini completely agrees with PETA. That is why Mario Negri animals are kept in a safe, clean, healthy environment, and the humans have to be decontaminated to visit the animals, as they are called "animals" at the Mario Negri Institute. We asked the head of the Animal Clinic, Giuliano Grignaschi, "Why don't you call it the "Mice and Rat Clinic?"

He replied, "Because they are as special as beagles or monkeys." Calling it the Mice and Rat Clinic would imply they are morally less important. "Silvio asked me to take up this position because he said he knew how much I loved my animals and how careful I am with them," Giuliano told us. "The Animal Clinic is fantastic. You should see it!" We suited up and did.

"The [new] Clinic completely reverses what has been done for years, carrying cages of animals to the researchers and their labs," Giuliano explained. "Instead, the researchers now come to the animals, and all the research equipment has been relocated with them. The animals used to get very stressed being carried to the researchers. And stressed animals produced much more variable results so the data were more inaccurate. Making the researchers come to the animals is much more humane and also produces much more accurate research results. Researchers don't like the inconvenience and the rules I have set out that they must observe. They must go through an elaborate and inconvenient process of being completely suited in sterile suits and go through a sterilizing air 'shower' . . . Researchers are coming into a perfect environment for the animals; so we have to make sure they keep it that way. It's not pleasant working for hours inside those suits.

The PETA material emphasizes that lab animals "are locked in cages and abused" (http://www.peta.org/). Short of the experiments, which we will get to next, the animals at Mario Negri live in a much safer, healthier, calmer, and more stable environment than living in nature. They never have to forage and not find enough food as they do in nature. Their chances of disease are much lower than among mice and rats living outdoors in nature. They get a perfect, full night's sleep, every night. Temperature, humidity, and ventilation are ideal for them. They never get cold in winter or swelter in summer. They eat regularly an ideal, tasty diet, we were told—not too rich or too lean. Caring for the animals is very expensive, the second largest budget item after the salaries of the researchers. The ideal conditions, food, and dedicated staff add up.

Garattini explained, "We have greatly improved the precision of measurements. What used to take 100 mouse brains to measure can now be measured in one brain, along with many better measurements. Further, with nuclear magnetic resonance, we don't have to kill a mouse at all to see what's going on inside . . . Years ago, we killed mice at 3, 6, 15, 30, and 90 days to study the progression of disease and drug intervention. Now, we can watch the progression using nuclear magnetic resonance tomography and don't have to kill any."

Giuliano told us that in 1972, 7.5 times more animals were used by one-third as many researchers as today. In *The Lancet*, Mario Negri Institute researchers reported that they halved the number of animals between 1980 and 1983, from 129,120 to 67,234.[24] Then it took 11 years to halve it again. By 1996, the Institute used only 24,781 animals. Yet the research staff published 53 percent more scientific papers from these in vivo experiments.

The usefulness of mice and rats depends on the disease and the strain of animal used. Based on years of data and study, specific strains are bred to more closely approximate the response in humans for a particular disease or intervention. An extensive data bank develops on which researchers can draw to make future experiments more likely to produce helpful information.

Concerning alternatives, Garattini has observed, "It is common knowledge that cell cultures *in vitro* do not retain all their properties and because they are freed from nervous and hormonal influences, they acquire some new properties. Therefore to limit research to *in vitro* techniques may be a source of considerable errors and artifacts."[25]

Finally, the PETA website quotes Michael Leavitt, the former Secretary of the US Department of Health and Human Services as saying, "Currently, nine out of ten experimental drugs fail in clinical studies because we cannot accurately predict how they will behave in people based on laboratory and animal studies." Ironically, nine out of ten drugs tests on human cells also fail. Thus, about 90 out of the 100 most promising drugs in vitro are found out in vivo to be more toxic or less effective than anticipated. Then 9 out of those remaining 10 successes in vivo fail in human trials, leaving only one in a hundred that proves effective and safe enough to be approved for patient care. Without the in vivo trials, however, all 100 "promising" drugs would have to be tested in humans, and 99 of them cause toxic reactions in humans.

In 2013, Garattini became Enemy Number 1 for the "animal liberation" associations because of his position against the Italian law on animals in research. Not only does Garattini receive death threats, but activists have rallied against him and depicted the Institute as the symbol of "vivisection," though its care of animals is the opposite. On social networking sites, one can easily find threats like: "We will make the Mario Negri explode" or "Professor: you will die with the same pain as you caused the animals you kill at the Mario Negri Institute."

Responding to the undiminished opposition to experimentation with animals, legislators wrote a highly restrictive bill that has substantial support. It goes far beyond the standards set by the EU and most nations for using animals in research.[26] The editors of *Nature Neuroscience* wrote, "This legislation, if approved by the [Italian] Senate and enacted, would prohibit the breeding or use of cats, dogs and nonhuman primates for experiments, with the exception of clearly defined translational (human health-related) research purposes. In addition, the statute mandates that anesthesia or analgesic agents must be applied during any procedure in which the animal may experience some pain, except in cases where anesthesia or analgesia are the subject of the study."[27]

Garattini explained his views about this pending law in an interview with Federico Tulli in the radical newspaper *Left* published on November 28, 2013.[28] He pointed out that there were "three aspects of the law, as it is now, that would prevent us collaborating with other colleagues in the European Union. The Italian version of the law has many restrictions compared to the other EU countries, where it has been enacted without any change in 22 cases out of 28 (among these, Great Britain, France, Spain, Belgium, Denmark and Sweden)."

According to the Italian version, *any* experiment on animals must be done under anesthesia, including an injection. The law also prohibits xeno-transplants, including the implantation of tumor cells in special strains of mice with very low immunological reactions in order to study the efficacy of an anticancer drug so that cancer research cannot go forward. The third restriction is "the prohibition of testing on animals any drug or substances that induce addiction. The controversy over animal research remains intense today, though the militant wing of the protest movement offers no alternative methods for developing better medicines for people with serious illnesses or pain. While the law has been approved by the Senate, questions raised by others have convinced the Minister of Health to have a moratorium up to January 2017 while the search for alternate methods will be pursued. Garattini points out that if opponents to animal research live by their beliefs, they should use no medications or cosmetics because both are tested on animals, and they should oppose public health programs to exterminate rats or other rodents."[29]

Giving to the Mario Negri Institute

In a widely respected treatise on trust, the Polish sociologist, Piotr Sztompka, identifies several kinds of trust that range from social to technological to organizational.[30] The vigorous, multidimensional efforts by Mario Negri leaders to fulfill their social mission by reaching out to various people and speak their truth about controversial issues has generated organizational trust in the Institute and personal trust in Garattini and other leaders. Although the Institute has never had a marketing department or fund-raising department, by the 1970s, people started donating to the Institute, not just checks, but stocks, works of art, apartments, summer homes, cars, and inheritance. By the 1990s, looking after and managing these gifts became a part-time job. There is nothing like the Mario Negri, though it can be replicated to advantage. One reason people give is that the Mario Negri is so frugal with the money it receives—low salaries, few frills, low overheads. All this, we believe, suggests that the Mario Negri Institute owes much of its excellent reputation to the fact that it does not try to please the general public. Its researchers make no efforts just to be popular, but they are dedicated to improving patient health through science without patents or profits.

Research Training at the Institute

Inherent in the Mario Negri Institute as a unique model of how first-class research should be done was the goal to teach both young and more established researchers the methods and strategies that Garattini and the pioneers had developed for themselves and by visiting leading laboratories in the United States and elsewhere. Not too many free-standing research institutes in the world have such an extensive and purposeful program in professional training but rather rely on universities. The pioneers drew on the Anglo-American models of having advanced students or fellows work side by side with senior researchers, learning by doing, coauthoring research papers, and even applying for funding for their own projects. These ideas were more or less implicit in Mario Negri's will—training should be grounded in research data and students should participate in the enterprise of science and learn through direct experience. Students had to be like apprentices. As Alfredo Leonardi wrote in 1981, "The comparison is not a paradox. In an artisan's workshop, the pupil [or apprentice], learns the job by doing the work and not only doing exercises on abstract patterns. Here it is the same. The student is immediately enrolled in the research team and is obliged from the very first day to face the practical problems of scientific experiments."[31]

Since 1965, more than 7,000 people of all ages and levels have spent a few months or more as trainees, and about 3,000 have completed a course after 2–3 years at the Institute. Scholarships are provided for all the students enrolled in the programs offered. About 90 percent of the scholarships are funded directly by the Mario Negri, while the remaining 10 percent are financed by foundations or associations like ARMR (the association for rare diseases profiled in Chapter 3), the Association of Friends of Mario Negri, the Monzino Foundation, the Associazione Italiana per la Ricerca sul Cancro (Italian Association for Cancer Research), and Fondazione ARTPer la Ricerca sui Trapianti (the ART Foundation for Research on Transplants).

From the start, training at the Mario Negri Institute (MNI) had four distinctive features: learning by doing, applying theory and concepts to specific problems, precise measurement, and full transparency for critical but constructive feedback. Cross-fertilization, open discussions, and interdisciplinary contact have always been strongly encouraged through the "Two O'clock Club" where young researchers present their work or a problem on which they want feedback; in the comfortable cafeteria staff of all ranks sit at long tables; and in the original research library, open at all hours, researchers used to meet to work and discuss things together, until literature searches went electronic.

Students and researchers work full-time in research programs using advanced equipment and learning the most modern methods, in regular contact with colleagues from different countries and disciplines. Besides its scientific value, this approach serves as an excellent basis for establishing good interpersonal relations.

At all levels of training there is a constant effort to relate abstract concepts to practical situations and specific problems, grounded in empirical facts and examples. Indeed, the philosophy of the "founding fathers" had two specific traits: the importance of empirical measurement and the importance of relating theory to facts and back to the hypotheses on which the theory was developed. This constant testing, then reconceptualizing, and open dialogue within the Institute is also expressed in the continuous efforts to engage the public, patients, and practicing doctors in dialogue about claims and myths affecting health and medicine. It is part of the Institute's organizational culture. Edgar Schein, the distinguished professor of organizations, stressed how an organization's culture can be influential but "invisible" at the same time:

> Perhaps the most intriguing aspect of culture as a concept is that it points to phenomena that are below the surface, that are powerful in their impact, but invisible and to a considerable degree unconscious. In that sense, culture is to a group what personality or character is to an individual.[32]

In the same years, another article that became very influential came out in the *Harvard Business Review*. In "How Bell Labs Create Star Performers,"[33] Kelly and Caplan demonstrated how productivity in a laboratory was not primarily connected to cognitive skills but work strategies. They identified nine strategies: taking initiative, networking, leadership, perspective, followership, teamwork, effectiveness, organizational savvy, and show-and-tell. In different proportions, all these dimensions are present in the MNI organizational culture based on highly organized project and informal interaction. The informal atmosphere rewards taking initiative and teamwork; leadership and followership are complementary qualities linked to the project pursued at any specific time. The fact that *Negri News* always published articles by Mario Negri researchers reinforces the organizational culture. Networking is facilitated by the design of labs, meeting spaces and the easygoing bar and long tables in the cafeteria. The Institute has always been an example of a future-oriented organization based on projects, where trainees have mentors but also are encouraged to develop their own ideas. This contrasts with many Italian and European universities.

The "School for the Kids"

In a project that put social mission ahead of advanced training, the first formal training program that the Mario Negri researchers established was a small school, Laboratoristi Biologici, to train teenagers for lab work. Between 1968 and 1976, early records show about 30–44 students were enrolled in any given year. Nicknamed "The School for the Kids," it took young boys and girls with at least eight years of schooling off the streets, away from gangs, and immersed them in a world where what mattered was precise measurement, technical mastery, and how to document the inner secrets of the body. They learned science, research methods, and the habits of disciplined study. They learned good work habits: arriving on time and dressing appropriately, taking responsibility for their work, and carrying out assignments properly. The concept, scope, arrangements, and range of subjects surpassed science training for teens in most of Europe or North America. Yet many of the kids were what Italians call "immigrants from the South"—families who had moved north from the poorer southern regions of Italy.[34] Even more miraculous, well-paying, stable jobs awaited them! Some of these students went on to attend high school, graduate, and go on to university. A few like Caterina went all the way to the top.

Caterina Bendotti first came to the Mario Negri Institute when she was 14 (in 1970), because she had finished eight years of schooling and was trying to find a way to get ahead. She still comes to the Institute every day, now as head of a laboratory. Her parents could not support her going to an academic high school; but the Institute had established a three-year course to give young teenagers the opportunity to qualify for a good job as a laboratory technicians. Moreover, the Institute paid her a little for her work in the lab as she apprenticed, "not very much, but enough to pay for my transportation. My parents were delighted: I was getting a good, practical education with no cost to the family."

She then qualified for a university education while working at the Institute, went to graduate school while still on the job, and finally added a PhD through the Institute's program with the Open University. She would never have gone so far, she told us, without the opportunities for working-class kids provided by this world-class research institute.

Caterina has good memories of The School for the Kids and its exceptionalism: "As we spent the afternoons in the lab I got home every evening at dinner time." She recalled, "There was practical work to do, experiments, but in the morning we did theory. Actually, most of that was the grounding for the experiments in the afternoon. We learned how the tools and labs functioned. The subjects were chemistry, physiology, theory, and techniques of laboratories; but we also studied English . . . Mr. Tognoni did a social science course applied to the contemporary world."

Caterina told us, "The school environment was very good. The third-year students made fun of us 'freshmen,' but the goad was the opposite of bullying. It was a typical high-school atmosphere. Girls were numerous, at least 50 percent. I was proud to be doing different things from friends in my

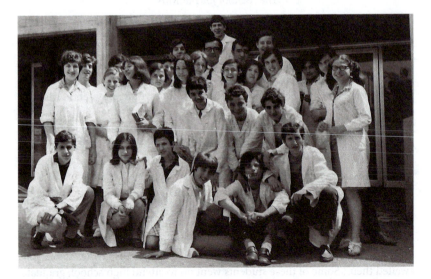

Photo 4.1   The "School for Kids," 1969

(a)

(b)

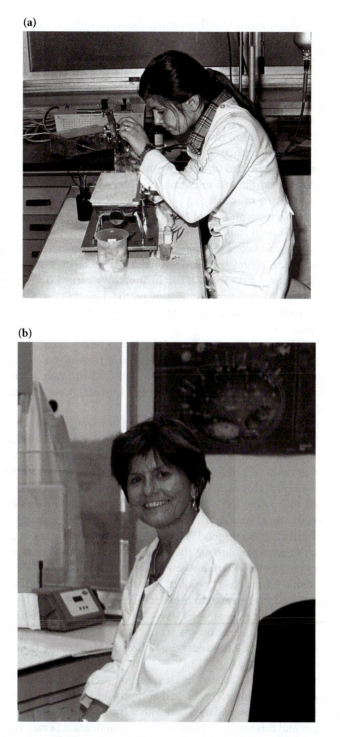

Photo 4.2   From "kid" to lab head: Caterina Bendotti (a) 1984 and (b) now

neighborhood at home. I told them about the work with mice and they were terrified, while I was proud of learning how to do it. At the time, I had no idea I would have become a scientist one day."

Attending that school must have made Caterina Bendotti feel a bit like Pippi Longstocking, the unconventional Scandinavian kid, getting an unconventional education at the Mario Negri, preparing her for unexpected events later in life.

After the three years in the School, Caterina received a small scholarship from the Institute and started work as a lab technician, the job she had been trained for. But she carried on studying in the evenings and at night courses to earn the five-year diploma in chemistry—*perito chimico*—a certificate that qualified her to enter university.

"When I finished high school Silvio [Garattini] said: 'You have done 30; now do 31.' This is an Italian saying implying 'you've got this far, now push on a bit further and take a degree.' The Mario Negri senior scientists always urged us to study, especially Silvio. Other ex-lab technician students and I took evening classes after work at the Institute. We earned our diplomas as worker-students. It was a very stimulating period: I lived in two worlds. I also attended university evening classes from 5 to 10 pm and eventually took a degree in pharmacy."

After her degree, Caterina followed the Mario Negri "internal doctorate" course in Biomedical Research. Then she won a postdoc fellowship to the Johns Hopkins University to learn more advanced research methods and do research for two years, together with her husband, also a researcher at the MNI.

At Johns Hopkins, they did not realize that any woman who could work full-time while getting advanced degrees was worth paying attention to. "I was the first student from another country in the lab and a woman"—twice over a stranger in the world of American male scientists. Faculty paid no attention, but she kept asking incisive questions. "They didn't realize how stubborn I was," said this petite, self-effacing terrier of a woman who would rise to international distinction. "And I had a terrible time with English, especially informal words like 'Sounsgood.' Finally I made them write it out and then I understood they were blurring their consonants." During her two years at Johns Hopkins, she learned many new research techniques.

"I am a total Mario Negri product. When I came back from the USA in 1988, I continued my research in the Mario Negri Laboratory of Neuropharmacology. It is hard to say at what level—we had few official distinctions at the Institute. I could decide on my research topics by myself, and I won a good number of grants. After some time I became Head of the Laboratory of Molecular Neurobiology."

But this remarkable ascent in defiance of sociological "laws" against working-class kids rising so far turned abruptly into a near-tragedy with an ironic twist: "In 2004 I was diagnosed with a lymphoma: a rare type. I study rare diseases and this was a very unusual skin lymphoma, a Sézary syndrome. I had the first symptoms in 2000, mostly an intense itch, but it took four years to find out exactly what disease I had. I asked Professor Rambaldi at the Bergamo hospital to be my doctor. He had worked at the Mario Negri, and I asked him because the hematological part of my disease had spread to my bone marrow. I did a lot of chemotherapy and other treatments but to no effect. In 2009, I decided for a transplant, after having discovered that one of my sisters was compatible. We transplanted some bone marrow, and it worked."[35]

Training PhDs

Although Italian universities did not have PhD degrees until 1980, the Mario Negri Institute started training university graduates and physicians in the late 1960s. Some tell their story in Chapter 2. The bold new Institute for research drew on the international reputation that the pioneers had already garnered and on their networks of colleagues in the rest of Europe, North America, and Asia, to organize research training and experience for postdoc (post PhD) visitors from abroad. A few years after postdoc training began, Professor Alan Cowan, now emeritus of pharmacology at Temple University, arrived in 1973 and recently recalled how his experience transformed his career:

The guard summoned me through the iron gate one wintry evening in January 1973. The dense Milan fog occluded the famous address—Via Eritrea 62—but, sure enough, ahead lay the legendary home of Italian pharmacology. I was there quite by chance. Destiny had selected me to drive our seminar speaker where I worked in Hull, UK. Unexpectedly, he invited me as a novice industrial pharmacologist to the Mario Negri Institute in Milan to learn about serotonin and brain lesioning techniques. The outcome was one of the first papers on buprenorphine, the oripavine that is still very much at the fore as a medication in the opioid drug abuse field, four decades on.[36]

The Institute was a vibrant, academic oasis in a rough part of the city. The impressive cast of foreign investigators benefited intellectually from the many provocative seminars, wonderful Pfeiffer Library and bonhomie of the on-site, residential International House. Scientific debates continued through impromptu lunchtime matches on the adjacent football pitch. Train journeys to Chiasso in Switzerland to post letters were endured with good humour amid the national mail strike in 1974. Luigi Valzelli, Daniela Ghezzi, Sergio Algeri and, of course, Silvio Garattini, are fondly remembered. Anthony Turner (from the UK), Charles Chidsey and Martin Adler (both from the USA) were also visiting scientists at that time. And it was Marty who, spontaneously, invited me to Temple University in Philadelphia and unveiled a new and totally unexpected career in the States. Serendipity with a capital S! The Temple-Mario Negri connection was solidified through the organization of an influential meeting of key opioid researchers at the Institute in 1976 and the subsequent editing of the proceedings ("Factors Affecting the Actions of Narcotics") by Marty, Luciano and Saro in the excellent Mario Negri Monograph series.[37]

A couple of years ago, while on vacation, I paid a nostalgic visit to the "old" Mario Negri—abandoned, decrepit and a sorry sight. No matter. I felt as if I was passing through pharmacological history, as if amongst the weeds I might catch a glimpse of my younger self. Ah, memories—they seem at the same time so vivid and remote.

In 1999, the Institute negotiated with the British Open University to confer a PhD to advanced students at the Mario Negri Institute so that they would have a degree that was recognized worldwide. PhD programs were also arranged with two Dutch Universities, Groningen and Maastricht. The International Graduate Program of the Istituto di Ricerche Farmacologiche Mario Negri trains students for research careers in pharmacology and toxicology, with special reference to oncological, neurological, cardiovascular, and kidney diseases. Other areas of training are environmental toxicology, organ transplantation, rare diseases, molecular pharmacology, public health, and clinical epidemiology. All students do not pay tuition and receive a modest fellowship.

A distinctive, perhaps unique, feature of research training at the Mario Negri was learning how to write scientific English and communicate research findings to an international level. Even in English-speaking graduate programs, students often do not receive formal training in writing articles for scientific journals. They may be native speakers and yet not know the customs or organizational styles of language that characterize effective science writing. The director of studies requires each student to present their data at departmental meetings and at the Institute's internal seminars.

After completion of the probationary period, PhD students were (and are) required to develop an original research thesis. They have regular meetings with their thesis advisers, one from the foreign university and one from the Institute, working in both English and Italian. They must present at least one Institute seminar in English. Two student representatives are responsible for the schedule of presentations at the "Two o'clock Club," and students also present in English at departmental seminars. After successfully completing all requirements and a thesis, students go before an external commissioner selected by the Open University. They are encouraged to spend some time abroad in a first-class research institute.

The organization and content of the PhD program and all the scientific and administrative activities of the Mario Negri Institute are certified according to high European standards (ISO 9001). The teaching and training staff of the school consists of the director of studies, internal examiners selected among the permanent scientific staff at the Institute, supervisors, and external examiners selected according to guidelines and specifications of the Open University (OU), Groningen, and Maastricht.

As an Open University Affiliated Research Centre, the Institute is visited periodically by a team appointed by the OU's Research School. In order to become accredited as a scientific partner, the Mario Negri Institute has to fulfill many requirements. A recent report stated that "Silvio Garattini himself works hard to oversee an effective and coherent research degree program, meeting regularly with staff and students, gathering and responding to feedback, and producing excellent and thorough program documentation."[38]

	2006	2007	2008	2009	2010	2011	2012	2013
Post-doctoral fellows	145	140	152	168	166	159	137	142
Pre-doctoral fellows (Laboratory Technician School)	28	24	26	27	17	15	8	6
Italian University PhD Students	41	35	34	50	61	51	52	41
Visiting scientists	21	25	23	19	19	18	16	15

Figure 4.3   Number trained

To date, 79 PhDs have been awarded, and 24 students are still in training. There is also a doctorate in research that the Italian Ministry of Research has offered since 2010. As of 2012, two students have graduated and 25 are still in training. Overall, Figure 4.3 provides an overview since the Institute reorganized its training courses. As one can see, the number of postdoc fellows rose between 2008 and 2011 and then fell back to around 140 a year. The number of predoctoral fellows has fallen steadily from 2006 to 2013. Visiting scientists, on salary from their home institution, and advanced researchers has declined from the mid-20s to the mid-teens. PhD students from Italian universities doing their thesis work at the Mario Negri has fluctuated within a steady range of 35 to 60. Such students were never allowed to even consider doing their university research at the Mario Negri after Garattini severed his relations with the University of Milan and the university system in 1961. Relations have warmed and normalized. These data indicate modest effects, since 2008, from the most severe and sustained recession in half a century.

Specialist in Pharmacological Research

The Institute also established a three-year course to train specialists in pharmacological research, in order to qualify graduates to work in industry, hospitals, or laboratories. In the usual Mario Negri mode of learning by doing, students work directly on experimental laboratory work, clinical trials, or epidemiological projects, while taking courses in statistics, methods, and scientific writing in English. If they contributed to a given project, they are entitled to be named as a coauthor. About 30 students take this course at one of two levels. The first is for young people coming from professional schools in chemistry, informatics, electronics, and the like who have attended 13 years of school and have a certificate. The second-level recruits graduates from universities in medicine, biology, chemistry, or pharmacy.

Each student receives a modest fellowship, and if they come from outside Milan, they can get a room in the residential facilities that have been a feature of the old and new labs. They can utilize the cafeteria for low cost or prepare food themselves. Fellowships are renewed each year. Students must present their work in English, pass a final examination, and present all their work to an external review committee in order to receive a certificate of graduation, validated by the Lombardy Region. Up through 2012, 664 students have graduated and 714 others left before finishing because they were recruited for a job. The Mario Negri Institute also offers a further two years' training in Advanced Pharmacology, and a few students continue through this training.

Master's Courses

In 2006, the Institute set up a first-level master's course in clinical research in collaboration with the University of Milan. This one-year course is open to medical doctors, nurses, biologists, biotechnicians, and pharmacists who are interested in learning the specific skills required to become clinical monitors in healthcare institutions and in pharmaceutical companies. First-level master's courses are for individuals who hold at least a bachelor-level qualification (three years of university or equivalent). The first-level master's course in clinical research requires full-time attendance, with classes in theory and practical activities.

In conjunction with the University of Turin, the Mario Negri's Center for Rare Diseases Aldo e Cele Daccò runs a two-year second-level master's course on rare diseases at Ranica. It aims to train participants about rare diseases, particularly the management of diagnostic and therapeutic paths, through the clinical assistance networks set up at Mario Negri and other centers for rare diseases.

For a second-level master's or PhD, candidates must have a university degree (five years at university), so this program is open to medical doctors, pharmacists, biologists, and psychologists. It is organized in collaboration with the National Center for Rare Diseases and the National Institute of Health in Rome (Istituto Superiore di Sanità). The Department of Health and the IT Center of the Piedmont Region also contribute.

The University of Maastricht, in conjunction with the Bergamo Hospital and the Mario Negri Institute, offers young Dutch medicine graduates and undergraduates the opportunity to spend a year at the laboratories in Bergamo and Ranica.

In conjunction with the University of Milan, the Institute also has offered since 2006 a master's degree program on clinical trials. The University selects the students for this one-year course and up through 2012, 51 have been awarded a degree. The Mario Negri Institute also offers a continuing medical education training program in clinical trials for physicians and nurses through the Lombard Region, which is responsible for all health-care services.

In each of the past dozen years, the Mario Negri Institute has organized a one-day educational symposium in Venice on Alzheimer's disease for clinicians and other interested participants.

Summer High School

For the past 24 years the Institute has organized a training internship called "Summer School" during June and July. It has admitted about 20 students in the past two years, coming from ten high schools based in the Milan area. A similar "Summer School" is organized in Negri Bergamo laboratories. As part of work-study programs, students leave home early and commute every day to do research all day long during an internship that gives them a taste of what real medical research is like. Ad hoc seminars are organized for scientists to explain the rules of science and how research is done. Francesca Fiorentino tells us about her experience:

> Yesterday, July 26, 2013, it was my last day at the Institute Summer School. I started the internship on June 10, as soon as I finished school. The first days were tough. I asked myself who had obliged me to wake up every day at 7, come to the Mario Negri Institute until 5.30 and cancel a month and a half of holidays! I was in a new environment which had been described to me as "very competitive." I had no idea what most of the instruments in the lab were and I was afraid to do something wrong as I was assigned to study what the researchers were already doing.
>
> Yet, I became steadily more passionate about research and the "job" I did each day. This was partly because people helped me and the guys in the lab (my tutors) created a pleasant and fruitful time for me. They explained and re-explained things I did not understand and taught me to use the devices I did not know about. They are nice people. They did not make me feel I was in their way. On the contrary, they involved me from the beginning in the lab activities and gave me the scientific knowledge I needed to understand their research project (not all the students were so lucky as to end up in such a nice a lab!).
>
> Obviously, being in a lab where real research is going on, sometimes there were moments when you had only to wait for things to happen; but I think this is something you have to take into account from the beginning. I personally found the seminars organized for us "summer students" at the institute very useful because they were held by researchers who not only explained the basis of the scientific concept they were presenting, but also described what kind of research they were doing and showed us the data they had produced up till then. I found this was the best part of the seminars so they helped deepen my scientific knowledge and explore the world of research, though as they were held after lunch I sometimes felt a bit tired.
>
> In these weeks I have met some very nice guys of my age, from different high schools, with whom I could discuss future university choices and other interesting topics.
>
> Just in case you have not yet understood, I liked the internship a lot. I really was touched by the world of research and these seven weeks let me enter it completely. I learned a lot both from the scientific side and about human relationships.
>
> Are seven weeks a long time? Yes they are. Even though I loved my internship the last week I was very tired. But I think they are needed. If the internship had been shorter I would not have had the time to see the end of any experiment nor would I have become so passionate.
>
> Would I suggest it to other people like me? Yes, Yes!—obviously for someone who loves science. Have nice holidays and thank you for the great opportunity!

To conclude, the Mario Negri Institute has been providing hands-on training students from eighth grade through postdocs for decades, drawing its

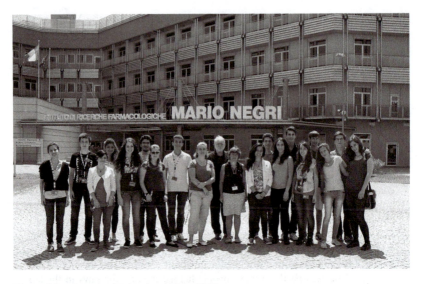

Photo 4.3   Summer high school kids, 2013

own rigorously designed and commercial-free projects that range from bench science to clinical trials and epidemiological studies of people's health, health care, drug use, and exposure to environmental hazards. These projects and the trainees contribute to the extensive programs to educate and engage the public about both the Institute's research and their own health behaviors.

Part II

Reconceiving the Aims of Pharmacological Research

5

From Measuring Environmental Toxins to Drugs as Contaminants

On Saturday, July 10, 1976, at 12:37 p.m., a large explosion occurred at a chemical factory in Seveso, 15 kilometers from Milan, releasing a whitish cloud over several small towns downwind to the south.[1] How toxic was the fallout? No one knew. Within the first days, however, many birds and domestic animals kept by residents in their small plots and homes began to die, and some children had to be treated in hospital for skin rashes or blisters from chemical burns.[2] The company, ICMESA, a subsidiary of the Swiss company Givaudan, which was owned by Hoffman-La Roche, immediately started to look into the accident. However, they kept workers *on the job,* and they did not communicate much with public officials or residents in the area about the explosion or subsequent risks. As Luciano Manara and Silvio Garattini wrote, "No mention of the TCDD [2,3,7,8-Tetrachlorodibenzo-*p*-dioxin] risk was made to the local authorities before the disaster and even after it. Roche took almost two weeks to admit that TCDD had escaped from the plant."[3]

Early samples taken surreptitiously by the company and secreted back to Switzerland for analysis confirmed the presence of 2,3,7,8-TCDD, or dioxin, famously known as an ingredient in Agent Orange in the Vietnam War and in herbicides. Developing an emergency strategy for defining which people, animals, and soil were exposed to what levels called for thousands of samples to be taken and assayed as soon as possible. Difficulties included the extreme toxicity of dioxin that posed serious problems and required special skills, and the reluctance of personnel to obtain and handle samples from the soil and dead animals. Also the distribution of TCDD in the area was extremely uneven and varied by tenfold within centimeters, because the particles from the cloud varied greatly in size and fell out at different rates.

As local, regional, and national government units started to mobilize, they and the companies became involved in a tangle of confused actions and inactions. Some gave assurances that there was no serious risk, while others warned ominously that everyone should leave their homes. Finally, the regional government commissioned the only two expert teams in the region with a gas chromatograph-low resolution mass spectrometer, and, therefore, able to measure traces in samples from the soil and elsewhere: the pharmacology department at the University of Milan and the Mario Negri Institute.

Although this was not the first time that the nation's most respected independent research institute had been asked to address a pressing public issue concerning pharmacology (see Chapter 7), it opened a new line of research that led to establishing a Laboratory of Pharmacology and Toxicology and to investigating health risks of other pharmacological agents in meat, burning waste, in rivers, and in the water supply. Ironically, the widening circle of research into other pharmacological agents has come full circle today to measuring prescription drugs as toxic pollutants that are constantly ending up in the water supply along with illicit drugs.

Given that 80 percent of new expenditures are spent on drugs with few or no advantages over existing ones (because regulators use minimal criteria for approving them), rather than on new drugs with superior clinical advantages for patients,[4] and given that undertested risks of harmful side effects have become a leading cause of road accidents, falls, hospitalizations, and death, tied with stroke as the fourth leading cause,[5] there is a great need to fix the way that new drugs are approved and prescribed that includes their environmental impact.[6]

Returning to the explosion, it occurred on Saturday at 6 a.m., about six and a half hours after the plant had closed for the weekend. Company technicians had switched off the superheated steam used to heat the reactor and they stopped the agitation of the contents, reasoning that the contents would slowly cool down without adding thousands of liters of water to stop the reaction.[7] But after they left, the temperature rose and blew a safety valve on a vent pipe. Exactly what chemicals went up in the cloud and how much dioxin will never be known. Various reporters and officials estimated a half pound, two pounds, even four pounds. Local police were informed. Officers of ICMESA told residents not to eat produce from their gardens. Over the weekend, officers of the company told the local mayors and a health officer that the chemicals were produced for herbicides but never mentioned dioxin. The local health officer then wrote a letter saying there was no significant risk of harm, an expert certifying safety because information of toxic risk had been withheld. Physicians do the same every day based on selective and biased information in medical journals that hides risks of harm.[8]

The company sealed off the plant and took samples from the surrounding area. On July 15, the company's chief chemist traveled to inspect the plant personally and "began to be concerned that abnormally high amounts of dioxin might have been produced."[9] Early samples came back with high concentrations of dioxin, more than one part per thousand rather than one per million, a thousandfold difference. He met with Roche's clinical research director, Dr. Reggiani. "Prior to the meeting, Reggiani had never heard of dioxin"!

Given dioxin's central rule in Agent Orange and the Vietnam War, this seems surprising. He called the plant doctor, who said the workers were fine;

but a few local children were developing skin rashes from chemical burns. They traveled to meet the dozen children affected, four of whom had swollen faces. Within a week, however, the swelling subsided. The Lombardy regional government and the national government became involved. Pregnant women felt vulnerable and feared giving birth to malformed babies. Some exposed women wanted to exercise their right to a legal abortion but encountered fierce opposition from religious authorities, political groups, and some doctors. Between 10 and 20 percent of pregnant women had an abortion. Otherwise, humans did not seem seriously affected, though long-term follow-up was needed.

Then the story broke in the Milan papers and subsequently throughout the world. While the press made Seveso into an international event and symbol, "the mass media seem to suggest that people resembling the pictures seen throughout the world of small children burnt by the cloud could be met at every street corner in the area."[10] The press came up with arresting headlines: "A Little Hiroshima" (*Irish Times*); "Gas More Potent Than Thalidomide" (*The Observer*). Equally misleading were Hoffman-La Roche officers stating at international meetings that the few dozen documented cases constituted all who were adversely affected.[11] The truth lay in between.

The workers, meantime, were kept uninformed and decided to strike, as they had done two months earlier, to force the company to issue information about plant health hazards. But the manager told them he really had no solid information to give them. This seems disingenuous, because government reports showed that the company had repeatedly failed to comply with checks on its discharge of effluents, and residents described repeated episodes of dead animals for which the company provided compensation, an admission that they knew and felt responsible.[12] The Parliamentary Commission of Inquiry into the Seveso explosion reported that substantial amounts of TCDD had contaminated the area for years. The team from the Mario Negri Institute concluded that the explosion "was the logical fallout of a production process where controls and safeguards were practically nonexistent, and which had been modified over the years to maximize output."[13] This Mario Negri assessment foreshadowed the theme of companies risking exposure of populations to toxins in order to cut corners on safety and squeeze out more profits. That still characterizes current "Seveso III" international policy.[14] Questioning in 1977 whether Seveso was an accident or a crime resonates with the authoritative modern histories of industrial pollution by the famous team at Columbia University, Gerald Markowitz and David Rosner.[15]

On July 20, Roche officers started calling other companies, and all replied: evacuate the residents. Meantime, pet rabbits and chickens kept dying. Vegetable greens wilted and turned brown. Fear of an invisible poisonous cloud spread throughout the land, and Antonio Maturo remembers how Seveso haunted the imagination and gave him nightmares about it as a boy. On July 20, eight adults were hospitalized. The regional government closed off the area from all traffic. Finally, on July 23, the first large-scale meeting of industry and government officials occurred, including leading scientists from the Department of Pharmacology at the University of Milan and the Mario Negri Institute of Pharmacological Research. The regional minister of health reported that all necessary actions had been taken and no families need be evacuated. Roche's clinical advisor bluntly dismissed the public health measures taken and said that "the population at Seveso had to be evacuated without delay."[16] Fear and controversy became so intense that he decided to escape back to Switzerland out of reach. Meantime, lettuce was still curling up brown, and rabbits and chickens were dying.

The teams from the University of Milan and Mario Negri quickly carried out the analysis of soil samples, and by Saturday evening, July 24, they had the results as well as a map that outlined the areas of highest concentration, 269 acres in Zone A, and 669 acres with lower concentrations in Zone B. Beyond that were 3575 acres in Zone R. On July 26, the first 225 residents were obliged to leave their homes by police and military troops called in. By August 2, another 511 were evacuated. They crammed into nearby hotels and suffered from being treated as if they themselves were contaminated. Intense debate swirled around whether to evacuate another 4800 people in Zone B, with the company pressing for it and public health officials deciding they could avoid it, except for women in the first trimester of a pregnancy. No one was to eat anything grown in the soil. Farms were sampled and if the assays proved positive for dioxin, all animals on the farm were killed. The Mario Negri team found dioxin in milk, and all milk production stopped.

From Clinical Pharmacology to Clinical Epidemiology

Silvio Garattini and Gianni Tognoni played important roles in persuading people to leave their homes in Zone A. At the Mario Negri Institute, however, they had played seminal roles in developing the Institute into a leader of fine-grained measurement. Garattini may have paid low salaries and stinted on allowing staff to make color slides because black-and-white would suffice; but he quickly bought the most advanced, new, expensive spectrometers, penny-wise as well as pound-wise. Tognoni led the Institute to expand clinical pharmacology into clinical epidemiology. "By the end of the 1960s," Fanelli explained recently, "we were measuring small traces of drugs in rats, mice, and patients, and we measured how different individuals metabolize the same drug differently. [personalized medicine] We also measured variations in how the same person metabolized a drug . . . The same techniques and methodological advances developed at the Mario Negri Institute could be applied to other man-made active agents from dioxin to digitalis in the widening field of pharmacology."[17]

Under the leadership of Professor Emilio Mussini, the young Roberto Fanelli and his wife did many of the assays. Garattini had hired Fanelli in 1965 with only a certificate in chemistry from a technical high school. But Garattini, who started the same way, may have seen something of himself in Fanelli. Like Garattini, he explained to us how easy and pioneering it was to bring techniques from analytical chemistry to pharmacology. "Back then," he explained, "pharmacologists didn't analyze drugs in the bloodstream. They didn't know the metabolic pathways of how a drug distributes itself—only its visible, observable effects . . . This emphasis led to our using mass spectrometry in pharmacology for the first time." Back from a year of advanced training at the Institute for Lipid Research at Baylor University, where leading researchers were developing the first computer-based instruments, Fanelli recalls the Seveso incident:

> It was a factory owned by Roche that made Agent Orange (trichlorphina). It's supposed not to have more than one part per million of dioxin. We don't really know how much more blew up in the air from the explosion of the factory, but probably quite a lot more.
>
> Within a few days, we were called for help, because garden plants were turning yellow. Then the manufacturer advised residents to evacuate their homes, especially in the more concentrated areas. They refused—it was quite disruptive after all. Then people's cats and pet rabbits started to die, which made them scared—like an invisible, odorless killer. Then kids' skin began to blister with caustic soda. I can get you photos . . . but people kept living in the area . . .
>
> Not much was known about the toxicity of dioxin in humans or different animals; so we were the first to measure it using our mass spectrometry instruments . . . In the end, there was an increase in cardiovascular events, but we don't know how much was due to stress and how much to the dioxin. We concluded in the end that humans have a low sensitivity compared to rabbits or cats, for example.
>
> The whole incident led to a stark realization by authorities and people of risks from chemicals; so this incident helped change the culture, as society increasingly began to label, warn, and restrict exposure to a wide range of chemicals.

Based on taking samples from the livers of dead animals, where dioxin was most concentrated, the Mario Negri team found more than two-thirds of rabbits and goats were positive but only 10–20 percent of horses and cows. Rabbit mortality was 32 percent in Zone A, 8.8 percent in Zone B, and 6.8 percent in Zone R. They did not trust their data on chickens or pigs.[18] Milk was contaminated. It took until May 1977 to put together a map where soil, animal, and human data could be grouped. The Mario Negri team found that the half-life of dioxin exposed to the sun on the surface was one year, but later they found that dioxin beneath the top-soil had a half-life of ten years.[19]

As for humans, there did not seem to be serious harm, though it was hard to tell close to the time. A long, 20-year, follow-up of adults exposed in 1976 found no significant differences in morbidity or mortality from a control population, and "no laboratory pathology was related to TCDD levels in both the acute and chronic phases."[20] The only effects were an increase in skin eruptions including chloracne, acne, and cysts, and a change in sex ratio related to paternal levels of dioxin exposure.[21] Risks of cancers are mixed and unclear.[22]

The legacy of Seveso and other chemical accidents has shaped European policy ever since—called "Seveso policy." "The Seveso accident has changed the way public opinion looks at pollution and the chemical industry, and a short video as part of a chart (http://prezi.com/ybkzdsrdlrqk/seveso-disaster/) provides an overview from 1976 up to "Seveso III" policy for 2015.

This work by the Institute and by the Department of Pharmacology at the University of Milan follows the great tradition of Giovanni Maria Lancisi, 1654–1720, the physician to three popes who researched the cause of malaria in Rome, concluded it was malaria, and in 1717 mapped "the noxious effluvia of marshes" outside the city.[23] He urged they be drained. He also analyzed other public health issues and mapped them.

Lancisi made these astute observations, inductions, and maps over 100 years before England's famed John Snow deduced that the cholera plague was water-borne and mapped the pattern of cases to show the cause was the Broad Street pump. English and American sources credit Snow's work as the beginning of public health, but Lancisi deserves the credit. For the Mario Negri Institute, involvement in the toxic fallout of Seveso built on this pioneering work of tracing the environmental contributors to illness in a population. It led some Mario Negri scientists to realize that they, like colleagues, had allowed clinical pharmacology to narrow its gaze to inside the body, "biochemistry, in-vivo and in-vitro drug metabolism . . . kinetics at the expense

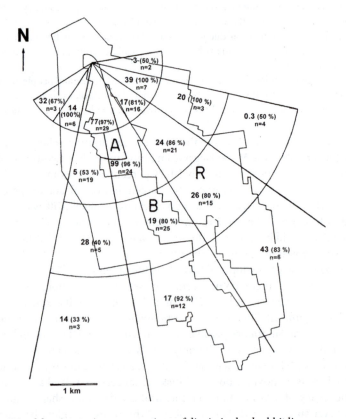

Figure 5.1 Mapping toxic concentrations of dioxin in dead rabbit livers

of the clinical side."[24] Publishing in *The Lancet*, Bonati and Tognoni urged a return to studies in how a drug is used in the community and a focus of therapeutic issues of safety and efficacy. The Seveso study, along with studies at the same time by Tognoni, Garattini, and others at the Mario Negri of how medicines developed in research were actually being used in practice prompted a growing realization that clinical pharmacology should concern itself with patient care and environmental factors.

Dioxin, Dioxin Everywhere . . .

This work measuring traces of dioxin, first in the soil and then in animals, went on for years and years, because dioxin is such a widespread chemical. Technically, Fanelli explained, there is little difference between measuring traces of medicines and measuring traces of pollutants. In animals, especially rabbits, anything accumulates and becomes more concentrated. Many grants centered on understanding in detail how dioxin was metabolized in different animals and how it affected them.

Then several years later a research group in The Netherlands showed that waste incinerators *produced* dioxin in their emissions. This meant all the world is exposed to dioxin! "Burning fuel for heat produces dioxin too, especially wood used by the poor," Fanelli added. "But then the rich burn more plastic, which is worse." The Institute's research in environmental epidemiology expanded. The work was much more complicated than Seveso, where there was only one isomer; incinerators emit more than 100 isomers. Yet little was known about them, and the Institute began a long series of studies about these new types of "dioxin." The crisis in Naples of uncollected piles of garbage that peaked in 2008, and continued to fester thereafter, led the Mario Negri Institute to further studies of "environmental pharmacology"—active agents not put in a pill and designed to help the sick, but toxic agents produced by society.

The discovery that dioxins were ubiquitous pollutants prompted a worldwide search for industrial sources of dioxin. Soon it became evident that almost every type of combustion was generating small amounts of dioxin. Even small amounts of organic chlorine compounds decomposed into dioxins during combustion. Ironically, the chemical industry was trying to demonstrate that dioxins were natural (i.e., good) compounds present in nature for millions of years and produced by forest fires. But the proliferation of dioxin has paralleled the rapid growth of the chemical industry.

At the Institute, the lab team studied how dioxin was formed inside waste incinerators and discovered that high temperatures were able to destroy dioxins in the waste; but the products of degradation then easily recombined to form dioxins again.[25] These findings led the incinerator industry to develop methods for catching dioxins after combustion. The lab team also contributed to explaining to frightened residents living close to dioxin-emitting industrial plants the risks they faced, and to describing the sources, transport, and presence of dioxin in the food chain.

Drugs as Toxic Residues in Meat

In the 1990s, Ettore Zuccato, head of the Mario Negri Laboratory in Environmental Sciences, made a shift from examining dioxin in foods to antibiotics in meat. Ranchers are allowed to use antibiotics only when a disease seriously threatens their animals. There are strict regulations. But 80 percent of antibiotic use is for their growth potential—antibiotics can boost meat volume by 30 percent. When eaten, however, they increase resistance in humans and also become toxic in our gut. Side effects can include increased risk of kidney problems and cancer. Antibiotic resistance leaves people defenseless against MRSA as an infection that causes more than 365,000 hospitalizations a year in the United States alone—a major issue today.[26] A typical compromise by many countries was to allow drugs in livestock to treat disease but prohibit their presence in meat at the end of the process by having a period of no drugs until their concentrations fall below the "maximum residue limit" for therapeutic use. The European Union began banning the nontherapeutic uses of antibiotics in animals in 1999 and completed the ban in 2006.

In 2013, David Kessler, the much-revered commissioner of the FDA from 1990 to 1997, sized up the scope of the problem produced by antibiotics in meat and what is known. Meat and poultry "are bellwethers that tell us how bad the crisis of antibiotic resistance is getting. And they're telling us it's getting worse."[27] About 80 percent of all antibiotics go to livestock, about 30 million pounds a year, or 136 billion grams. Dr. Kessler wrote that they "are often fed to animals at low levels to make them grow faster and to suppress diseases that arise because they live in dangerously close quarters on top of one another's waste." This disgusting way of growing animals at factory farms is spurring a movement back to old-fashioned, small-farm methods with no drugs. Still, using antibiotics for animal growth remains widespread, despite a voluntary initiative by the FDA to restrict their use.

Medicines as Toxic Waste

Fanelli, Zuccato, and other Mario Negri researchers also turned in 1995 to measuring traces of prescription drugs in rivers and wastewater. They found small but measureable amounts that come from the excreted residue of drugs that people take, plus drugs on the skin being washed away and drugs thrown away in the toilet. (See Figure 5.2) "The point is that the half-life of many drugs is very long—10–20 years; so the presence of active drugs is growing fast," said Zuccato. "We found traces of hundreds of drugs." They published the first major article, in *The Lancet* in 2000,[28] and generated international attention.

In 2011, the WHO completed a report stating that "appreciable adverse health impacts to humans are very unlikely from exposure to the trace concentrations of pharmaceuticals that could potentially be found in drinking-water."[29] But Sonia Shah reported that birds and fish are affected. Momentum

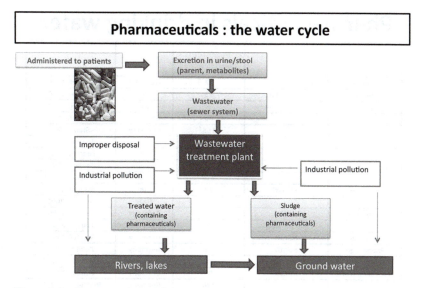

Figure 5.2   How prescription drugs get into our water

is building for "green pharmaceuticals" that do not harm the environment.[30] For example, the levels of antidepressants found in some wastewater alter the genes responsible for developing fish brains, and "females produced fewer eggs and males become aggressive killing females in some cases."[31] The drugs used in the study were among the most common found in sewage: Prozac, Effexor, and Tegretol. The MistraPharma multiyear project has developed the "critical environmental concentration (CEC)" measure that would harm fish.[32]

In 2012, a five-month, 14-part investigation by the Associated Press found that nearly every body of water sampled in the United States, in small and large cities and in watersheds, tested positive for prescription drug residues, though in tiny amounts.[33] More worrisome, water filtration systems do not deal with this form of toxic waste, and water companies do not report their presence to customers. Bottled water companies do not test for drugs in their water at all. Thus, increasingly, both public and bottled water are likely to have prescription drug residues in them.

What reports like these do not mention that Fanelli and Zuccato emphasize is that pharmaceutical companies use maximum doses in their clinical trials to get more positive results faster so they can run shorter trials, save money, and increase evidence that their drugs should be approved as "effective." The FDA and EMA rules allow—even encourage—clinical trials to be designed this way. In most cases, however, the higher the dose, the greater the toxic side effects. These high doses then go into the label and become the recommended dosages for doctors to prescribe. As a result, drugs approved look more effective and less toxic than they really are. A large percent of label changes involve lowering the dosages as clinicians learn what the most

Pharmaceuticals in drinking water

Compound	Therapeutic group	Maximum conc. (ng l^{-1})	Country	Reference
Bezafibrate	Lipid regulator	27	Germany	Stumpf, 1996
Bleomycin	Anti-neoplastic	13	UK	Aherne, 1990
Clofibric acid	Lipid regulator	+	UK	Fielding, 1981
		70	Germany	Stumpf, 1996
		165	Germany	Stan, 1994
		270	Germany	Heberer, 1997
		5	Italy	Zuccato, 2000
Carbamazepine	Anti-epileptic	24	Canada	Tauber, 2003
		258	USA	Stachelberg, 2004
Diazepam	Anxiolytic	10	UK	Waggot, 1981
		23	Italy	Zuccato, 2000
Diclofenac	NSAID	6	Germany	Stumpf, 1996
Gemfibrozil	Lipid regulator	70	Canada	Tauber, 2003
Ibuprofen	NSAID	3	Germany	Stumpf, 1996
Phenazone	NSAID	250	Germany	Zuhlke, 2004
		400	Germany	Reddersen, 2002
Propyphenazone	NSAID	80	Germany	Zuhlke, 2004
		120	Germany	Reddersen, 2002
Tylosin	Antibiotic	1.7	Italy	Zuccato, 2000

Jones, 2005

Figure 5.3   List of prescription drugs in our water

effective dose is. But chances are 1 in 5 that a new drug will produce serious enough adverse reactions to prompt regulators to add a severe warning or have the drug withdrawn.[34]

According to Jan Vandenbroucke, an internationally distinguished professor of pharmaco-epidemiology, toxicity of widely used drugs like statins steadily increases because companies increase dose or efficacy levels with each new drug in a class so that it can be marketed as stronger or faster or "more effective." For example, newer statins start at levels five times higher than the first ones (e.g., 25 instead of 5). Risks of toxicity rise accordingly. This winding up of the dosage level tested also narrows the range of dose-choices for doctors and their patients. The minimum or floor level of prescribing narrows upward, and billions in marketing gets doctors to shift to these more powerful and toxic, newly patented variations, which find their way into the environment.

The criteria used by the EMA and FDA for concluding that new drugs are effective, compared to a placebo and often using a surrogate end point, mean that independent reviewers judge 90 percent of new drugs as little or no better than previously approved drugs.[35] Yet effective marketing has led to doctors writing one billion more prescriptions in the United States than a decade earlier.[36] Toxic reactions in patients are more likely to result as are toxic residues in the water supply at higher dosage levels than are therapeutically necessary.

The Mario Negri group studying environmental contamination by pharmaceuticals wrote a review of their work and others in 2006, saying,

"Pharmaceuticals are widespread contaminants, entering the environment from a myriad of scattered points."[37] Thus, "hundreds of tons of pharmacologically active substances can enter sewage treatment plants each year." Patients and animals are the main sources, and several drugs are excreted unchanged or as active metabolites in high percentages and often disposed of improperly in wastewater. Most wastewater treatments do not remove them effectively (though some do). With long half-lives, they accumulate, even after drugs are withdrawn as dangerous.

In other parts of life, people regard pollution as a price for real benefit, like pollution from burning fuels to heat their homes or drive their cars. But in the case of drugs, the evidence presented indicates that the health gains are limited compared to the increased risk of harm from prescription drugs.

The EMA requires companies to measure the environmental impact of each new drug; but Zuccato finds they do so in a simple, minimal way, and the EMA never uses it as a criterion for judging the merits of a drug. In the case of drugs used by tens of millions, like statins taken to reduce heart attacks and death in people with no risk except high cholesterol, independent studies find modest evidence of real clinical benefit, and yet the billions of pills contaminate the water supply for years. "If we continue to add more medicines," Fanelli warns "we will get into trouble and have to abandon a given water supply." The European Water Framework Directive of 2000 established standards for the "good chemical status" of surface waters that were strengthened by a 2008 directive. Proposed amendments by critics like the World Wildlife Fund, who find the standards inadequate, would add more substances to be controlled, including prescription drugs.[38]

Illicit Drugs as Toxic Waste in Drinking Water

The Mario Negri environmental health sciences team drew on its studies of therapeutic drugs to search for *illicit drugs* in both wastewater and drinking water. Some team members had found that amounts of pharmaceuticals roughly reflected the amounts prescribed to a population.[39] Since illicit drugs are consumed worldwide in comparable amounts, they wondered if their consumption could be measured the same way. They developed new methods for measuring based on high-pressure liquid chromatography—tandem mass spectrometry. They completed the first investigation of cocaine and its metabolite, benzoylecgonine, and found they were "in concentrations for a population of 5 million that were equivalent to about 4 kg of cocaine per day. This would imply an average daily use of at least 27 ± 5 doses (100 mg each) for every 1000 young adults, an estimate that greatly exceeded official national figures."[40] Four kilos is about 40,000 doses or 200,000 lines of cocaine snorted on average a day.[41] The researchers are confident about the accuracy of their measures and methods because with prescription drugs they matched records of prescriptions. Zuccato showed us a chart for Milan, and we could see that use is low until Thursday, when it increases.[42] Then it increases sharply again

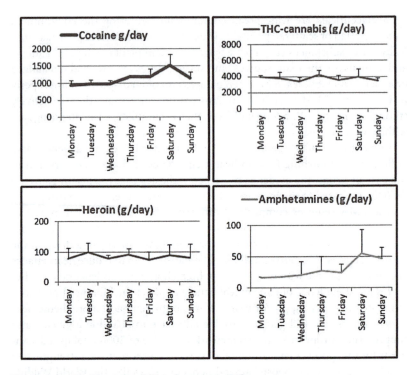

Figure 5.4 Weekly cycle of illicit drug use in Milan

on Friday, peaks on Saturday, declines half-way down on Sunday, and plummets back on Monday to the level it holds till the next Thursday

When the authors were ready to publish, Zuccato told us,

> We first sent it to *Nature*, then to *Science*, and the editors rejected it right away, saying it was too "specialized." They recommended that we submit it to a specialty journal. They didn't get it! We also submitted it to a couple of medical journals, but their editors thought it was not "medical." The article finally came out in a minor journal . . . I was starting my vacation when I received hundreds of calls from journalists all over the world and had to come back to address them. It got featured in *Nature News, Science News, The New York Times, The Times*, and elsewhere.

The Mario Negri team next developed more elaborate methods for detecting and measuring a range of 16 illicit drugs, including amphetamines, morphine, cannabinoid derivatives, methadone, and some of their metabolites. Using complex techniques, they measured them in solids both in wastewater and later in surface water.[43] Removal in treatment plants varied, with plants in Milan removing 97 percent of the illicit drugs detectable in untreated wastewater. Illicit drugs have since been measured in rivers in the United States, Germany, Spain, Ireland, and Belgium.[44]

Modified methods can measure local drug consumption in real time and in small populations, such as a school or college or residential area like a military base. Drug testing in the United States started in the 1960s to discourage the use of illicit drugs, which cause about 40 million serious illnesses and injuries a year.[45] Many schools have advocated drug testing but met resistance, both active and passive. The Mario Negri group modified its methods to use another approach, measuring changes in two 50-gallon tanks in consumption and types of drugs in a school or residential population, by the hour and the day of the week. Residues from as little as one whole dose can be detected this way, such as Adderall as a source of amphetamine.

Since its founding, senior researchers at the Mario Negri Institute have pioneered methods for measuring adverse effects and benefits of drugs within specific organs in a person's body. Since Seveso, they have developed ways to look at adverse effects at a societal level and developed a global model for how clinical pharmacology can improve human health and the human condition. The next chapter describes an entirely different manifestation of this vision.

6

Pioneering Ethical Trials for Integrated Research

In 2013, the editors of *The Lancet* expressed the frustration of patients and doctors everywhere at the continued lack of published or even disclosed evidence concerning the benefits, and especially the risks of harm from new drugs and vaccines like the flu vaccine.[1] They drew on an assessment by Iain Chalmers and Paul Glasziou that estimated that 85 percent of the billions spent on commercialized biomedical research is being wasted because of four deficiencies:

1. Researchers do not investigate questions relevant to patients and their clinicians because they do not ask them what matters to them.[2]
2. Half the time, no systematic review of existing evidence is done, and studies fail to protect themselves against forms of bias.
3. Disappointing results are underreported and over 50 percent do not publish results in full.
4. Over half of planned study results are not reported, and 30 percent do not describe interventions sufficiently to be useful.

This disturbing assessment stems from commercial distortions of research and trials from being dedicated to better patient care to more patents and greater profits. It underscores the global need for a new paradigm for how governments and health-care systems should fund, choose, and regulate innovation in terms of real patient improvements, a paradigm that leaders of the Mario Negri Institute for Pharmacological Research (MNI) articulated in an institutional set of ethics in the early 1960s and more fully developed in the 1980s. Good clinical pharmacology, they wrote in a declaration that transformed their own work, must be a joint undertaking with clinicians and patients, using the entire health-care system as "the natural laboratory of clinical pharmacology."[3] Not research by researchers in their own sphere aimed at maximizing patents and publications, but collaborative, open investigations of concerns or questions that matter to doctors and patients, with trial designs "applicable to the majority of patients affected" without

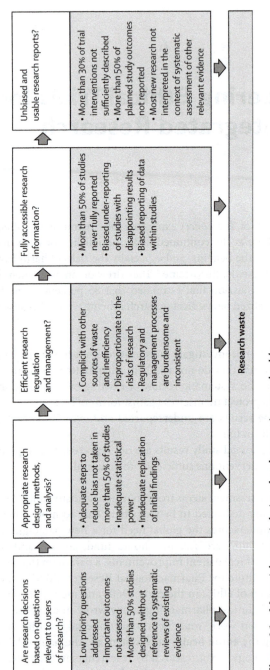

Figure 6.1 Most trials are misdesigned and cannot improve health

Acknowledgment: Reprinted from *The Lancet*, Vol. 374, Iain Chalmers, Paul Glasziou, "Avoidable waste in the production and reporting of research evidence," 9683, July 2009, with permission from Elsevier.

exclusionary criteria, and "perceived as relevant by the professionals who are meant to apply them." To carry out such practice-based trials, paradoxically larger but less costly than commercial trials, one must build "a permanent network of research-conscious and research-oriented clinicians" as partners and coauthors.

And this is exactly what the Mario Negri did, 30 years ago. What the *Lancet* editors bemoan as noble goals now faded have remained in full force at the Mario Negri Institute as a real utopia, despite highly commercialized research practices all around them.

What researchers at the Mario Negri Institute continue to do can be done by other research institutes if they decide to insist on scientific integrity and transparency. This is a conscious, and conscious-raising commitment. The more groups or institutes that do it, the easier it will become to have patient-relevant research with unbiased, clinically meaningful results, fully accessible to all. Ben Goldacre's chapter on Bad Trials in *Bad Pharma* can become an account of past practices.[4] We would even argue that today's deeply troubled pharmaceutical giants would profit.[5] Besides being more clinically relevant, unbiased, and scientifically valid, Mario Negri trials cost a fraction of industry trials, and far fewer are needed. Among the more than 165,000 clinical trials registered today, fewer than 10 percent provide clinically useful information for patients and their doctors. This means most of the millions of people volunteering as subjects are exposing themselves to risks without clear clinical benefit—by design.

Through generous American and British support in the 1960s and 1970s, continued awards from the National Institutes of Health, the US Army, the US Department of Agriculture, and many contracts from others that included major corporations that agreed to its terms of independent, transparent science, the Institute grew enough to undertake its first clinical trials in the 1980s. These pages describe how researchers at Mario Negri worked with specialty associations to organize national networks of colleagues to become code-signers and coauthors of practice-based, unbiased, fully transparent clinical trials. Instead of building commercial networks of paid specialists, why not build science-based networks of volunteers? This approach to trials involved educating these national networks of specialists about clinical research methods and reviving their initial interest in using medical science to help their patients. The Mario Negri Institute has turned "research and development" into "research in practice."

Randomized, double-blinded clinical trials (RCTs) are "the Gold Standard" for scientifically validating that an intervention improves patients' health, only if outcomes are used that matter to patients.[6] Observing that principle disqualifies about 90 percent of all clinical trials today, because funders almost never ask patients or their doctors what really matters, and much of the time they use surrogate or substitute end points instead of real clinical ones.

Doing what is best for patients has three implications for how Mario Negri has carried out clinical trials. First, it has led to testing clinical treatments other than new drugs. These are as just as important, perhaps even more so, because current undertested therapies are what patients actually receive, for better or worse. Second, practicing doctors serve as advisers to the research trial team, if not members. Third, trials should be conducted on samples that reflect the patient population who will actually be taking a drug (or other intervention), not on samples that Ben Goldacre accurately characterizes as "freakishly perfect 'ideal' patients"[7] that exclude those most likely to have a serious adverse reaction and include those most likely to have a positive response in order to make the results look much better than they are in real practice.

Through these practices, illustrated below, the Mario Negri Institute has raised the quality of clinical medicine for a nation, and an institute, like it could do the same in other countries. This contrasts with taxpayers paying billions through high prices for thousands of trials not needed for regulatory approval and designed to gather good-looking but clinically unreliable results about additional uses in order to get more people taking more drugs. These costly practices also contribute to the global epidemic of toxic side effects from drugs that usually have few advantages to offset their risks of harm.[8]

In 1983, the first megatrial trial, known as GISSI, began, and its publication in 1986 galvanized the medical world and medical practice. "It was a bombshell," declared Eugene Braunwald, the Hersey Distinguished Professor at Harvard Medical School and editor of the *American Heart Journal*.[9] Braunwald, as a giant in American and international cardiology, was the first to see the results of the Mario Negri trial in a satellite symposium, and he quickly requested the key slide to feature it in his main lecture at the September 1985 meeting of the American Health Association.[10] Just as when Garattini's research generated international attention in the 1950s and when the NIH kept awarding the Mario Negri Institute grants and contracts in the 1960s and 1970s, so the quality of the Institute's research during the 1980s reaffirmed its place in the front ranks of research centers. This first, breakthrough, trial depended on the Italian Association of Hospital Cardiologists (ANMCO) persuading 88 percent of the nation's cardiac care units to participate in a huge trial that showed beyond a doubt the benefit of administering a single large dose of streptokinase (SK) as soon as possible after symptoms of an acute myocardial infarction (AMI).

The GISSI trial design shows that it takes a village—if not a whole healthcare system—to reduce the devastating effects of heart attacks on patients' lives. Family, workers, police, shopkeepers—everyone needs to know the signs of a heart attack to get that shot of SK into a person as quickly as possible. On the research side, it takes the involvement of a nation's doctors to design trials pertinent to real patient care.

The GISSI-1 trial is credited with saving millions of lives through the world. Within the first year, 99 percent of cardiac units in the country were administering SK to patients who came in with symptoms of a heart attack because it was *their* trial about *their* practices.[11] Subsequent years turned to educating everyone who might come into contact with someone having a heart attack to get them quickly to a cardiac unit.

What Mario Negri did would be as if the Salk Institute of medical research in San Diego parlayed its outstanding laboratory research to organize large trials with the chapters of the American College of Cardiology throughout California and the Western states to test a drug in their practices. If it did, it still would not reach the equivalent population that the Mario Negri reached in the GISSI trials. Other nations, especially ones that have universal health care and need to provide good care within a reasonable budget, from little Taiwan to the immense United States, need one or more institutes of research integrity like Mario Negri to both attract research dollars and improve care for all their patients. The cardiologists, or nephrologists, or other specialists in a whole state, like Vermont, or Pennsylvania, or Oregon, or in a whole nation like Mexico, or Poland, or Thailand, could learn from Mario Negri and do the same. The benefits to society are presented in Figure 6.2. The quality of care increases because these kinds of trials test real efficacy and safety in practice and so many practicing doctors participate. They make important contributions to clinical epidemiological methods and knowledge, including the assessment of markers. They may have implications for both the organization and economics of health care.

Benefits from Doing Mario Negri Trials

- Ethical dialogue with providers about what kind of trial would be best for patients

- Methodological dialogue with providers about how best to design a trial for patient benefit

- Discussing all past literature to decide what outcome measures would be best

- Assessing with providers clinical diagnostic and outcomes markers

- Discussing quality of care and quality of life outcomes measures

- Determining with providers the practice-relevant population to sample

- Designing with providers the practice-based methods & measures that least interfere with practice

- Developing strategies to put results into practice and into training

Figure 6.2   GISSI trials benefit patients, doctors, and society

GISSI-1 Origins

The first GISSI trial resulted from four parallel developments. During the 1970s, the Lombardy Region suspected they were wasting money paying for drugs; so they contracted with the Mario Negri Institute to create a scientifically based approach to prescribing drugs. How its researchers responded provides a blueprint for others that will be described in Chapter 7. They first established a Regional Center for Drug Documentation and Information in order to find out what doctors were actually prescribing. Then they organized networks of practitioners to discuss what their survey found, and they developed methods for assessing the clinical effectiveness of drugs.

The second antecedent to the GISSI trial stemmed from seminal articles by Richard Peto in 1976 and his development of large trials at Oxford. In these articles, a leading British statistician laid out in sentences as readable as an introductory textbook the reasons why large clinical trials were necessary in heart disease, cancer, and other debilitating disorders. Imagine an article in the *British Journal of Cancer*, 25 pages long and double-column, but as readable as the Science section of the *New York Times*. Peto wrote a second article, even longer. He pointed out that even with a trial involving 60 patients (as many as a large hospital could organize alone for a serious condition), if 7 of 30 died from one treatment and 14 of 30 died from another, it may mean nothing beyond chance. In a second sample of 60 patients, the results might be reversed. "However," Peto wrote, "most small trials could, with profit, be larger if the organizers attempted collaboration with other hospitals."[12] In large trials, Peto recommended comparing only two treatments, making them as different as possible. Yet most trials compare two similar treatments. That may be important for the funders to sell more drugs; but such trials are not important for patients and waste a great deal of money. This same basic error is repeated today, nearly 40 years later.

Silvia Marsoni, an internationally distinguished research oncologist and a clinical member of the Mario Negri team for years, explained during a 2013 interview the revolutionary importance of Peto's work. Before the mid-1970s, clinical pharmacologists worked with basic scientists to find drugs that would make a big difference, like reversing the course of a disease or curing it. But such drugs are rare, and others can provide a smaller benefit in a larger number of patients, only we do not know that the small gains are taking place. Large trials make small gains for many patients visible and prove the benefit is statistically secure or "significant."[13]

Peto's team urged that medical studies focus on establishing the benefits of relatively simple, practical treatments for common conditions.[14] Clinicians need to know how effective they are, the duration of their benefit, and what factors matter. Major interventions with a striking benefit are so clear that one knows they work by observation. But establishing the impact of moderate gains on common problems is more subject to debate, even though they can have greater benefit if proven effective. The outcome needs to be simple, like death, because patients with the same condition vary greatly in whether they survive and for how long.

Several different mechanisms may affect an outcome. In treating heart attacks for example, Peto's team found 126 clinical trials that had been carried out in several different ways to treat heart attacks; but not one of the trials was large enough to establish a reliable, statistically significant result. If a simple trial of about 10,000 patients were organized, however, one that could include all the variations among patients and how their doctors treat them, except for the intervention being tested, then one could establish the value of an intervention that improves patient health by 15–20 percent rather than by 80–90 percent. This requires strict control of both systematic and random errors, Peto wrote. It also requires a simple, quick protocol that doctors can employ in their usual practice. Such large, simple trials can also be inexpensive.

Third, cardiologists made advances in understanding heart attacks and how to save more patients from death. It wasn't until 1980 that Marcus Wood and colleagues abandoned autopsies and set out to perform coronary angiography in live patients within 24 hours of an MI and found total occlusion in 87 percent of their patients.[15] Wood's demonstration of coronary thrombosis during AMI set the stage for a large-scale, randomized mortality trial like GISSI. Meantime, investigators had found in small trials that the early administration of SK reduced in-hospital mortality.

Finally, Italy decided to transform Italian health care into a National Health Service and end the frustrations, fragmentation, and inequalities of universal health care through national health insurance run by the usual mixture of private insurers and public programs to cover the "uninsurable." Its development was more halting and difficult than when the British created their NHS, based on the impressive coordination of all services during the 1940s in face of a German invasion. In Italy, many patients and specialists continued to use private practice, and doctors played both sides by having a salaried job with the NHS and a private practice as well. But the Mario Negri team and Italian leaders in cardiology realized that a national trial could be a strategy "that considers the NHS as the natural laboratory to test challenging hypotheses" and "provide[s] active and explicitly theoretical education and field training to cardiologists . . . as a school of methodology."[16]

Prior to GISSI, the first double-blind trials by Mario Negri were conducted by Tognoni, Garattini and colleagues between 1976 and 1978.[17] Then they and Italian cardiologists joined Richard Peto, Peter Sleight, and their team in Oxford who were developing ISIS-1, the first in a series of large-scale, multisite clinical trials on how to improve survival after a myocardial infarction. Maria Grazia Franzosi, young physician who rose to become head of cardiological research at the Mario Negri, coordinated ISIS-1 in Italy. Starting in 1983, the Italians decided they wanted to conduct a similar study in Italy and called it GISSI, the Gruppo Italiano per lo Studio della Steptochinasi nell'Infarto Miocardico.[18]

Mario Negri staff worked with ANMCO, the Italian Association of Hospital Cardiologists, to "transform routine clinical activity into an experimental exercise and to become a cooperative, public health-oriented network."[19] Leaders of ANMCO, which represented ordinary hospitals rather than academic hospitals, and Mario Negri researchers traveled the country by second-class rail to meet with colleagues in most of the coronary care units in Italy so that "a large number of physicians across the country were actively participating in the conceptual development, implementation, and reporting of the research findings."[20] Chiefs of coronary care units trusted Professor Fausto Rovelli, a cardiologist at Milan's largest hospital and a founder of GISSI.[21] They explained why the trial was important to their practice and their patients, answered questions and asked for feedback from their practice experience, getting them to volunteer time from their busy practices to help out and involving them in all phases of a trial.

Although academic leaders were skeptical that organizing a large trial through coronary care units (CCUs) at community hospitals could succeed, the collaborative team from ANMCO and Mario Negri motivated cardiologists at nearly all the CCUs to recruit 11,806 of their patients who were admitted within 12 hours after onset of a suspected heart attack (AMI). (Later, more than 94 percent received a confirmed diagnosis of AMI.) The recruitment, monitoring, and clinical reporting was done on a voluntary basis so that no physician or CCU was paid for participating. Exclusion criteria were kept to a minimum and did not include old age or sex. The trials were made part of practice: "The protocol did not require modification of diagnostic and therapeutic practice."[22]

The team set up a complex but largely voluntary organization to sustain this national network, with a coordinator in each region, coding and reviewing teams, a scientific advisory board, an ethics board, a coordination and data monitoring group, and a central steering committee.[23] The design was negotiated with practicing cardiologists to draw on their routine care and to differ from it as little as possible. "The transformation of routine care into a randomized scheme of treatment countrywide was a major cultural decision," wrote the leaders, one that showed that a "change in attitude of a professional society combined with the availability of drugs and care for all NHS patients entering CCUs could become a uniquely powerful tool for testing a scientific hypothesis . . . A trial is no longer perceived as a 'foreign' body searching for a place in the busy routine, but is recognized as part of the general framework in which all patients without contraindications belong naturally."[24]

Besides conceiving and implementing trials as an integral part of clinical practice, the Mario Negri leaders followed their ethic of doing what is best for patients. As Tognoni put it when we interviewed him in 2013:

> The development of an epidemiology focused not simply on incidence/prevalence of disease but on how patients are cared for and on the documentation of unmet needs. A trial is the recognition of an unmet need . . . [the] tool for making clinicians aware of their uncertainty and ignorance and ready to take collectively the responsibility of looking for an answer.

	GISSI-1	GISSI-2	GISSI-3	GISSI-Prev	GISSI-HF	GISSI-AF
Enrollment	1984-85	1988-89	1991-93	1993-96	2002-05	2004-07
Publication	Lancet, 1986	Lancet, 1990	Lancet, 1993	Lancet, 1998	Lancet, 2008	NEJM, 2009
No Centers	176	223	200	172	351	114
No Patients	11 806	12 490	19 394	11 379	6 975	1442
Total costs	350 000 €	4M €	6M €	4M €	20M €	3,7M €
Cost per pt	30 €	320 €	309 €	350 €	2 800 €	2 680 €
Regulatory approval	SK by FDA	—	Lisinopril by FDA	n-3 PUFA by IMH and EMA	n-3 PUFA by IMH (ongoing)	—

Figure 6.3   Features of six GISSI trials

A central randomization team assigned patients either to receive intrave-nous streptokinase (SK) to dissolve blood clots, or not (in the control arm). By keeping the design simple but rigorous, the staff for this large trial con-sisted of only two senior and three junior investigators, a data manager, a half-time biostatistician, and three secretaries. The scientific and monitoring center not only organized the trial but also served as an information center to answer questions and provide support for clinicians and patients. Total costs were $350,000 or $390 (€300) per patient for a 24-month study![25] As shown in Figure 6.3, the average cost of subsequent GISSI megatrials rose to about $420 (€350) per patient in the mid-1990s and $3,700 (€2800) in the early 2000s, a fraction of what drug companies said trials cost them, though there are good reasons to suspect they inflate their unverified trial costs to justify high prices.[26]

The trial aimed to provide clear answers to questions raised about the ben-efits of SK in many small trials that had produced variable results. After 21 days, 19 percent fewer patients receiving SK died than patients who did not, and the extent of benefit correlated strongly with how promptly treatment began. Compared to the control group, the chance of death was 50 percent less for patients receiving SK in the first hour after onset of symptoms, 26 percent less for patients receiving SK in less than 3 hours, 20 percent less for those receiving SK in 3–6 hours, and 13 percent less in those receiving treat-ment in 6–9 hours. Women benefited as much as men, but as the tougher sex, women were less likely to die than men!

The first data from the GISSI trial was presented in September 1985. The data were very clear, but there is a prejudice against small countries, even when they produce top scientists and researchers, Tognoni explained to us. We rarely get important work written up in *The Times, The Guardian,* or *The Observer.* They assume nothing important happens outside the big countries and themselves—another small country. In the 1970s, Tognoni said, when we initially asked the international Boston Surveillance Network on drugs made up of Harvard, Stanford, and other major universities if we could join, they as much as said, " 'Who are you? Are you kidding?' But all that changed after GISSI."

Tognoni recalled, "When Eugene Passamani, then the Chief of the NIH Division of Clinical Trials saw the 1985 results, he doubted the data and its quality. He said 'I can't believe these findings. May I come and see the data for myself?' He came and interviewed me personally for three hours and scrutinized the data to verify its quality. Meantime, we had convened a meeting with WHO-Europe and with ISIS-1 at Oxford to make a confidential presentation. Dr. Passamani asked if he could come. We said, 'Of course.' "

Then Tognoni flew to present the GISSI findings at the American Heart Association meeting, and the keynote speaker was Eugene Braunwald, the world's leading authority on cardiology and founding editor of *Braunwald's Heart Disease*, (now in its ninth edition). When he concluded his speech, he added that "Everything I've said today is now up for discussion because the Italians have shown us . . ." Tognoni concluded, "It was a formal recognition that our work in this little, minor country was valid and worth paying attention to."

Because cardiologists at nearly all their units participated from the start, 99 percent of all the nation's CCUs were using SK as a routine treatment within one year, an extraordinary example of putting research into practice. Research-in-practice meant research into practice. The potential for a whole health-care system "to be a natural and readily available laboratory is often not recognized and therefore badly underused," wrote the Mario Negri leaders.[27] GISSI's "demonstration of the capacity of a health service to produce reliable scientific results was itself a major achievement."[28]

Reframing Informed Consent

In the same spirit and ethos, informed consent takes on an entirely new meaning and function, not just to explain a trial design to a person so that he or she will sign a release, but also to share power and asymmetric knowledge:

> to focus on information and communication and participation for the care provider/investigator and the patient . . . Too many clinical experiments fall short: trials of non-innovative or "me too" drugs; trials with weak scientific bases; trials that are market-driven; and trials that do not make sense even though they comply with GCP [Good Clinical Practice]-like requirements.[29]

In those cases, it becomes even more important (though less likely) to tell patients they are being asked to participate in a trial that is unable to produce statistically valid results or unable to improve their care. If the millions of Americans and Europeans who agree to participate in trials each year were honestly told how few of those trials could improve actual care, they probably would not. Ironically, most of them think they will get better care or even be cured. If this were true, aside from the first-class diagnostic work-up that trials provide, the trial could not be randomized and blinded. Yet "informed consent" often does not include disabusing patients of their false hopes. Others participate for the money, another distortion of good research that has led to low-income serial trial "volunteers," bad pharma leading to bad medicine.

The follow-up study to GISSI-1 concluded that "The beneficial effect of a single short-term intravenous infusion of 1.5 million units of SK in prolonging survival . . . clearly extends beyond the hospital phase to at least 12 months."[30] Remarkably, this follow-up study tracked down 98.3 percent of the 11,712 patients in the original study, before computers. And a ten-year follow-up traced information on 93 percent of all of the randomized patients in GISSI-1. It found that benefits of that one shot of SK continued into the tenth year and noted the GISSI trial was "widely recognized as the opening of the thrombolytic era."[31] Advantages in survival from receiving a single dose of SK remained proportionate to how soon patients received it after first symptoms of an MI. Thus shortening the time became clearly established as critical, and that has meant shortening the time from first symptoms to getting a patient in the hospital door by informing anyone who might be contacted, as well as older people who might mistakenly think they have "indigestion" or feel "faint." Better to get to the hospital and *then* ask, "Am I having a heart attack or just heartburn?" In fact, a later Mario Negri trial underscored the importance of shortening time for people who live alone or are very old, or who experience symptoms at night or have a doctor who does not respond with urgency to a call.

This first megatrial by GISSI appears to have reduced death from cardiovascular disease more than the much-celebrated development of coronary care units (CCUs) in the 1970s. Although widely credited with sharply reducing deaths, randomized controlled trials of CCUs "did not show a consistent advantage over non-invasive ward care or simple rest at home."[32] Moreover, the national network of interaction and training transformed the community of providers into a community of researchers. Salim Yusuf, the distinguished cardiologist at McMaster University, wrote, "No longer was clinical research the exclusive prerogative of a limited number of academics, but instead the larger community of practicing cardiologists, physicians, and allied health workers . . . More important, this shifted the emphasis in research to seeking answers primarily to satisfy the intellectual pursuits of a few select academics, to addressing issues of practical importance, relevant to the health of patients."[33]

Looking back on that period, Professor Braunwald at Harvard also recognized the culture that the trial had created: "The GISSI 'culture' has created enthusiastic investigators who wish to ask important questions, cooperate enthusiastically in patient enrollment, and insist on the acquisition of data of high quality. Thus GISSI serves as a model for other national and international clinical research groups."[34] It considers the entire health-care system as a natural laboratory and provides the basis for practitioners constantly learning from field-based training about their own practices.[35]

Commercial Clinical Trials

In order to appreciate how greatly Mario Negri trials differ from most trials, consider how they are done now and how badly society needs to draw on the Mario Negri approach to stop the flood of new drugs with few advantages for patients and to stop misleading information being published in medical journals that shape clinical guidelines and practice. First, most commercial trials use many kinds of exclusion criteria to rule out the people most likely get the drug but have an adverse reaction, and include those most likely to show improvement on surrogate or other substitute outcome measures.[36] Then they take random samples of this biased population. As a result, new drugs that doctors prescribe based on results from most "randomized trials" of such selected populations may be worse for patients than well-established generic drugs.[37] Billions are invested in doing these trials in sophisticated, costly ways that Mario Negri researchers not only refuse to do but widely oppose as unethical.

Second, a large number of trials use surrogate or substitute measures instead of measures that are important to patients. But most surrogate end points, even when they correlate with clinical outcomes, do not accurately predict clinical benefits.[38] Using surrogate end points instead of real clinical outcomes to "prove" a new drug is "better" in a shorter time at lower cost also violates Mario Negri's ethical principles and its cardinal rule.

Third, most newly approved drugs treat conditions or risks already treated by established drugs.[39] In studies dating back 40 years, few are found to be clinically superior by independent review teams of physicians and pharmacists.[40] This happens because regulators do not require evidence of real patient benefit but rather allow companies to test their own products against a placebo, when an effective treatment already exists, or using a surrogate end point when a real one can be used, or using a "noninferiority" design to prove the new drug is not too much worse. Mario Negri researchers think these trials are unethical in every sense—unethical to recruit patients to them, and unethical to use as a benchmark for approving a drug for general use.[41] They violate Mario Negri's principles explained in Chapter 1 and its guiding principle—do what is best for patients.

Fourth, big-budget commercial trial designs create a dependency by everyone involved on having to constantly raise funds that can distort or corrupt the true scientific mission of a good trial to benefit patients. Companies seek out or hire global clinical trial companies known as CROs to hire clinical specialists who recruit patients for a bounty fee or for generous pay and monitor their patients during the trial. Although trials cost companies billions, those costs are income and profits for everyone involved. Companies almost brag about how staggering the cost, and they use their claims of staggering costs to justify charging high prices. All these bounty fees, retainers, and other forms of pay are unnecessary, corrupt trials, and invite scientific compromise. From the start, Mario Negri researchers have avoided all this.

Fifth, prevailing practices in most commercial trials keep clinicians largely in the dark about the design, the rationale, and the analysis of a trial. The authoritative research of Jill Fisher indicates that each party and layer knows only about its specific job and therefore has no responsibility for the rest, a kind of blinkered ethics where each horse can only see what's straight in front of him.[42] As a result, she finds that contract ethics—carry out the instructions correctly—replace clinical ethics to do what is best for one's patients. "Don't ask questions—just take your check and get on with your part of the job." In the United States, doing trials generates additional income for practicing specialists. Doing these trials is often regarded as a sign of status and enables practices involved to offer treatment options to worried patients, even though these "options" randomize the drug they are testing to see if it is effective and, therefore, these are not real treatments.

Finally, commercial bias has been found at every stage of trials: the trial design, the choice of dosages, protocol design, the analysis of data, and the way results get written up (or left out) in published articles about the results.[43] Mario Negri trials avoid all these biases by adhering to principles of research integrity and independence. They are designed to test the clinical effects of a therapy, not to generate positive results for regulators so the therapy will be approved for marketing. The Institute's data is open for public inspection, and Mario Negri researchers publish all negative as well as positive findings. They write their own research articles, free of ghost management, publication planning, and ghostwriting that can seriously bias what doctors and patients can read and know.[44]

In May 2012, we asked Dr. Maria Grazia Franzosi, as head of the Department of Cardiovascular Research and a key staff member of all the GISSI trials from 1984 to the present, if clinical trials at the Mario Negri Institute differ from commercially run trials. "Yes, absolutely," she replied.

> We can compare different drugs made by different companies, and we choose what we test based on medical science, not potential sales. We almost always use hard clinical end points that matter to the patients. Doing trials this way requires more patients, more cost, and they are less likely to show success than trials using surrogate end points. But they produce information useful to doctors and patients. We sample an inclusive population, rather than excluding the elderly, or women, or minorities. Thus results from our trials more accurately document how well a drug will work once put into use. We also do not carry out "equivalency" trials because we think they are unethical. The increased use of these trials by companies wastes a great deal of money and works against the interests of patients. Finally, we keep ownership of the data and make it available to anyone.

GISSI-2, 3, 4, and Beyond

The formation of large networks among specialists to carry out large trials about critical issues in medical care spread rapidly from its beginnings by

Richard Peto's group at Oxford and the Mario Negri Institute. Close on the heels of the GISSI-1 trial, the ANMCO Research Centre, together with Gianni Tognoni, Maria Grazia Franzosi, and colleagues at the Mario Negri Institute organized GISSI-2. They worked with 233 of what by then had become the nation's 250 CCUs (coronary care units) to recruit 12,490 patients, plus another 8,000 included in an international arm. They tested how the newer, pricey intervention from Genentech, TPA, would compare to Hoechst's much cheaper drug, SK, and whether following up with heparin 12 hours after beginning either would improve clinical outcomes further.[45] This trial was supported through a main grant from Boehringer Ingelheim Italy SpA, ICI-Pharma Italy, and Italfarmaco SpA, as well as the Italian National Research Council, but was run by the Mario Negri Institute and the National Association of Hospital Cardiologists (ANMCO). Commercial support of scientific trials that are entirely controlled by the Mario Negri researchers holds important lessons for how research teams at universities and elsewhere can keep control of the science, the data, and the analysis while negotiating with companies about sponsorship.

Even before the trial was reported, evidence leaked that TPA performed no better than SK. As the *Wall Street Journal* reported, Genentech's shares began "Taking a Pounding from Analyst's Leak of Study of Clot Drug."[46] Genentech's vice president of research countered with a promise of three new trials soon that "together will conclusively demonstrate TPA's clear-cut benefit." No credible researcher would make such a statement—how could he know the outcomes of scientifically valid trials before they were completed? In fact, the claim was not supported: The trials found no differences between the four combinations of TPA or SK, with or without heparin.[47] The president of Genentech immediately told the *Wall Street Journal* and investors that GISSI-2 was confusing and inconclusive, a frequent response by companies when well-designed trials find their drug less beneficial than they claim.[48] This misleads investors as well as doctors and the public by creating doubt, the subject of the book, *Doubt Is Their Product*.[49] Health-care systems asked themselves, why pay eleven times more for TPA than SK when there is no clinical advantage?

The big news of GISSI-2 lay buried in the baseline mortality rate for all 12,490 patients in both arms of the trial: because the national network of cardiologists had so quickly and thoroughly implemented the lessons of GISSI-1 that the baseline for GISSI-2 has changed as national mortality had declined by a third. Advocates of single-payer health care could emphasize this added advantage to the benefits of this equitable, free-choice, and cost-effective way or organizing health care.

During the same time, researchers at Oxford and the Mario Negri Institute worked with a much wider set of international networks to organize a trial to compare the outcomes of using SK or aspirin, both, or neither. With a control placebo group for each intervention, this megatrial involved allocating patients at random to one of eight comparison groups.[50] One of the resulting landmark articles ends by listing paragraph after paragraph of the participating cardiologists as unpaid coauthors in networks from Australia, Austria, Belgium, Canada, Denmark, Finland, France, Germany, Ireland, Italy, New Zealand, Norway, Spain, Sweden, Switzerland, the United Kingdom, and the United States.[51] Only those few with staff functions received compensation.

In all, these volunteer cardiologists registered 17,187 unpaid patients who had entered 417 hospitals up to 24 hours after onset of an MI, with a median time of 5 hours. This trial population represented the real-life population of patients with suspected heart attacks, because statistically the researchers were able to recruit with "only a phone call and no forms, [and] the use of ancillary treatments was not restricted."[52] Eric Topol has pointed out that one needs both smaller trials to test out a specific intervention "with maximum precision by a pre-specified protocol and an effort made to control all other confounding factors," and also mega "simple" trials, so large as to obviate the need for detailed data and controls.[53] In combination with GISSI, the British ISIS-2 trial found that the combination of both SK and aspirin was significantly better than either alone (or none), reducing mortality by 42 percent compared to a 25 percent reduction by SK alone. Thus the scientific effort to find effective (and inexpensive) interventions to save lives moved further forward.

Other important unanswered questions led the GISSI research team at the Mario Negri Institute, now headed by Dr. Franzosi, to design GISSI-3 with 19,394 patients randomized to test whether or not early administration of lisinopril (the ACE inhibitor Zestril or Prinivil) or glyceryl tri-nitrate (GTN) could prevent deterioration after an MI. The sample was drawn from the entire range of people who experience an MI, with an emphasis on the more vulnerable elderly patients and women.[54] GISSI-3 found that while a six-week treatment with GTN did not produce a statistically significant benefit, lisinopril lowered the risk of death by 11 percent. However, both together "produced significant reductions in overall mortality"—15 percent in patients who were already receiving the proven effective treatments from GISSI-1. Thanks to the ways in which the GISSI trials had changed medical practice throughout the entire health service, national mortality from MI dropped significantly further, from 8.8 percent during GISSI-2 to 7.1 percent. The prescription of beta-blockers increased substantially, as shown in Figure 6.4, while the prescription of calcium antagonists decreased. The trial was funded by Zeneca and Schwarz Pharma. GISSI-3 changed practice worldwide. "Before GISSI-3, [ACE-inhibitors] were used for hypertension or heart failure but not in patients with acute MI. After the trial produced favorable results, they were given to more than 80% of patients with acute MI."[55]

One preventive measure for heart disease was using angiotensin II-receptor blockers (ARBs) such as valsartan (Diovan—Novartis) to prevent recurrent atrial fibrillation. Some smaller trials had indicated a benefit. Using the GISSI organization and network, Novartis funded the largest randomized, double-blind trial to test this use.[56] The drug reduced mean systolic blood pressure nearly four times more than the placebo group. However, "the mean heart rate

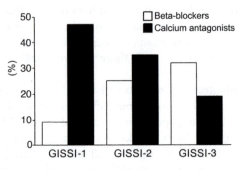

Figure 6.4   Impact of GISSI-3 on clinical practice

was unchanged from baseline values at 8 weeks and at the end of the study," and the same proportion of patients in both groups (51–52 percent) had a recurrence of atrial fibrillation. In other words, there was no evidence that reducing high blood pressure in these circumstances saved lives. Published in the *New England Journal of Medicine*, the study concluded, "Our findings do not support the original hypothesis of a beneficial role of blockers of the renin-angiotensin-aldosterone system in the prevention of recurrent atrial fibrillation."[57]

This example illustrates the importance of being able to do independent trials on prevailing practices that do *not* help patients. It is also an example of a surrogate end point that does not make a clinical difference. It reflects the principles and culture of the Mario Negri Institute to follow the facts, not the funding, in publishing nonpositive or negative results.

In GISSI-4, or GISSI-Prevenzione, centered at Mario Negri-Sud, a large randomized trial tested whether giving patients who have survived a recent MI omega-3 polyunsaturated fatty acids (n-3 PUFA) or vitamin E, or both, or neither would affect mortality. The trial of 11,324 patients did follow-up clinical assessments at 6, 12, 18, 30, and 42 months for a total of 38,053 person-years that also included a questionnaire about food eaten. Researchers found that vitamin E did not affect mortality, but PUFA significantly reduced the risk of a combined end point of death plus a nonfatal MI or stroke by 10 percent and the risk of cardiovascular death by 17 percent.[58] Support was provided by Bristol-Myers-Squibb, Pharmacia-Upjohn, Società Prodotti Antibiotici (SPA), and Pfizer. This was "the first clinically controlled confirmation of the possible anti-arrhythmic activity of n-3 PUFA" as secondary prevention in a post-MI population.[59]

In GISSI-Atrial Fibrillation, scores of investigators, led by Tognoni and Franzosi in Chieti and Milan, enrolled 1,442 patients with serious cardiovascular or diabetic histories to see if valsartan (Diovan) could reduce recurrence of atrial fibrillation. While other studies showed it reduced surrogate end points like blood pressure, this 52-week study used a hard, clinical end point and found no reduction in atrial fibrillation or other clinical benefits to patients.[60]

An overall perspective of these Mario Negri trials was provided by Peter Sleight at Oxford: "Professor Silvio Garattini and colleagues have for many years emphasized the need to carry out trials in which the design, execution, analysis, and publication are independent of industry (although, as in many trials, industry has been a willing collaborator and sponsor)."[61] Besides maintaining scientific objectivity, this approach has enabled these trials to be done at less than one-tenth the cost per patient. The widespread involvement and organization of specialists and the resulting huge data set also enable the trials to establish unbiased guidelines and influence general cardiac care.

The methods used to maintain research integrity with commercial funding are nicely described in a GISSI trial, funded by SPA-Italy, Pfizer, Sigma Tau, and AstraZeneca. "The GISSI-HF group coordinated the study, managed the data, and undertook analyses, under the supervision of the [independent] steering committee, who designed the GISSI-HF study. None of the funding sources had a role in the trial design, conduct, data collection, analysis, data interpretation, or writing of the report."[62] The median age of participants was 67, and 42 percent were over 70, a faithful reflection of actual patients treated. Patients taking omega-3 fatty acids had fewer hospitalizations and deaths. Data were stored at GISSI, and all members of the steering and writing committees "had full access to the database and final responsibility for the decision to submit for publication." This summarizes the ways in which the Mario Negri Institute has retained its scientific integrity and protected itself from widely recorded sources of bias by companies in medical science, knowledge, and publication.[63] If Mario Negri researchers can do it, so can research teams elsewhere. Today, the GISSI series, internationally respected and a source of national pride, will continue with new trials investigating why certain subpopulations respond differently. It continues to bind cardiologists together to work on clinical problems.

In any given year, Mario Negri researchers are involved in over 100 clinical trials with more than 85,000 patients enrolled. Funding comes from national agencies (32 percent), followed by pharmaceutical companies (22 percent), scientific foundations (15 percent), public programs, including the European Commission's research program (11 percent), associations (6 percent), hospitals/local health units and regional institutions (4 percent each), and charities, institutes of excellence, medical technology companies, universities, and donations (1 percent each). Trials are also registered in the United States at Clinicaltrials.gov (www.clinicaltrials.gov), the European Union's Clinical Trials Register (www.clinicaltrialsregister.eu), and the International Standard Randomised Controlled Trial Number Register (www.controlled-trials.com/isrctn).

The Institute has started its own registry to further increase transparency and independent accountability. A registry is valuable for five reasons: "planning new studies, promoting collaboration among researchers, facilitating patient access and recruitment into trials, preventing trial duplication and inappropriate funding, and identifying therapeutic needs that remain neglected."[64] Registries prevent authors from reporting different primary outcomes from those initially intended and avoid the loss of scientific data.

GISSI's Scientific Offspring

The GISSI approach has spawned several offspring within the Mario Negri Institute, not to mention beyond it. We have already described in Chapter 3 the REIN, Remission Clinic, and Benedict trials. Other valuable trials are too numerous to describe, but more recent published trials are listed in Appendix 2. Several trials were carried out by international networks of specialists that reflect the international influence of Mario Negri's pioneering work. For example, the International Stroke Genetics Consortium (ISGC) and the Wellcome Trust Case Control Consortium 2 (WTCCC2) studied genetic factors that might contribute to stroke. They identified a variant in HDAC9 associated with large vessel ischemic stroke, which they reported in *Nature Genetics* in 2012.[65] The Mario Negri Institute is an active partner in many such international networks and collaborations.

Another network began when Luigi Naldi, a young research fellow at the Mario Negri Institute, submitted a proposal in 1986 for organizing a clinical network to study skin disorders. Inspired by what GISSI had accomplished in cardiology, Naldi used an investigation of the lichen-hepatitis syndrome as the basis for proposing the network to the Italian Society of Dermatology and Venereology. A total of 50 dermatological centers have become involved in a series of trials, and members of the network have led sessions of methods and studies at 24 annual meetings. Students and research fellows have done their training at the GISED network center. It has become part of international research networks for cross-national studies.

In the early 1990s, Gianni Tognoni and Vittorio Bertele' established a network called ICAI that grew to involve more than one hundred angiology and vascular surgical centers to address the terrible condition of critical leg ischemia. It kills more people than several cancers, and no effective drug has been found. But one promising possibility was prostaglandin E_1. The organizers used the classic Mario Negri approach:

- Engage the clinicians in an epidemiological survey of clinical needs and practices.
- Lead surgeons to prioritize the working hypotheses.
- Plan educational training on clinical trial methodology.
- Develop a trial on a shared, high-priority issue.

The group ran the largest pragmatic trial ever done in this clinical setting, which was reported in the *Annals of Internal Medicine*.[66] They found the drug provided a short-term benefit, which decreased over time. One problem with the trial reflected the ethics of the Mario Negri Institute. The investigators cross-checked the data and discovered that 18 patients or their relatives followed by five centers had reported their outcomes incorrectly. The investigators and the external safety and monitoring committee excluded all 226 patients recruited by those five centers from the main study, just to be sure the quality of the data would not be compromised. In most trials, just the data from the 18 would be excluded, or kept in despite knowing their data were inaccurate.

A notable network that began way back with GISSI-1 consisted of general practitioners. Cardiologists wanted to see a network of GPs organized, Tognoni explained, because they realized how vital GPs are for detecting signs of a heart attack and getting patients quickly to a hospital. But it wasn't easy, first because the law did not allow clinical trials through GPs, only through specialists, and, second, because it took longer to persuade them to participate. Tognoni and his colleagues at Mario Negri even wrote about "lessons from a failure" after they carefully signed up 806 GPs to participate in a trial through meetings with over 90 percent attending; yet only 63 started recruiting patients.[67] The fact that those 63 followed the trial protocol faithfully proved it was sensible; so what went wrong?

One factor concerned possible damage to the doctor-patient relationship. Imagine your doctor has been treating you for hypertension and one day he says, "I'd like to take you off the medication I recommended for you, first to see how high your blood pressure is when untreated, and second to see how much good your medication is actually doing. It's all part of a clinical trial to put my practice on a more scientific footing." This hardly builds confidence, and it casts doubt on whether your doctor diagnosed and treated you correctly in the first place. Nevertheless, Tognoni and others at Mario Negri persisted in developing general practitioners as a critical research network, where over 90 percent of all patient problems are first addressed, in persuading legislators to change the law about GPs doing clinical trials, and in carrying out important trials.

In a profound essay, Tognoni and his colleagues on behalf of general practitioners articulated the core issues.[68] Research is an expression of care. It cannot be separate, parallel, or occasional (as it is for commercial testing) and be clinically real. The greatest risk in clinical medicine is to dissociate care from research about how effective that care is. Yet this is what usually happens. Rather, research into treatments must be nested within practice, and primary care is the most representative of a people's risks or illnesses. These in turn reflect the state of the economy and the rights of patients in that society. They should not be "recruited" so much as invited as persons with needs and rights to help provide answers to unsolved questions and uncertainties as part of a collective authorship in a research project of shared objectives and outcomes. For example, a new study has involved 324 GPs and 2,417 patients who experience depression, two-thirds of them for more than a year, to document prevalence and response to treatment. Only 16.6 percent were judged to have fully recovered, 42.7 percent partially recovered from their depression, 33.1 percent did not improve, and 7.6 percent worsened.[69]

The network of GPs has also provided the basis for the first large randomized control trial (RCT) entirely conducted by General Practitioners in Italy, on the preventive role of omega-3 fatty acids in patients with multiple cardiovascular risk factors or atherosclerotic diseases but no previous myocardial infarction. The Risk and Prevention Study, led by Gianni Tognoni and Carla

Roncaglioni, enrolled 12,513 patients followed for five years by a network of 860 GPs throughout the country. The average age of patients was 64 years and 60 percent were males. There were two main results of the study, published in May 2013 in the *New England Journal of Medicine*. The first one is scientific, with relevant public health implications: For people who haven't had a heart attack, the study provides no evidence that omega-3 fatty acids prevent cardiovascular diseases or death. As news websites put it, fish-oil supplements do not reduce the risk of heart attack, heart failure, or death. The second result is just as important: For the first time and with the largest study in the field, the work of Italian primary care clinicians has been recognized at the highest level of scientific literature and become an international reference in a key area for cardiovascular prevention.

Studies of Breast Cancer Treatment

In parallel with its famous trials in heart disease, Mario Negri began studies of cancer care in the late 1970s, led by Alessandro Liberati together with Gianni Tognoni, Carlo La Vecchia, and Fabio Colombo. As in the project with the Lombardy regional government on prescription patterns, the first task was to obtain an accurate picture of current practice patterns for the treatment of breast cancer as "the commonest malignant tumor in Western countries besides non-melanotic skin cancers."[70] The investigators found that across 31 hospitals the stage of disease was recorded for only 44 percent of all patients. Toxic side effects from chemotherapy were often not noted, even though 35 percent of women dropped out of chemotherapy. Chemotherapeutic protocols were recorded for only 37 percent of all cases. Radiation dosage was not recorded for 56 percent of the women. Follow-up data existed for only half the patients. These deficiencies were similar to reports of unprofessional—one could say irresponsible—record-keeping found in the United States and Great Britain as well. They violated established standards of practice. Once again, the study found that when doctors are left to practice autonomously, they will do what each thinks best, and from the perspective of science-based medicine, "best" will not be good.

Follow-up studies found that 36 percent of breast cancer patients were diagnosed more than three months after the appearance of first symptoms, and proportionately more of the women diagnosed more than three months after symptoms had stage-III or stage-IV cancer. The doctors were more likely to provide thorough information to women who were younger or more educated. They also provided *less* information to women who had larger tumors than women who had smaller ones. The Mario Negri team also looked into causes for the delays and found that the hospitals were a significant factor.[71] Doctors who used a structured protocol or worked at larger, more organized hospitals provided more thorough information to their patients. Compared to a standard protocol, doctors did not give women thorough information 61 percent of the time, though they thought their communication was thorough

69 percent of the time. Throughout the literature one finds that doctors think they are providing better, more science-based care that is not affected by commercial influences than clinical researchers find they are.[72] Studies like these by an independent research institute can significantly improve the quality of clinical practice in a country.

The national network of cancer centers and oncologists organized by the Mario Negri Institute and others is called GIVIO. Led by Alessandro Liberati—now sadly missed—as head of the Laboratory of Clinical Epidemiology at Mario Negri, the GIVIO team moved on to analyze the benefits of providing a program of intensive follow-up surveillance. Does it detect metastases in women already treated for breast cancer, compared to routine follow-up with an annual exam?[73] Women wanted the intensive surveillance program, which included bone scans, chest x-rays, and liver echographies. Both they and their doctors thought that closer surveillance would detect cancers earlier and reduce the chances of dying. But rigorous trial data showed that the mean time to detection of distant metastases was nearly the same: 53 months using intensive testing and follow-up compared to 54 months using routine surveillance. Even the duration of symptoms before detection differed only by 3 percent between women given routine follow-up and those receiving intensive, frequent follow-up. These women also rated the changes in their quality of life, and on average it did not differ between intensive and routine surveillance, perhaps because intensive follow-up may have reassured some but made others more anxious. For intensive surveillance "induces additional tests because of the dubious results of tests performed by protocol."[74] In sum, this randomized trial of practices found that routine surveillance saves a great deal of money, staff, and effort without harming patients.

Clinical trials of drugs and cancer care continue at the Mario Negri Institute up to the present, with results published in the best medical journals. For example, a large international network involving Mario Negri researchers carried out a meta-analysis of trials to study whether statins reduce the incidence of cancer or death.[75] They do not. Another important international network of oncologists from a dozen institutions had more members from the Mario Negri Institute than any other center for a study of erlotinib as second-line treatment for certain patients with advanced, non-small cell lung cancer.[76] Using a comparative, superiority design, they found that standard chemotherapy did significantly *better* than high-priced erlotinib, which had looked very effective compared to a placebo. These examples illustrate world-class cancer research currently being done at the Mario Negri Institute to find answers relevant to clinical practice.

Saving Patients on the Brink of Death

In the beautiful nineteenth century Villa Camozzi, the youthful Guido Bertolini heads up the Clinical Epidemiology Laboratory with nearly irrepressible enthusiasm for the Italian Group for the Evaluation of Interventions in

Intensive Care Medicine, GiViTI. Building on earlier work by Tognoni and Liberati, Bertolini and his group have persuaded chiefs and staff of intensive care units (ICUs) to improve their care of critically ill patients and to give them the right tools to identify trouble spots in their very complicated work by doing research on their own practices. In fact, it was a dozen ICU specialists who came to Mario Negri in 1991 to ask if it would act as an external, trusted third party in evaluating their work so they could improve it. After its central role in Seveso crisis and in organizing networks of specialists for the famous GISSI trials describe in this chapter, the Mario Negri Institute was the acknowledged authority in clinical epidemiology and highly trusted as a private, nonprofit institution of great integrity.

Since 1991, initially under the guide of Giovanni Apolone as head of the Laboratory of Clinical Epidemiology, Bertolini worked with his staff and the intensivists to build and consolidate the GiViTI network, which now has 428 affiliates. In 1992, to show ICU doctors what Mario Negri's research paradigm in clinical epidemiology could do, Bertolini and Apolone collected an epidemiological profile of ICU patients, demonstrating a high variability in the care and the outcome of critically ill patients among Italian hospitals. From then until 2002, GiViTI carried out many influential projects that have improved clinical care for patients. In 1994, they showed how analgesia and sedation were underused in ICUs, so that many patients were unnecessarily suffering from a suboptimal treatment. In 1995, a project dedicated to critically ill children revealed that the lack of pediatric ICUs caused higher than expected mortality among the youngest patients, inappropriately treated in adult ICUs.

A three-stage study of resource consumption in ICU (1995–99) was able to identify different diseconomies in the organization of the units, and even to develop a new two-dimensional representation of the relative cost of treating different clinical conditions, comparing expenditures per surviving patient with patients who died. In 1999, Bertolini coordinated two important international projects on the incidence and treatment of bloodstream infection and ARDS (acute respiratory distress syndrome). In both cases GiViTI recruited far more patients than other national ICU networks and became internationally recognized as one of the most important and reliable in intensive care medicine. All these projects stemmed from several lines of research initiatives that in due time improved patient care.

In 2002, Bertolini with his team launched a new generation of projects known as Margherita, or "daisy" in English. They developed a software package that has a core (the center of the daisy) of all key data needed to evaluate ICU performance in terms of quality and resource expenditure against clinical outcome. Petals radiating out from the core represent selected studies of data to address certain clinical questions or responses to a trial. In 2002, 95 ICUs responded and began collecting data on 23,285 patients. The network grew steadily to 2010 and has leveled off to about 240–250 ICUs and more than 80,000 acutely ill patients benefiting from this program of continuous quality improvement.[77] The system is efficient and inexpensive. Mario Negri does not pay the ICUs, and the ICUs only reimburse expenses to the Mario

Negri: All funding comes from winning competitive bids for Italian and European funds, as well as a few companies, a total of about €500,000 a year.

The quality of ICU care has steadily improved so the mean performance has improved, and the Margherita research team calculates that 2,500 seriously ill Italians who would have died in the past five years have not, because continuous quality improvements have been implemented. Variations among ICUs have lessened as ICUs performing less well have moved up toward the mean. The quality of care for the most acutely ill patients has improved across regions as well.

Each ICU owns its own data and gets its own report, with the Mario Negri project team producing subreports that can pinpoint where clinical care can be better. As trust and transparency grow year by year, more ICUs are sharing more of their results with each other. The Mario Negri team runs short courses in statistics and other topics for ICU specialists throughout the country. In these ways, the ICU project is like a continual observational trial, as intensive care treatments across centers reveal what works better or less well, and the results are fed back to the specialty teams. It reminds one of Deming's Continuous Quality Improvement model that transformed post–World War II Japan into a model of high quality.[78]

An important contribution of the project is to develop superior and current methods to estimate the probability of death or survival that is much superior to the APACHE, MPM, PRISM, SAPS II, and other models that are based on old data from the 1990s and on US health care, where avoidable deaths has ranked among the lowest among 19 advanced health-care systems in affluent countries.[79] "We never mix patients with other countries, particularly with the United States," Bertolini wrote us in August 2013. "If you apply SAPS II to the patients admitted to your ICU in 2012, you get the number of deaths a selected number of European and North American ICUs would have observed if they had treated your patients in 1993!" Instead, the current death rate is established for each ICU, based on about 120 variables that describe each patient's characteristics and clinical history as well as present condition so that one is comparing similar patients treated today as closely as possible. Then, each year, Bertolini rebases the entire model—a lot of work but a great advantage.

In 2011, Margherita started moving ahead as Bertolini developed prognostic models that can be reliably used in subgroup analyses to pinpoint problems in performance. "In a very recent example (2013), we showed an ICU that they had serious problems with patient with acute hypercapnic respiratory failure. They reviewed the ventilation strategy and improved the outcome." Again, they are able to monitor their clinical outcomes over time. In another case, the Margherita comparative system recorded that mortality was steadily lower than expected and worsened for weeks, then months! What was happening? The system alert led to a desperate search, and the ICU figured out what was happening. When two surgical units merged with lots of infighting among the surgeons, the quality of surgery suffered and their patients died more than expected.

In this framework, an exciting new advance is the Calibration Belt, the first statistical tool in the world that can compare quality of care in an individual ICU to the group with 80 and 95 percent confidence levels across the full range of expected mortalities. One can pinpoint a problem right away. The Calibration Belt also plays a significant role in developing prognostic models for better clinical management. So far, the press has not paid much attention to this remarkable contribution that improves care for very sick patients and saves lives.

In the future, Bertolini and his hand-picked team will be applying their methods to specific diseases and to other settings. One development since 2012 called Margherita3 drills down to assess how single treatments affect patients.

This Mario Negri project is going international. In 2010, the European Union recognized the exceptional achievements of GiViTI and funded a large project called Promoting Patient Safety and Quality Improvement in Critical Care (PROSAFE) to have the Mario Negri team teach other European countries how to carry out advanced epidemiological monitoring of patients admitted to ICUs. Work is under way in Poland, Hungary, Slovenia, Cyprus, Israel, and Greece.

Margherita constitutes an original national and international contribution by the Mario Negri Institute. Since it started, the British NHS, Australia, Germany, and other countries have developed ICU networks. In the United States, a national ICU network that systematically uses epidemiology to improve patient outcomes and save lives is likely because private hospitals and units compete against one another rather than work collaboratively. Each claims it is "the best," which ironically makes it impossible to know what "best" means or how to save more patients. For example, in 2013, the famous Harvard surgeon-writer, Atul Gawande, wrote how a health-care corporation he called "Big Med" was upgrading ICU performance across its hospitals.[80] But he described "corporate" implementing intrusive methods of surveillance that offended the ICU staff, a sharp contrast to the collaborative Mario Negri approach of persuading clinicians to join up in a shared undertaking based on trust and ownership of the process. In the end, there was no evidence that Big Med's efforts actually helped dying patients survive or get better. Unfortunately, Gawande did not mention the much more systematic and effective project at the Mario Negri Institute based on motivating a network of doctors to improve their own performance, available at minimum cost and with no patents or copyright to any health-care system or nation in the world. Recently, Bertolini's team has won a six million euro EU project to establish the fate of patients with brain trauma.

The Mario Negri research principles and practices can inspire other labs and research teams to join together into international networks of ethical, science-based, principled clinical trial organizations that can end surreptitious biasing in trial design, operation, coding, and reporting. A 2012 Cochrane review of trials concluded that "Independently sponsored trials should focus on testing innovative and essential treatments, as well as comparisons with existing effective treatments, thus shifting the resources spent on drug and device trials away from trials with a marketing purpose to those that are clinically important."[81] For more than 30 years, the Mario Negri Institute has shown how this is done, carried out as part of the health-care system itself and integrated into clinical practice. If only new medicines were tested against existing effective treatments using patient-relevant criteria, and funded by the medical service systems that will use them rather than the companies keen on selling them, most of the distorting practices of Big Pharma would disappear.

Part III

Promoting Good Science for Better Medicines

Science-Based Initiatives against Dangerous or Useless Drugs

Researchers at most centers for either pharmaceutical or pharmacological research keep their heads in the lab and do not consider it their business how companies promote the drugs they develop or how doctors actually prescribe them, even if they know about the distorting commercial practices often featured in the lay and medical press. But since the Mario Negri Institute is dedicated to basic and clinical pharmacology for better patient care, its leaders pioneered ways to replace "bad pharma" with "good pharma" by reducing the thousands of medicines that drug companies put on the market after World War II without evidence of patient benefit and with risks of harm. They worked to eliminate bad drugs and limit doctors to prescribing good ones more rationally. This chapter describes some remarkable efforts by research leaders at the Institute to apply clinical pharmacology to whole regional, national, and international formularies for prescribing.

Selecting Beneficial Medicines and Eliminating Harmful Ones

After World War II, many small Italian companies and several pharmacies decided to manufacture and sell drugs, not unlike the proliferation of nostrum manufacturers in the nineteenth and early twentieth centuries.[1] Most concentrated on marketing, and few did much research or testing of new drugs. Thus the mission of health care and good pharma to improve patient health or to keep them from getting worse was corrupted by the pursuit of large profits. Leaders at the Mario Negri Institute began to root out the institutional corruptions of medicine and government.

Separating the Wheat from the Chaff

Before the advent of the Italian National Health Service in 1978, a system of public health insurance called INAM was funded through deductions from workers' salaries. Prescription drugs on its list were paid from taxes and free to patients. On several occasions and particularly in TV debates, Garattini criticized this national health insurance scheme for reimbursing many useless, even dangerous drugs that wasted workers' money. Finally, in 1971, INAM decided to set up a committee to revise its formulary of reimbursable drugs. Made up of pharmacists, professors of pharmacology, and clinicians, the committee included Garattini, who led the pharmacological review of benefits and harms from these drugs.

The committee identified 365 drugs that were useless or dangerous and published their names in the newspapers. All parties who benefited from their sale came out of the woodwork protesting. Pharmacists, who were paid by fee and volume, saw that their incomes would drop, even though the nation would save a lot of money. Doctors felt their autonomy, choice, and judgment in prescribing these drugs was threatened, and patients felt deprived of drugs they "knew" helped them. Pharmaceutical companies opposed the threat to sales and profits. What all these parties wanted, it seemed, was to sell drugs and market hope, regardless of how much good or harm the drugs actually did, like the peddling of nostrums that Oliver Wendall Holmes had in mind when he proposed feeding them to the fish.[2]

The INAM committee was convinced and proposed to remove these drugs. But union representatives blocked it because they feared that drug companies would cut jobs. Garattini publicly resigned, causing a national debate. Charges and countercharges of alleged corruption flew back and forth. The press published sympathetic articles with headlines like "Harmful pharmaceuticals are sold with the imprimatur of the Ministry of Health," and "Chaos on ineffective pharmaceuticals still high." INAM delayed action by sending all the documents to the Ministry to "double check" the committee's work. Although the proposal was endorsed by the Council of Health, the minister did not remove the useless and harmful drugs from the formulary.

The debates made clear how important a national formulary would be for promoting rational and cost-effective prescribing, and this contributed to the wider movement to change the inefficient, dysfunctional mixture of public, nonprofit, and for-profit insurance organizations that made up national health insurance, similar to what Obamacare is cobbling together in the United States.

Eliminating Useless Drugs

Spiraling costs of medicines led the health assessor for the Lombardy Region to ask the Mario Negri Institute in 1975 to develop a positive list of effective medicines for the region's hospitals.[3] This request stemmed from the Institute working with Lombardy hospitals to develop formularies. Meantime, the proliferation of drugs and multiple brands for the same active ingredients increasingly disturbed the National Commission of General Practitioners. By the mid-1970s, more than 400 pharmaceutical firms had developed 14,176 products with 7,812 brand names they promoted.[4]

Responding to the region's requests, the Mario Negri team first established a Regional Center for Drug Documentation and Information in order to find out what doctors were actually prescribing. Then they surveyed prescribing practices, based on what each doctor thought best. They found that of the 14,176 pharmaceutical products on the market, three-quarters of all prescription drugs were "useless, irrational, or even dangerous."[5]

Ironically, the drugs with least therapeutic value were being promoted under the most brand names, evidence that widespread marketing was prevailing over good medical care. Tognoni observed that "drugs did not seem to be selected for use on the criteria of reliability and worth, and because the pharmaceutical products were listed and indexed only by their brand names, the national formulary did not aid more rational prescribing."[6] This pattern was widespread throughout Europe and the United States. It raised fundamental doubts about the basis on which doctors choose what to prescribe.

Tognoni emphasized how important it was to involve the prescribing doctors.[7] The Mario Negri team began discussing with doctors the fact that different ones among them were treating the same kinds of medical problems with different drugs, each based on his experience and belief of what was "best." This process led to developing a formulary of safe, effective drugs in the mid-1970s. It excluded fixed-dose combinations, a marketing favorite but not clinically responsible, and it established the methods for creating a list of "essential drugs" for the world.[8] Through participation, practitioners continuously learned how to think like evidence-based applied scientists, rather than basing clinical decisions on their personal practice, selective memory, and promotional information from sales reps.

A working group of the GPs from their Commission drew on the scientific knowledge of clinical pharmacology at the Mario Negri Institute to prepare of list of effective active ingredients for practitioners. Led by Gianni Tognoni, they concluded that only 1,398 of the 7,812 brand names in the national formulary were based on 352 active ingredients with documented therapeutic value. However, since so many of the other drugs were well known, established, and used, thanks to the extensive marketing by the drug companies, "applying stringent criteria for selecting effective drugs would have required too many basic changes in common therapeutic practice." This sobering assessment reminds us that during what is now remembered as "The Golden Era of Pharmaceutical Innovation" between 1955 and 1975, pharmaceutical companies largely developed so many me-too and minor variations and so distorted good prescribing practices that correcting them had become impractical.

The GP working group's model report for 1978 included guidelines for prescribing, warnings against irrational prescribing practices, and a detailed discussion of "widely prescribed classes of drugs of doubtful value." It was the first time an organization representing a majority of primary care doctors had taken the initiative to critique their own prescribing practices. The national medical association embraced the report while industry spokespersons criticized it for curbing the freedom of doctors to choose the drugs they thought best. Freedom to choose without good evidence, however, is unprofessional, violates professional ethics, and may harm patients. Throughout the 1980s, this formulary for general practice kept being used and refined.

Within a decade of its founding, then, the Institute had been asked to apply its scientific expertise to separate the wheat from the chaff and help keep national and regional pharmaceutical costs from spiraling. As research programs at pharmaceutical companies developed scores of me-too or minor variations every year and then spent millions to get doctors to prescribe them, important therapeutic advances were being developed too, but at the rate of one real advance for every ten "me-too" or minor variations.[9] This pattern dates back to at least the 1950s, when the distinguished American physician Henry Dowling observed that pharmaceutical companies were putting on the market 200–400 "new" medicines each year, with only about three of them offering a real clinical advantage.[10] All of them, however, were marketed as "better" by attractive sales reps with expense accounts they were expected to use to get doctors to write more prescriptions.

Improving Medicines for Critical Care

As part of a Regional Center for Drug Information they had helped to set up for the Lombardy Region, Gianni Tognoni and colleagues at the Mario Negri undertook a collaborative study in 1978 of the powerful drugs that staff at intensive care units (ICUs) use to treat acutely ill patients.[11] As the authors put it:

> Pharmacological treatment of patients admitted to [an] ICU is supposed to be based on strict criteria of drug selection and use. The pressure of difficult cases and of the often hectic workload could perhaps be borne better if simple rules are followed such as avoidance of useless drugs, reliance on solidly documented and updated therapeutic schedules, controlled evaluation of newly proposed regimens, [and] careful integration of drug treatments into the global management of patients.

The Mario Negri team persuaded colleagues at 15 ICUs to undertake a self-study. By the late 1970s, medicine regarded itself as advanced and sophisticated. Many good medicines were available, and board-certified specialists gave orders about what to prescribe. But the study found overuse of two or more antibiotics per patient, questionable selection of cardiovascular drugs, frequent and unjustified use of two routes of administration (like an injection and an infusion), underuse of beta blockers, wide use of insulin as an add-on, and use of corticosteroids for supporting circulation and shock, all in response to company marketing campaigns.

The ICU teams also frequently prescribed vitamins, liver extracts, and "fortifiers" without evidence to justify them. Building on this self-assessment, the ICU clinicians then agreed it would be important to undertake a double-blind, placebo-controlled trial of steroid therapy in shock patients. The protocol was designed by a team with representatives from all the centers. The trial documented the inaccuracy of long-accepted criteria for diagnosing shock and administering steroids.

These and other findings from the larger study were used for training. The overall project transformed the consciousness of busy specialists prodding them to gather data about their practices and critically assess them. This 1978 study became the basis for the development of network-based self-studies described at the end of Chapter 6. As the authors concluded:

> The application of simple techniques of drug utilization review has once more proved a useful, inexpensive tool for creating favorable conditions for wide-scale improvement in therapeutic practice.

It also illustrated how leaders at the Mario Negri were developing an integrated approach of researching not only the mechanisms of action of drugs in different parts of the body, but also the mechanisms of prescribing in clinical practice.

Developing the Essential Medicines List with WHO

Soon after the Institute staff completed the hospital formulary in 1975, the director of the division that oversaw drugs and devices at the World Health Organization, Vittorio Fattorusso, paid a visit to the Institute. Garattini and Tognoni discussed their methods for developing evidence-based formularies with him and explored the idea of a list of "essential drugs" that could be useful for all nations that wanted to promote rational, cost-effective prescribing.

Dr. Fattorusso liked the idea, developed it further, and in 1977 called the first meeting of the WHO Expert Committee on the Selection of Essential Drugs, an extension of a WHO committee that was already in place. Garattini served on the committee, and Gianni Tognoni served as an adviser.[12] The director-general of the WHO emphasized the project would be "totally independent from commercial interests and from individual donor decisions."[13] Committee members observed that "by the 1970s, effective medicines . . . existed for nearly every event and major illness we know."[14] This view may seem dated and quaint, but the physician-historian James Le Fanu concurs.[15]

The Committee could draw on national lists of effective drugs dating back to the 1950s and 1960s from Peru, Cuba, Tanzania, and especially Sri Lanka.[16] By 1975, there was a call for a list of effective, affordable drugs, and, in 1976, a list of national practices based on lists was assembled. Garattini and Tognoni brought to the process their methods for developing therapeutic formularies with GPs and hospitals. After the report, Fattorusso established the Drug Policies and Management Unit at the WHO.

Today, the Essential Medicines list is widely emulated and adapted to national contexts around the world.[17] Still, this effort pales before the billions spent on promoting patent-protected minor variations. As a result, drugs consume more than one-third of the health-care budget in some developing countries, even though generic, postpatent drugs could be used for a fraction of the cost. Even in Canada, with its sophisticated system for grading new drugs, 80 percent of the increased expenditures for medicines goes to new drugs with few or no advantages, rather than to the few superior new drugs.[18] A well-selected list improves the quality of prescribing, lowers costs, reduces harmful side effects, and stimulates serious, real innovation.

Developing a Cost-Effective National Formulary

The transformation of universal health insurance in Italy to a National Health Service (NHS) in 1978 established a stronger, single-payer foundation and culture for applying the Mario Negri Institute's commitment to evidence-based superior medicines through research. NHS principles center on good care available to all, with minimal payment barriers or insurance companies, coordinated through one's personal, primary-care doctor. However, the new NHS adopted the large, loose drug list used by INAM that senior researchers at the Mario Negri Institute had tried to repair in 1972–73 and the tradition of copayments. As drug reps kept "educating" doctors throughout the 1980s about the benefits of prescribing many drugs for many uses with little evidence, Tognoni, Garattini, and others at Mario Negri kept criticizing the old formulary as wasting precious funds and even being harmful to patients.

A single-payer NHS is not without problems, such becoming bureaucratic. General reforms in 1992–93 tried to address the low public rating of the NHS and its bureaucratic character by decentralizing operations to the regions and instituting competition based on quality—what Margaret Thatcher famously called an "internal market" within the single-payer framework. Rapidly rising costs had to be capped to meet EU limits on national debt; so the government imposed a series of expenditure caps and set about cutting the rapid increase in pharmaceutical expenditures. Then a unique opportunity—a series of corruption scandals that destabilized the government—enabled reformers to do much more by promoting evidence-based, rational prescribing.

In 1992, scores of politicians and government officials were found to be systematically taking bribes and using public money for private purposes.[19] These included the minister of health, the head of the Pharmaceutical Division, the president, and most members of the Inter-Departmental Committee on Pharmaceutical Pricing, as well as the president of the trade association. Many officers of drug companies went to jail along with government officials. Duilio Poggiolini, the director of the drug department at the Ministry of Health, which decided which drugs would be covered by the National Health Service, was arrested along with his wife for taking bribes worth 20 billion lire (10 million euros) from pharmaceutical companies.

The Ministry of Health abolished the scandal-ridden committee, established a Commission on Pharmaceuticals (CUF) as a technical, nonpartisan authority, renounced its own power over pharmaceutical policy, and transferred power to the CUF. Composed of experts named by the regions and the

New drugs increasing level of innovation

1. Drugs showing increased efficacy
2. Drugs showing less or different adverse reactions
3. Drugs specifically studied for special populations, such as children and/or old people
4. Drugs in fixed combinations showing better efficacy than individual components alone
5. Drugs leading to increased patient compliance
    a. Longer duration
    b. Oral administration
    c. Spray or patch administration
6. Drugs showing a therapeutic effect in a population unresponsive to available drugs
    a. For patients resistant to, as an example, anticancer or anti-HIV drugs
7. Drugs showing a therapeutic effects not available with other drugs (given in order of preference)
    a. For diseases having a high social impact (AIDS, cancer Alzheimer's disease)
    b. For correcting bad habits (alcoholism, drug abuse, smoking)
    c. For rare diseases
    d. For diseases not present in Europe

Figure 7.1   How to select better drugs

Minister, CUF was granted sweeping powers to decide which drugs should go on a positive list, which should go on a negative list, and which should be delisted as over-the-counter. On a television show, the minister said that strong, swift action had to be taken to restore even a modicum of trust. When a journalist said, "The only way to solve this problem is to put Dr. Garattini in charge," she did. Aided by technical subcommittees set up by Garattini, the Committee worked feverishly from September to December to evaluate the entire national list of NHS drugs. The CUF made decisions about them based on the best evidence available and the criteria listed in Figure 7.1.[20]

In 1994, the old positive list from 1978 was abolished and replaced by three copayment classes based on explicit criteria: (A) essential and chronic-disease drugs free of charge; (B) other therapeutically effective drugs for a copayment of 50 percent; and (C) drugs not reimbursed by the NHS as unnecessary. Hospital-only medications made up a fourth H-class and were paid in full. Specifying full reimbursement for drugs when used for the conditions they had been tested on minimized off-label prescribing. Doctors remained free to prescribe any drug for any condition; but only evidence-based prescribing deserved the use of taxpayers' money. This simple idea to reduce waste of money and exposure to harmful side effects from ineffective uses has still not been discovered in the United States, 20 years later, outside of places like the Veterans Health Administration or Kaiser-Permanente that also have a single payer–like set up.

Under Garattini's leadership, the CUF elimination of useless or dangerous drugs and the restructuring of how taxpayers' money should be spent resulted in about 3500 useful drugs being promoted from class B to class A and another 1000 being demoted from class B to class C, where they joined other unnecessary drugs. Based on the best evidence available in 1994, 4,152 drugs were judged not worth covering, 4,171 were deemed worthy of full coverage, and 705 worthy of coverage with a 50 percent copayment by the patient.[21] Sales of some drugs dropped 50 percent or more.[22] Interferon-B, for example, dropped from being the fifth most prescribed drug to the forty-seventh. The national drug bill dropped from the equivalent of 6.5 billion euros to 4.5 billion euros, a savings of 30.7 percent. Garattini and others toured the country to explain to doctors why some of their favorite but ineffective or hazardous drugs had lost NHS coverage. This, however, did not deter them or their patients from continuing to use them privately, but no longer at taxpayers' expense.

Pharmaceutical companies were outraged and claimed, as always, that such policies would undermine "innovation." In fact, the reforms rewarded real innovation for clinically superior drugs and discouraged prevailing research on developing me-too drugs. Industry leaders also claimed that the changes would lay off thousands of skilled researchers and cut R&D budgets, never mentioning that most R&D focused on developing minor variations of little benefit to patients. From the 1970s to the present, about 90 percent of all new drug products developed by patent-dependent companies have provided few or no advantages over existing drugs.[23]

The trade association charged that members of CUF would be legally responsible for any adverse outcomes. Science journalists, who were used to writing about new breakthroughs "at exotic locations with all expenses covered by the companies themselves," wrote hostile, critical reports.[24] Farmindustria, the Italian Association of Pharmaceutical Companies, trumped up charges that Garattini had financial ties to some companies whose drugs made the A-list, at the expense of others. They claimed he favored companies that had contracts with the Mario Negri Institute, and the Senate held hearings. In fact, many of those companies withdrew their contracts with Mario Negri to punish the Institute for Garattini's evidence-based culling of the national formulary. No evidence-based objection to the assessments, however, was raised.

At the Senate hearings, Professor Garattini proved his independence from the companies; but the president of the Senate Committee accused him of disrespect for not wearing a tie! Then Senator Lavagnini rose to say he did not understand why a scientist like Professor Garattini, who had brought such distinction to Italy, was being accused by the president of conflict of interest when the president himself presently had two secretaries being paid by pharmaceutical companies! The Committee exploded in an uproar, while Garattini sat at the witness table watching. On several occasions, Garattini was asked to be the minister of health or to run for Parliament. He always refused, explaining that once one belongs to one party, the other parties will criticize your ideas or facts, even if they are right. To be credible, one must be independent of all parties. "Besides, I would have been fired within 15 days!"

In addition to the deep cultural and political shift from commercially based evidence to scientifically based evidence of efficacy, Garattini's revolution succeeded in moving the oversight of medicines from the Department of Industry to the Department of Health. That is, medicines were treated as a social good for better health, rather than as commercial goods for market expansion. He invoked two principles: Drugs are not commodities but rather medicine to reduce risk and suffering in patients, and costs should be minimal. With distrust of politicians at an all-time high, the minister of health renounced his powers over medicines and said she would accept what the Commission decided, thus shielding it from interest-group pressures.[25]

Because of the reforms, Italy went from being one of the highest paying European nations for drugs from public money to one of the most frugal. The CUF was also granted jurisdiction over pricing after 1997, with specific financial targets for keeping pharmaceuticals a fixed percentage of the entire health-care budget. This concentrated power in a single agency within a single-payer system. To discourage the proliferation of therapeutically similar drugs under new patents and new brand names, with different prices, Garattini established the principle of "same prices for same drugs," that is, for the same active ingredient.[26] He also established the need for a solid scientific and technical infrastructure, which has grown over time.[27]

Despite such tough measures, the percentage of the budget going to drugs has crept up, and some kinds of drug use have increased beyond evidence-based prescribing.[28] From 1996 to 2001, the price index rose about 3.5 percent a year, and new product expenditures rose 2.4 percent a year.[29] Total growth in pharmaceutical expenditures increased 9.5 percent per year. But the countervailing powers behind a single-payer system are the Ministries of Health and Commerce and the Treasury, which loathes budget growth. As the Treasury asserted more power, the price index from 2001 to 2006 declined by 3 percent per year, and new product expenditures rose only 1.4 percent per year. Total growth in pharmaceutical expenditures increased only 2.2 percent a year. Copayments were abolished in 2002, but some regions reintroduced them.

Garattini believed that these revolutionary changes to cost-effective drugs should be applied to all European and other nations: rewarding of clinically effective drugs based on scientific evidence, regarding medicines as the domain of the Ministry of Health rather than Commerce, and independently overseeing the market for a social good. In 1993, he and his son Livio, a health economist, published in *The Lancet* a prescient analysis of the 50 most widely sold medicines in the UK, Germany, France, and Italy.[30] Only seven were common to all lists, and the rankings varied widely. These differences imply that doctors are not prescribing on a scientific, rational basis. The study found that only about half of all pharmaceutical expenditures went to effective medicines in France and Italy, due to commercial pressures, compared to 70 percent in Germany and 95 percent in the UK. The research team concluded that the newly established European Medicines Agency should reduce such nonrational differences and harmonized prescribing around good evidence.

Mario Negri's Relations with Industry

During these decades, from the 1960s through the 1990s and beyond, the Institute's laboratories and research units have continued to work on basic and applied research problems with pharmaceutical companies as well as with governments, foundations, and others. With companies, the Institute has sought open, scientific collaboration, particularly on experiments to elucidate the mechanisms of action of active ingredients, as a prerequisite for their maximal use.[31] Such collaboration, without promotional or marketing goals, is maximized by the Institute not patenting discoveries and not participating in royalties when companies patent. "Interest in patents," Garattini writes, "promotes a tendency to secrecy and limits collaboration, a practice which is in contrast with the objective of science in medicine."[32] For clinical trials, the Institute's researchers require "complete freedom in all the necessary steps: the preparation and registration of the protocol, the selection of centers, monitoring, collection of results, statistical analysis, and publication."

Believing in medicines as a social good means the Institute opposes using brand names because they confound good clinical use, especially when several brand names are invented and promoted for the same medicine. While the Institute recognizes the need for patents, it opposes their extension, especially the 1992 law that prolonged patent protection and thus high prices that taxed health-care budgets. Although the industry insists that longer patent protection and data exclusivity promote "innovation" through more research, there is little evidence that they do, especially if one means clinically superior drugs for patients rather than new paths to the same result as strategies for getting around another company's patents and increasing market share.[33]

Even though the Mario Negri Institute is dedicated to discovering better medicines and how to make medicines work better, it has always strongly promoted what are called "generics" because they are postpatent, established drugs whose risks of toxicity and adverse drug interactions are much better known, and cost-effectiveness is much greater. As a noncommercial research institute, Mario Negri knows that the many scientific advances in understanding the body and diseases we read about every month rarely translate into specific drugs effective against specific targets. Not recognizing this sobering reality results in wave after wave of illusory expectations fed by industry-based news sources, from biotechnology to the genome.[34] Thus the model for a nation's or the world's prescribing drugs should be based primarily on postpatent, proven drugs, with patents and high prices reserved for superior new drugs when they are found.

As much as possible, Mario Negri policy analysts think that drug development and trials should be publicly funded. The goals of pharmacological research should focus on unmet needs identified by patients and their doctors, quite different from companies setting priorities to maximize sales and profits. For similar reasons, clinical trials should be funded by public or independent sources. They should address important clinical questions in ways that contribute to better care. At present, most of the 185,000 clinical trials worldwide appear started to produce marketing material and to sign up specialists as product advocates. They distort medical knowledge. Most of these trials use, as Ben Goldacre put it, "hopelessly small numbers of weird, unrepresentative patients, and [are] analysed using techniques which are flawed by design, in such a way that they exaggerate the benefits of treatments."[35]

Being Transparent about Risks of Harm

Few stories of pharmaceutical maleficence has so rocked Europe as the Mediator scandal that started in 2009. French regulators withdrew Mediator (benfluorex) in late 2009, and its manufacturer, Servier, withdrew it worldwide as evidence of hospitalizations and deaths of women accumulated.

But researchers and leaders at the Mario Negri Institute knew of and spoke out against the serious risks years earlier. Although they first helped develop the company's progenitor for Servier, they publicly spoke out against the serious risks once they learned about them. The Institute's autonomy and insistence on transparency of all results—harms as well as benefits—allowed it to speak out once the risks were known.

Roberto Invernizzi, head of the Laboratory of Neurochemistry and Behavior at the Mario Negri Institute, told it this way:

> There has long been a search for anti-obesity drugs. The first were amphetamines, but they had significant toxic side effects. We did important, early research for Servier during the 1960s and early 70s in developing fenfluramine as an alternative. It sold very well. But some years later, physicians and patients became concerned about its side effects, which caused heart valve disease and pulmonary hypertension [the Phen-Fen scandal].[36]
>
> Then Servier kept a derivative, benfluorex, or Mediator, on the market *without testing for its side effects*. It was obvious to us researchers at the Mario Negri that side effects would be about the same as fenfluramine because they were pharmacologically so similar. Garattini wrote a letter to the Italian minister of health in 1998 recommending its withdrawal as a dangerous drug. That's what makes this Institute different. The Italian minister withdrew it and expressed his concern to the French minister; but benfluorex remained on the French market.

As *The Lancet* reported, "Italian regulators started to question the safety [on the basis of the Mario Negri letter in 1998] and raised their concerns with the European Medicines Agency (EMA)."[37] Subsequently, benfluorex was withdrawn from several countries. In France, however, it appears that Servier manipulated the regulators by registering Mediator for diabetes in order to avoid scrutiny of it as a diet drug. Then Servier marketed it heavily off-label for weight loss. Servier also paid members of the French regulatory body as consultants.[38]

These two strategies resulted in Mediator staying on the French market long after Mario Negri had publicly warned against its toxic side effects. The contrast in ethics between the Mario Negri and Servier could not be greater. Because the drug was not withdrawn in France as dangerous and Servier marketed it aggressively, millions of women took the drug for an untested and unauthorized use, thousands of them required hospital treatment, and 500–1000 died unnecessarily.

Since 2009, the wake-up call of the Mediator scandal has led the French to pass a new law that requires new drugs to be compared with existing therapies. It also sets terms for much greater transparency and renamed its regulatory agency the National Agency for the *Safety* of Medicines and Health Products.[39] Numerous lawsuits charge Jacques Servier with lying to doctors and causing involuntary homicides and injuries.

An authoritative review in 2010 by the French inspector general concluded that Mediator should have been withdrawn a decade earlier in 1999. That would have been just a year after Professor Garattini and Mario Negri researchers persuaded other countries to withdraw it.[40] Equally worrisome is the lack of action by the powerful EMA until 2010, a year after the French withdrawal. As national representatives to the EMA, Garattini and Bertele' tried to reform its rules and culture so that unsafe and ineffective drugs will be identified early. Had the EMA followed Garattini's recommendations for greater independence from the pharmaceutical industry it regulates, the EMA might have acted more quickly to protect patients and the public.

Fostering Independent Research on Drugs

In response to a campaign led by Garattini, Liberati, and other senior researchers, an Italian law was passed in 2003 requiring that all pharmaceutical companies contribute 5 percent of their yearly expenditures for promotional activities (from seminars to trade fairs to gifts and software) to a national fund for independent research.[41] In 2005, Nello Martini, director of AIFA and other advocates for independent research got the minister of health to issue a decree that set terms of eligibility like those of Mario Negri. AIFA, Italy's regulatory body, can commission and fund independent research on questions for which it needs answers. Researchers must have complete control of their study design and all parts of the research project. They must be free of conflicting interests, with no patent ownership, and all results must be published. Research like this is important, as the Committee wrote, because less than 1 percent of biomedical research funding goes to research on how to treat patients better, because commercial trials often exclude large populations like the very old, children, and pregnant women, and because many important clinical questions do not interest companies.

During the first five years, the Research and Development Committee was chaired and shaped by Garattini. The Committee consulted widely among researchers, government officials, clinicians, the public, and drug companies for suggestions of what areas or questions need to be addressed: orphan drugs for rare diseases and drugs for nonresponders; comparative studies of benefits and risks; and pharmacovigilance studies to better define the benefit-harm ratio.

The Committee received 1,217 letters of intent from researchers and funded 151 of them. An international peer review group grades applications and oversees results. The comparative trials that met their high standards cost an average of one million euros, and the pharmaco-epidemiological studies averaged 100,000 euros. These studies investigated important questions of no commercial interest to companies, such as whether earlier, shorter treatment of breast cancer would be equally efficacious with less risk of toxic reactions and lower cost.[42] The studies, funded in every region of the country, strengthened research capacity and had several benefits for pharmaceutical companies. While the funding source was not ideal, it enabled the nation and its health service to get answers to important clinical questions, especially about how two or more patented brand names compare or how they compare to older, postpatent drugs. Mario Negri's involvement is one more way in which it has fostered independent, transparent research at the national level to identify good medicines for patients with real needs.

Nurturing a National Cochrane Center

While Garattini, Bertele', and other leaders of the Mario Negri Institute worked from the 1970s to the present decade to base the approval and use of medicines on independent, transparent, scientific, and clinically relevant evidence, a parallel movement was developing in health care as a whole, inspired by the British doctor Archie Cochrane. During World War II and after, Cochrane became convinced that most health care was practiced without scientific evidence about which interventions were best for which patients. He first organized a trial of yeast to treat an outbreak of famine edema while he himself was suffering from chronic hunger in a German prisoner of war camp.[43] After the war, he studied coal dust exposure among Welsh miners and learned about randomized control trials from the great statistician Austin Bradford Hill. In 1972, Cochrane published a little book about how to assess which health services are effective and efficient.[44] It became in international bestseller and launched what came to be called evidence-based medicine and comparative effectiveness research. At one point in 1979, Cochrane admonished the medical profession for not organizing "a critical summary, by speciality or subspeciality, adapted periodically, of all relevant randomized controlled trials." And he observed that obstetrics and gynecology was the least scientific specialty in medicine.

Iain Chalmers, a young obstetrician working in Cardiff, had been inspired by Cochrane's writings and had come to know him personally. This led

Chalmers to plan a response to Cochrane's unflattering challenge to obstetrics. He and about 100 colleagues from around the world embarked on a search for published and unpublished reports of randomized trials and prepared systematic reviews of them. These were published at the end of the 1980s in a 1500page, two-volume book, but also a paperback summary written for the users of maternity services, and an electronic publication issued twice a year to update and amend the reviews. This project became—in essence—a pilot of what was to become the Cochrane Collaboration.

In 1992, Chalmers received news that the first director of Research & Development of the British National Health Service had approved funding for "a Cochrane Centre," "to facilitate the preparation and maintenance of systematic reviews of randomized controlled trials of healthcare interventions," and this was announced in an editorial published in the BMJ.[45] In 1993, the Cochrane Centre convened a meeting of 90 or so colleagues from about ten countries whom he thought would be interested in extending the principle of electronically published systematic reviews to all of health care. Among those invited was Gianni Tognoni, a pillar of the Mario Negri Institute whom Chalmers had come to know in the late 1970s after he had been invited to contribute to a conference convened by the Mario Negri Institute on the epidemiological evaluation of drugs and a book based on it.[46]

Among the staff at the Mario Negri during the 1980s, it was Tognoni's protégé, Alessandro Liberati, who had developed a particular interest in systematic reviews and meta-analyses. He had spent some time in Boston with Tom Chalmers, one of the pioneers of the application of these methods in medicine, and Liberati coauthored one of the earliest of such studies.[47]

Liberati first came to the Mario Negri Institute the way that several other talented researchers began, as a conscientious objector choosing the Institute as an alternative to military service while completing a degree in preventive medicine at the University of Milan. He soon directed the Laboratory of Clinical Epidemiology, and in 1992 he contacted Chalmers after reading about the creation of the first Cochrane center. Although Liberati was in the United States at the time, Chalmers called him to suggest that he was the obvious choice among Italian health service researchers to establish a Cochrane center in Italy. Liberati accepted the challenge, and Il Centro Cochrane Italiano became established in 1994 at the Mario Negri Institute. Garattini provided a wealth of expert colleagues, rooms, heat, light, phones, Internet, and the invaluable services of the nation's leading scientific librarian, Vanna Pistotti.[48]

The center soon had its own staff and addressed questions about interventions in cancer and intensive care. Organizing disease review groups was a prime task and produced a systematic review of antibiotic prophylaxis in critically ill patients. The Italian and other Cochrane centers around the world have supported the 52 Cochrane Review Groups and contributed to transforming the practice of health care by helping to put practice on a scientific basis. Liberati became one of the pioneers of evidence synthesis, was invited to serve on the editorial boards of the *Annals of Internal Medicine* and the

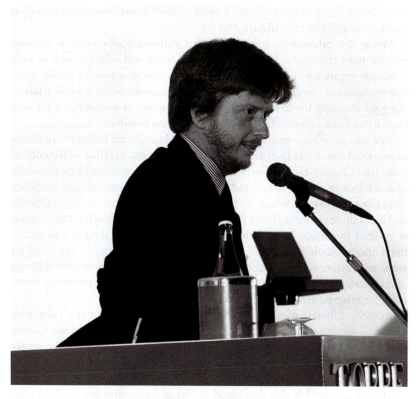

Photo 7.1   Alessandro Liberati

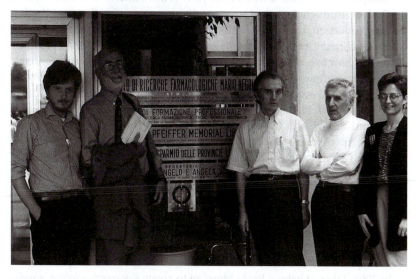

Photo 7.2   Alessandro Liberati, David Sackett, Gianni Tognoni, Silvio Garattini, and Kay Dickersin opening the Italian Cochrane Center, 1994

BMJ (*British Medical Journal*), and helped to develop such research evaluation methods as PRISM and GRADE.[49]

While the mission and focus of the Cochrane Collaboration is more specific than the Mario Negri Institute, its ethos and ethics match it well, especially regarding clinical trials that test for clinical outcomes in real practice populations. Both organizations believe in randomized control trials as the gold standard for determining the effectiveness of an intervention, and both strive to be as institutionally independent as possible.

In a way somewhat analogous to how the Mario Negri Institute organized networks of specialists in order to design and carry out practice-based clinical trials (see Chapter 6), the Cochrane Collaboration organizes large networks of specialists in groups supported by Cochrane centers to evaluate evidence from trials and other sources, and to author their systematic reviews. Liberati and his staff, together with the Mario Negri Institute, supported the creation of reviews by groups to evaluate treatments concerning alcohol and addictions and multiple sclerosis.[50] Much later, the Collaboration extended its scope to evaluate screening and diagnostic tests because they expose millions of essentially normal people to their risks and to the risks of follow-up treatment for false-positives as well as confirmed cases.[51]

In 1998, Liberati moved to the University of Modena in the Faculty of Medicine as a professor of biostatistics; but the Italian Cochrane Centre remained at the Mario Negri Institute. Among its many activities, the center translated into Italian *Clinical Evidence*, a well-known point-of-care summary for clinicians of best evidence for practice, which is available online to every practicing doctor.[52] It also developed the basis for continuing medical education using a free, e-learning system called ECCE. An average of 14 units are completed by Italian doctors each year. While American doctors update themselves through heavily commercialized courses for their continuing medical education, this collaboration between the Mario Negri Institute, the Italian Cochrane Centre, and the Italian Medicines Agency (AIFA) provided a model of how to educate practicing doctors and reinforce their professionalism without commercial bias and at much lower cost. By 2008, Italian health professionals had accessed almost 100,000 abstracts of Cochrane Reviews. As the recession took its toll on funding, however, the program was closed.

Liberati shared with Garattini and other leaders of Mario Negri a strong commitment to reach doctors, patients, and lay audiences. In 1995, the Cochrane Collaboration had established a Consumer Network, and most of its review groups involve consumers.[53] In 1997, Liberati called for

> a transparent process where the views of all the relevant stakeholders are equally considered. With very rare exceptions—the case of the AIDS advocacy movement is an exemplar—patients and consumers have no voice in how research is prioritised, funded, and monitored.

In 2006, Liberati helped Paola Mosconi to create *@PartecipaSalute*, a website, newsletter, and organization to bring patient and consumer associations together with medical and nursing associations as well as researchers in order to dialogue about key issues concerning health care and strengthen patient empowerment.[54] The founders wrote that "the medical and scientific community still fails to see patients and consumer groups as partners with 'equal rights and weight.'"[55] Liberati, who was suffering from a decade of multiple myeloma, wrote with increasing urgency about the neglect of the patient's perspective in clinical trials. In 2011, for example, he searched and found 1,384 studies on multiple myeloma, but in only ten (0.7 percent) was overall survival the primary end point, and not one was a head-to-head comparison of different drugs or strategies—so many patients recruited to so many expensive trials, designed not to be relevant to patients and doctors seeking better care.[56] One of the most important "findings" in Cochrane reviews is how many trials are discounted because they do not meet the criteria of rigorous evidence. Liberati wrote:

> Pharmaceutical companies avoid research that might show that new and expensive drugs are no better than another comparator already on the market . . . Researchers are trapped by their own internal competing interests—professional and academic—which lead them to compete for pharmaceutical industry funding.[57]

Although patient groups concerned with myeloma donate millions to research to develop drugs that will help them, the trial-and-approval system we have described does not support that goal well. Liberati called for a new governance strategy that would "bring together all the stakeholders . . . to promote better care." Since Liberati wrote these words in 2011, policy leaders have moved rapidly toward patient-centered research. The United States has founded PCORI, the Patient-Centered Outcomes Research Institute, to address "the long-lingering disconnect between patient needs, patient engagement, and research."[58]

After Liberati's untimely death (http://www.cochrane.org/alessandro-memory-book), Il Centro Cochrane Italiano moved to the University of Modena. Professor Roberto D'Amico now directs it, but several staff at the Mario Negri Institute continue to do projects with the center, including Vanna Pistotti. The center keeps growing, from 1,017 Italian reviewers and 722 authors in 2012 to 1,243 reviewers and 798 authors in 2014. Over 230 reviews have been authored by Italian reviewers. Italy ranks third among non-English speaking countries in the number of contributors. They contribute to some of the 52 Cochrane review groups that draw from 31,000 reviewers worldwide in more than 120 countries.[59]

When it comes to medicines, the Cochrane Collaboration of centers and reviewers constitutes an attempt to compensate for the EMA, the FDA, and other regulators whose methods and criteria of review embody industry biases and do not protect the public against biased medical knowledge when companies design their own trials to test their own products. The FDA and EMA are not financially independent of the industry they are to regulate in order to protect the public from unsafe and dangerous drugs. The Cochrane Collaboration not only offers a model of institutional integrity parallel to the Mario Negri Institute that avoids these biases, but its leaders have become major forces for reducing or eliminating forms of institutional corruption through independent evaluations that serve as a counterforce to the evidence put forward by companies to "educate" doctors and patients.[60]

8

International Campaigns against Harmful Regulations and Practices

Good pharma, that is, the development of clinically better and safer drugs based on patient outcomes, requires a good regulator because the regulator sets the terms for approval and subsequent use. Soon after Silvio Garattini and research staff from the Mario Negri Institute developed a science-based formulary for Italy, the government appointed him in 1997 as one of two national representatives, together with Vittorio Bertele' as an expert, to the newly formed European Agency for the Evaluation of Medicinal Products. (Ironically, the word "Evaluation" was later dropped and the agency renamed EMA for the European Medicines Agency.) This agency reflected the goal of the pharmaceutical industry to replace as much as possible each nation in Europe reviewing new medicines with a consolidated review procedure for all EU countries.

The Corruption of Mission

What Garattini, Bertele', and other Mario Negri researchers found as they took up responsibilities in London to review new drug-candidates for use by all Europeans was that the European Parliament and Commission had allowed institutional rules, procedures, and barriers that distort or corrupt the stated mission. The concept of institutional corruption provides a helpful framework for describing the issues, concerns, and actions taken in the campaign for better regulations that would promote good pharma, because it focuses on the distortion and compromise of a societal institution's mission, often built into the laws and regulations.[1] We will start with the compromises of the EMA's mission, how they put patients at avoidable risks for serious harm, and the need for an independent body to monitor those risks in use. Then we will describe Garattini and Bertele''s campaign against secrecy that allowed the regulators and companies to get medicines approved without

patients or their doctors knowing what was going on. Garattini and Bertele'
also identified ways in which the EMA allows low-grade evidence and
unethical trials to be used in approving new drugs, and they campaigned
for specific measures to eliminate them. Orphan drugs particularly suffer
from poor, loose regulation that approves many with little evidence that they
actually help patients with rare diseases get better. Finally, we will turn to the
Mario Negri vision for what a good-pharma regulator would look like if, for
instance, the European oversight of medicines were recast as an independent and proactive set of practices, shorn of conflicting interests and based
on good scientific evidence that new medicines are better for patients than
existing treatments.

To set the stage, let us start with the mission and mandates of the new
European regulator. They were

> "to promote the protection of human . . . health and of consumers of medicinal
> products" and to carry out "scientific evaluation of the highest possible stan-
> dard . . ." under the aegis of an independent Committee . . . in order to provide
> "the best possible scientific advice on . . . the quality, the safety, and the efficacy
> of medicinal products."[2]

The EMA is also required "to make provisions for . . . the intensive monitoring of adverse reactions to those medicinal products through community
pharmacovigilance activities, in order to ensure the rapid withdrawal from
the market of any medicinal product which presents an unacceptable level of
risk under normal conditions of use." This includes coordinating the responsibilities of Member States in "the provision of information about medicinal
products, monitoring the respect of good manufacturing practices, good laboratory practices and good clinical practices."[3] Intensive monitoring of adverse
reactions and "rapid withdrawal" sound reassuring. However, partial and passive monitoring is more common, followed by long-delayed withdrawal, if at
all. The Danish authority, Peter Gøtzsche, reports that prescription drugs are
the third leading cause of death.[4]

Protection of health by an independent reviewing body that provides the
best possible scientific advice is certainly what doctors and their patients want
but not what the European Parliament or European Commission provided.
Garattini and Bertele' found that nearly every one of these terms had been
compromised. The EMA's own industry-friendly criteria for approval contain
little to protect public health, and the EMA contributes regularly to the epidemic of adverse reactions that Europeans experience. Evaluations fall well
below the highest possible scientific standards. The Committee is not independent, largely by its own doing. Finally, the EMA cannot provide "the best
possible scientific advice on . . . the quality, safety, and efficacy of medicinal products" because it allows biased trial designs and evidence on which
it approves many drugs. A good-pharma regulator would send them back
and write, "When you have unbiased, scientific evidence about this drug,
we are happy to review it." But then a good regulator would not have staff

salaries dependent on company fees for reviewing what evidence the company chooses to send.

Like the FDA in the United States, the EMA is a classic example of "institutional corruption" as articulated by the Edmond J. Safra Center for Ethics at Harvard University. The first and most obvious way to corrupt a regulator's mission is for the government to underfund and understaff it against a multibillion dollar industry with a long history of unethical behavior promoting drugs that are less beneficial and more harmful than they claim.[5] CDER, the division of the FDA that reviews drugs and safety issues, has about 1,300 staff and $300 million for a population of 300 million in one country. Only 5 percent of the FDA budget goes to addressing the widespread harmful side effects discussed in the Introduction.[6] The EMA has a staff of less than 1,000 and a budget of about $300 million for a population of 500 million spread across 28 countries. Funding is too low for the EMA to do its own studies. Responding to pressure from the pharmaceutical companies who pay large fees to have their drugs reviewed for approval, both the FDA and EMA now emphasize accelerated reviews. This may sound good, but it means less evidence that new drugs are safe or effective before patients take them. The risks of harm are high, from one in five new drugs likely to produce serious adverse reactions in the years after a full-length review, to one in three when reviewed more quickly.[7]

Behind the low funding, staff, and capacity of the EMA lies a history of each nation wanting to retain its regulatory staff and ability to review new medicines, to decide whether they should be reimbursed, and if so at what price to reflect their added value to patients. Thus the EMA was originally regarded more as a coordinating body for all the national regulatory agencies; but over time, central review has become more prevalent. National regulatory agencies then compete for substantial fees to carry out the evaluation of each drug. As the Mario Negri leaders pointed out, the whole arrangement is rife with conflicts of interest that serve the corporations, but compromise the protection of health as the EMA's mission.

Compounding the conflicts of interest that undermine the EU's mission is the alternate, mutual recognition route to approval. For drug classes that do not require central review, European law allows any company to circumvent the central review by choosing the weakest or most friendly national body to review its drug. After that country approves it, a company may ask other countries to mutually recognize the approval. If it does not, the matter is referred to CHMP, the scientific committee of the EMA whose opinion becomes binding on all member states. Since a review might be critical of the drug, however, companies can "withdraw the application in any member state at any time during the evaluation . . . [thus] eliminating member states whose objections might head to a referral, a negative opinion and no market anywhere in the European Union (EU)."[8] One might call this Pick-and-Choose Approval—a good distance from the EU standard of "scientific evaluation of the highest possible standard." In this way, companies can maximize sales of a drug approved on the weakest review of safety and efficacy.

This double procedure puts the EMA staff and leadership on notice not to be more scientifically rigorous than the most industry-friendly national regulator, or a company can choose this alternate route and the EMA will lose the review fees—its main source of income to pay for staff. It would be as if each state in the United States also had a regulatory body in addition to the FDA, and the rules allowed all states to accept the approval of the most industry-friendly state, bypassing the FDA altogether. Competition for company fees has a further corrosive influence by putting a company's interests and priorities above those of patients.

The Mario Negri leaders at the EMA strongly opposed this double route and succeeded in contributing to the revised legislation in 2004 that avoided this risk by increasing the classes of drugs that should undergo the centralized procedure and by making the EMA arbitration compulsory in case of disagreement among the member states in the mutual recognition procedures.

The lack of public funding for these regulators undermines their ability to protect and promote health and safety. For decades, companies did not fund the FDA; but starting in 1992, Congress set up a system of large fees that companies paid to the review teams at CDER. Today, about 80 percent of CDER's budget at the FDA comes from company fees. In Europe, company fees pay for about 85 percent of the EMA budget. Garattini and colleagues at the Mario Negri Institute have long held that "if the [EMA] is an organization of public interest, the EU should support it independently of industrial funding."[9] If industry fees are necessary, they should come in at arms-length to the European Commission, "independent of the activities undertaken, the products and the companies involved," the opposite of specific fees from individual companies for specific work on specific medicines.

Garattini and Bertele' found other conflicts of interest everywhere they turned at the EMA. For example, the companies test their own drugs and write up the results in a dossier on which the reviewers wholly depend. That is, companies create the "facts" about their own drugs and also control the interpretation of those "facts." With some exceptions, the EMA approves new drugs that provide few advantages over existing ones. Most doctors and patients have no idea that the risk of serious harm is so high.

Equally unacceptable and self-corrupting in undermining the regulator's mission to protect the public's health is the "unwritten rule that allows the industry to 'suggest' one of the two experts (who are always accepted) responsible for assessing the dossier of a new pharmaceutical product and, if it is approved, to follow it once it is on the market."[10] Together with another Mario Negri researcher assigned as an expert to EMA, Bertele' and Garattini campaigned against this rule that turns the allegedly independent review into an "inside job."[11]

Another example of regulatory bias was the rules of the EMA and CHMP, the review body on which Garattini and Bertele' served. They allowed companies to take as much time as they wished to pull together their responses to questions or concerns about a drug under review, but limited CHMP to only two months to evaluate the responses (which can be hundreds of pages) and one further month to decide whether to approve or not. The bias to approve rather than give priority to safety is built into the language that "approval may only be refused if a drug does not demonstrate . . . evidence of its efficacy, or it does not show adequate safety."[12]

The primary purpose of developing and approving drugs, Garattini and Bertele' wrote in 2000, is people's health. "No other purpose, not even defending jobs, can claim higher priority."[13] Yet the principal objection when Garattini and research teams at the Mario Negri Institute demoted dangerous and useless drugs in Italy was the possible impact on jobs, revenues, and profits. Every state wants to attract pharmaceutical companies, with their high-paying jobs. Should regulators then help patients to take more drugs of questionable benefit and risks of harm in order to generate more jobs?

Garattini also campaigned against the EMA being governed by the director-general for enterprise and commerce in the European Commission rather than the director-general of health (SANCO). "This anomaly, which heavily influences the policy of the EMA and its scientific advisory committees, raises the suspicion that pharmaceutical products are considered more significant for the market than for individual and public health."[14] Just as it had in Italy (see Chapter 7), the Mario Negri Institute opposed subjecting the EMA and drug safety to the oversight of the director-general dedicated to economic growth and more jobs rather than to improved health. The campaign finally succeeded in 2009 when political governance of the EMA was transferred to SANCO.

Exposing Patients to Risks without Offsetting Benefits

Garattini, Bertele', and other researchers at the Mario Negri Institute have been particularly outspoken about how the EMA's own criteria and procedures for approving new drugs without evidence that they are better or safer for patients than existing drugs undermine its mission to protect (and promote) health and consumers. Instead, these practices lead it to approve "a flood of clinically unjustified copies . . . simply because they are 'equivalent' to their comparators." Differences between them are hard to tell from their labels "so it is impossible to make a rational choice based on their risk-benefit profiles."[15]

How can the EMA provide "the best possible scientific advice on the quality, the safety, and the efficacy" of drugs when it requires no evidence about how a new drug compares to ones in use? The same applies to the FDA, which leaves it up to sales reps to "educate" doctors about how new drugs are better.[16] This lack of comparative data means the EMA and FDA fail also to require "the best scientific information." In fact, they allow companies to design trials that cannot provide valid scientific evidence and then accept that evidence for review, as we shall soon see.

Reflecting the Mario Negri's principles laid out at the beginning of this book, the authors write, "it is pointless—besides being scientifically and ethically inappropriate—to approve drugs on the basis of questionable clinical equivalence or non-inferiority to others already on the market."[17] Moreover, the regulators do not tell patients or their doctors that new drugs may be worse, especially when tested for so-called acceptable inferiority. The FDA criteria for approval are little different. During a 2013 interview, Garattini said, "Only question matters: 'Is this medicine better for patients than existing treatments?' Conveniently for the drug companies, this is the one question that regulators do not usually ask or answer."

"Acceptable inferiority" should clearly be stated as the absence of documented benefit and possibly a risk of harm. And the lack of cost-effectiveness as a criterion implies that cost is no issue. This leaves the real work up to each country to assess the actual *clinical* benefits or harms to patients and what the drugs are worth.

In cancer, for example, nearly all the drugs approved by the EMA and FDA provide little or no new clinical benefit and yet are priced so high that they threaten affordability.[18] In the United States, the high prices that companies charge for cancer and other "specialty drugs," even though about 90 percent of them provide few or no advantages for patients, are so strapping state health budgets that education budgets are being reduced. Patients are made to pay 20 percent of these drugs, priced at $50,000–$500,000 a year.[19] Paying out $10,000–$40,000 in cash drives many patients' families into poverty, without clear evidence of benefit. In Europe, ever-rising prices are "increasingly undermining the affordability of national health services."[20]

The regulatory framework set up by the European Parliament and Commission for approving new medicines that ignores price, value, and cost-effectiveness sends the wrong signal to research-oriented drug companies to develop more clinically minor drugs for disorders already effectively treated, like the fifth or eighth statin. Since companies succeed time and again through intensive marketing to get doctors to prescribe new medicines with little or no advantage to patients, or even inferior to existing products, why should they undertake much basic research to develop superior drugs?[21]

Approving new medicines or variations based on their being slightly better than placebo when effective medicines already exist not only deprives patients in the control arm from receiving the beneficial drug but also may be used to avoid documenting harms to patients. In a recent Mario Negri analysis of ten pivotal trials for the treatment of multiple sclerosis, 2,405 patients suffered an estimated 630 more relapses than they would have if an effective treatment had been used in the control arm to test if the new drug was superior.[22] In cases like this, which the EMA does not appear to examine, patients suffer, and the trial does not produce clinically useful information it needs to help patients with MS get more effective treatment and to avoid wasting taxpayers' money.

The Need for an Independent Safety Board

Given how few new drugs provide additional benefits to patients, the first priority of a good regulator should be "the *protection* of health and of consumers," not the promotion of possibly effective drugs whose efficacy and safety in patients is unclear from short trials and small samples. An "optimism bias" has supplanted the precautionary principle at the EMA (and FDA), to first do no harm. Five-sixths of all trials have inadequate statistical power because they are too small to reach conclusive results.[23] People who agree to enter clinical trials put themselves at risk of harm, with little or no possibility of benefits for themselves or anyone else except investors seeking profits. Most of the huge, $70 billion in "unsustainable" research costs by companies is wasted by their own choosing on such trials.

Like other leaders in the United States and Europe, Garattini and Bertele' called again for a separate, independently funded safety board to oversee postmarketing pharmacovigilance. An independent safety board would undertake proactive pharmacovigilance and work with companies on their activities. It would commission and fund independent studies on critical issues of safety. And it would collect all relevant information and carry out meta-analyses.

When the antidiabetes drug Avandia (rosiglitazone) was finally withdrawn in 2010 after 83,000 heart attacks had been attributed to it, GSK had more than 13,000 law suits against it from injured patients and was accused once again by government officials of knowing beforehand how serious its risks were, and Garattini and Bertele' called for root changes to eliminate the institutionally corrupt practices that so compromise the mission to protect the public from harm.[24] "Safety questions can be answered only by large, long-term studies," they wrote. Revenue from sales at prices 50–100 times the cost of manufacturing[25] can easily fund such trials; but one can hardly expect companies focused on huge price mark-ups to evaluate and monitor safety well. In the case of Avandia, the EMA should have known about its tragic risks four years before its withdrawal. Thousands suffered unnecessarily, as they have in other cases such as Tambocor (flecainide), cerivastatin [Baycol], or rofecoxib [Vioxx].[26]

Regarding pharmacovigilance more widely, major reforms were passed in 2010 to improve and coordinate it; but the Mario Negri team at the EMA found them seriously flawed. Rather than setting up an independent safety board, the European Parliament voted to have the members of the committee that approve new drugs also decide whether evidence of adverse events warrants a serious warning or withdrawal.[27] It entrusts the EMA with four conflicting roles: prosecutor, defense attorney around evidence regarding the profile of new medicines, trial judge when it concludes for approval, and appellate judge when it assesses evidence that the drugs it approved are harming patients. How can members of the European Parliament justify such a conflict-ridden arrangement?

The Mario Negri authors and others suspect the new framework for pharmacovigilance is being promoted in order to justify approving still more medicines with less evidence about their safety in order to speed up approvals.[28] They call for independent reviews of data, commissioned independent studies on critical safety issues, and independent implementation of the risk management plans that companies put forward in order to get early approvals from the EMA.

If we fast-forward to 2013, leaders of the twenty-first century EMA paint an enlightened, sophisticated picture of new procedures to get more "lifesaving" drugs to patients faster by requiring even less evidence that they have beneficial patient-oriented outcomes.[29] The whole argument rests on claims by EMA officers that companies are developing impressively "innovative" and beneficial new medicines, especially for people with "life-threatening" disorders. However, independent evidence up through 2013 shows the opposite: a steady decline of clinically superior drugs, from about 15 percent of all new approvals in the 1970s to 8 percent since 2000.[30] Yet the risks of their harming patients are substantial. In their articles about their twenty-first century vision, EMA leaders ignore the several million hospitalizations and 197,000 deaths a year in Europe from prescription drugs.[31]

In a 2013 assessment by Garattini and Bertelé, we see that the EMA is still serving the interests of companies rather than the public or patients by approving "a catalogue of products to be made available on the market" without considering their added value for patients.[32] The authors maintain that the EMA (and FDA) should require evidence that "new medicines prolong survival or improve patients' quality of life compared to available treatments or are effective in non-responders to current therapies."

Ending Bad-Pharma Secrecy—"Garattinization"

Based on the Mario Negri Institute's ethics, its leaders have persistently criticized the EMA's culture of secrecy and its key role in protecting company interests at the expense of patient and public benefit. Until recently, keeping the clinically relevant results of trials secret has been a central function of the industry-funded EMA. When Garattini and Bertelé arrived in 1997, the process of reviewing new drugs to ensure they were safe and effective, centered on an inner circle of colleagues coming to a gentlemen's consensus in private, without any disclosure about the debates or concerns about a drug. Worried members could not vote or record doubts about safety, the poor quality of evidence, or countervailing evidence—effectively a cover-up by the public regulator institutionally built into its practices. Serious questions about the quality of data, possible bias in trial evidence, lack of information about risks of serious harms, and other concerns were also minimized in the company-written leaflet or label. Having the company and not the regulator write up the label or product summary is another conflict of interest that has long served corporate investors rather than patients.

Garattini and Bertelé demanded that voting replace consensus, an upsetting idea, and staff at the EMA started talking about the "Garattinization" of European regulation—demands for transparency in all aspects of evaluation, for patient-centered outcomes, and for evidence of comparative effectiveness.

For years, companies have managed how trial results are selected or hidden from doctors and patients. As a result, positive results have been 3–5 times more likely to be published than negative ones.[33] In published medical articles, the research results that make up medical science are skewed by the marketing departments of pharmaceutical firms and the teams of writers, editors and statisticians they hire to ghost manage refereed articles in the medical journals.[34] They also publish positive results more than once so that in systematic reviews, positive results are double or triple-weighted while negative results are zero-weighted. Even conscientious doctors get misled. Yet regulators, who have all the trial results from what companies submitted to them, do not regard reviewing the accuracy of professional literature as their responsibility and say nothing when ghost-managed medical articles misrepresent the evidence submitted to the regulator.[35]

Keeping some trial results secret, or not disclosing important details, turns regulators into agents of corporate campaigns to market their new, high-priced drugs as more effective and safer than they prove to be in practice. Secrecy had allowed billions in taxpayers' money to be wasted and millions of patients to be exposed to the adverse side effects of these drugs, because the EMA and FDA had kept silent about trial results not published, or distorted in medical journals. Company-sponsored authors of medical journals are about three times more likely to conclude in favor of the company's product than independent authors do.[36]

Complete secrecy was also long allowed for any drug that companies withdrew or that regulators rejected, so that researchers and clinicians could not learn from their flaws or risks. In the EMA's first ten years, it evaluated 395 products but issued only seven negative opinions because companies withdrew drugs whose reviews were not going well before evaluation was completed so they could put all their clinical and other data behind the EMA firewalls of secrecy.[37]

The Mario Negri campaign for transparency of data about drugs withdrawn or rejected contributed to a change in policy. Since 2004, the EU has jumped ahead of the United States and the FDA by making available the assessment reports on drugs that the EMA rejects or companies withdraw, together with their reasons for the negative opinions or withdrawals. This is a major step toward "good pharma."

The postmarketing commitments to testing agreed by the companies are also now included in the assessment report EPAR (European Public Assessment Report), but only if the CHMP wants to record those follow-up measures. Actually, the EPARs seem to report only the "specific obligations" required for "conditional approvals." Information about whether the companies fulfill those commitments remains poor, and there is no report about the results of trials done. These practices are unethical, put patients at risk, and undermine the justification of early, conditional approval based on follow-up testing as protecting patients from harmful or ineffective drugs. These complicated fudges contrast with the Mario Negri model of full transparency. Good science can only advance by making all results known, as the Mario

Negri Institute has done since the 1960s. If this one research institute can realize full transparency, even when funded by pharmaceutical companies, then certainly society's regulator can and so can other research institutes or universities.

When the EMA was finally transferred in 2010 from the Enterprise and Industry Directorate of the European Commission to the Health and Consumer Policy Directorate, Garattini and Bertele' reviewed the extent of secrecy at the EMA and called on the Health Directorate "to end the secrecy surrounding approval decisions."[38] Figure 8.1 compares the secrecy of the EMA with the transparency of the FDA. The figure lists five ways in which the industry-funded EMA had long helped companies keep secrets from patients, doctors, and researchers: the registry of ongoing and completed trials, drug information held by the agency, records of meetings with industry, minutes of advisory committee meetings, and minority opinion statements.

There is still quite a way to go in informing doctors and patients. As of 2014, the EMA summary of product characteristics (the SPC or label) "does not mention when a drug is approved by majority vote," because a consensus could not be reached. The assessment report is now available with the reasons for the minority opposition, another contribution from the Garattinization era.[39] However, one has to dig for it in the less accessible parts of the evaluation on the EMA website. Institutional resistance manifests itself in many layers and degrees.

Product summaries or SPCs also do not contain information about how a drug compares clinically to others in its class and therefore are not useful for helping doctors decide which drug to prescribe to which patient. The EPAR also does not contain the reports by the two members of the Committee selected to assess the new drug or the manufacturer's replies to questions raised. Nor does it reflect the possibly different views within the Committee

Comparison of the regulatory systems		
	EU (EMA)	USA (FDA)
Register of ongoing and completed clinical trials	Not accessible	Accessible
Drug information held by the Agency	Not accessible	Accessible according to the Freedom of Information Act (FOIA) (5)
Records of meetings with industry	Not available	Available
Minutes of advisory committee meetings	Not available	Available
Statements of the minority	Not available	Available

Figure 8.1   Transparency in the European and the American regulatory systems, 2013

about any critical aspects of the dossier in the early stages of the procedure. Rather, it aims to provide a summary overview focused on general consensus. The EPAR is also subject to revision by the company, which may raise objections and negotiate amendments on the basis of alleged commercial confidentiality.

The case for transparency rests in part on how extensively the public contributes to the corporate development of drugs. First, companies draw on extensive research done at public expense. Second, the company's own R&D costs are heavily subsidized by the taxpayers. Third, clinical trials depend on public participation by volunteers. Fourth, the public pays for nearly all the drugs sold. The public "therefore has the right of access to all relevant information." This includes

> the original data, the rapporteurs' initial reports, the discussion between the Committee for Human Medicinal Products and industry, and the minority opinions . . . Abolition of secrecy by EMA would boost the regulatory authorities' credibility and show that patients' health has priority over industrial interests.[40]

This Mario Negri campaign has been joined by others, especially from the Cochrane Collaboration (see below) and the AllTrials campaign (http://www .alltrials.net), and resulted in substantial increases in transparency after years of resistance by EMA officials.[41] In 2012, the EMA announced a new proactive transparency policy, giving broad public access to clinical trial data, and, in April 2014, the European Parliament voted in favor of a proposal to make clinical trial data public.[42] But transparency is being blocked or undermined by some companies. The UK Parliament is still trying to get just the results of all the data from trials of one product,[43] and in May 2014, the EMA seemed to have reversed itself by restricting public access to screen-only reading, without being able to download, print, distribute, or transfer thousands of pages of information. The battles over simply knowing how clinical trials, done for public safety, turn out continues. Beyond that lies the Mario Negri vision of a fully transparent regulatory process to promote good pharma.

Allowing Low-Grade Evidence from Big Pharma

If full transparency were realized tomorrow, it would not address the deeper problem of how biased the trials are and how low-grade the evidence is that the EMA and FDA accept from trials that companies design with only one treatment arm, or too small to produce valid statistical results, or without a control, or based on end points that do not measure real patient-oriented outcomes.[44] For example, in a study of all new chemical entities approved by the EMA up to 2003 conducted at the Mario Negri Institute's Laboratory for Policy, *only 3.3 percent had clinical evidence of being better than existing medications*, as shown in Figure 8.2. The EMA invoked "exceptional circumstances for 14 of 75 new chemical entities."[45] That means almost one in

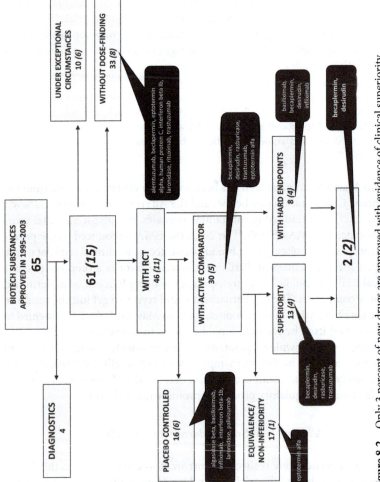

Figure 8.2 Only 3 percent of new drugs are approved with evidence of clinical superiority

every five drugs was approved without evidence. The Mario Negri authors write:

> While there is noisy propaganda claiming the superiority of new drugs, the evidence supporting these claims is often scanty and poor . . . There are several reasons, including the poor dossiers presented [by companies] for the approval of new drugs, the lack of comparisons aimed at showing superiority of new drugs, the bias frequently involved in clinical trials and the conflict of interests.

The point, of course, is that the EMA accepted such poor evidence rather than turning it back as insufficient for evaluating the company's drug.

Companies complain relentlessly about the too-stringent requirements of the EMA and FDA, and about the huge costs of testing; but in fact companies choose to mount far more trials than required by regulation and to spend billions on scientifically flawed trials that are by design unable to produce objective and valid results.[46] As a result, billions of the public's money are wasted on new drugs with few or no advantages over better-established drugs. We have a thick file of evidence that pharmaceutical trials in the United States are just as likely to be unscientific, putting patients at risk for no possible benefit.

For clinical trials to benefit patients, they must be designed to test whether a new drug is better *for patients*, as measured by outcomes that patients' rate as important. Instead, surrogate or substitute measures are used that the Mario Negri Institute opposes. In diabetes, for example, instead of seeing how much a new drug reduces blindness or amputations, regulators allow companies to test new drugs for their effect on blood pressure, lipids, albumin excretion, or C-reactive protein.[47] These make trials faster and cheaper but much less informative about real patient outcomes. The dominance of surrogate outcomes in trials starts a vicious chain reaction as the evidence gets into clinical guidelines, quality of care measures, and pay-for-performance targets so that millions are prescribed drugs that do not make them healthier but expose them to risks of harm. The good-pharma model of the Mario Negri Institute prevents any of this from happening.

Other kinds of low-grade evidence include add-on trials, which by their nature "do not allow assessment of the intrinsic efficacy and safety of new agents and their value as alternatives to available treatments."[48] Yet the EMA allows them as evidence, and a Mario Negri study found they "had an important role in the approval process of the newer antirheumatic agents," especially using the fudge-population of so-called partial responders. Another low-grade and biased practice is stopping trials early because the benefits are "so obvious." Yet this practice is well known for statistically skewing trial results because of an early run of positive results, and it prevents anyone from ever knowing how effective the new drug really is. In all these ways, the EMA fails to fulfill its mission to set and enforce high scientific standards for safety and efficacy, and it fails to protect the public from serious harm. Allowing these trials and flawed evidence means that medical care is based on *Bad Science*, as Goldacre detailed in the book he wrote before *Bad Pharma*.[49]

It takes years or decades to correct for the misleading or inadequate measures and findings allowed by the EMA and FDA. The variety of different end points measured, measurement scales, different dosing, and different trial designs arise from allowing each company to decide how it will test its drugs, rather than managing a coordinated regulatory process aimed at informing patients and their doctors how new drugs compare to existing ones.[50] It means that little of what could be called "medical science" gets established.

The twice-biased medical knowledge—once through trial designs, practices, and reports that the EMA and FDA allow, and then again as company-sponsored teams select, hide, or rearrange trial results into articles for medical journals[51]—becomes the basis for science news, reports, guidelines, and textbooks. The EMA (and FDA) fail to monitor this process of "ghost management" or to notify the public that company-sponsored authors have altered, switched, or omitted in published articles the trial results submitted to them. They limit their role largely to the product summary or drug label (which the company writes), even though most doctors and patients do not learn about drugs from the labels but from the billions spent on marketing materials and "education." Companies run elaborate networks of leading specialists to promote drugs for unauthorized uses "off" the label, which the EMA and FDA also fail to monitor or discipline. Yet off-label prescribing undermines the very purpose of the EMA or FDA in the first place to base prescribing on scientific evidence of safety and effectiveness.

Allowing Unethical Trials

For years, Mario Negri leaders have pointed out that recruiting people to non-inferiority trials or trials that deny participants best available is unethical.[52] By contrast, EMA officers state that "the most common primary objectives for pivotal clinical trials are to demonstrate superiority to placebo control or to demonstrate non-inferiority or equivalence to an active control."[53] They state that "it is not necessary for the benefit-risk profile of an experimental medicine to be at least as favorable as the benefit-risk profile of any or all established medicines in order to receive marketing authorization." But why not? These objectives, the Mario Negri leaders point out, "may allow drugs on the market that are in fact less effective or less safe than those already available." They also violate the ethical principles of the Declaration of Helsinki, which restrict the use of placebo to trials where no proven current intervention exists. Otherwise, people in the control arm are deprived of an effective drug. They may suffer unnecessarily, as did patients with multiple sclerosis described before. Good Pharma, "the active control trial to demonstrate superior efficacy over an established medicine should be the rule, not just an exception."[54] Superiority trials using patient-relevant end points, like those used by the Mario Negri in Chapter 6, "would serve to define the new medicine's place in therapy." For Good Pharma to prevail over Bad Pharma, one needs much more than full transparency of the results from dysfunctional and unethical trials. One needs to disallow such trials.

Another good-pharma change would address three-arm trials. The EMA claims that trials with a placebo arm and a noninferiority arm are "the scientific gold standard." But if the comparator drug is established as effective, a placebo arm is unethical.[55] "In short," the Mario Negri authors point out, "the three-arm trial represents a contradiction in terms and may be an unethical experimental design."[56] The public would be shocked if it knew that the EMA and FDA approve drugs because they demonstrate "inferiority within certain limits." Yet this happens every month of every year. Further, the drug's impact on the length or quality of patient life is not measured so it becomes "impossible to balance what one loses and what one gains."

The Declaration of Helsinki went under revision recently, and the problem lay in a new fudge-statement that placebos can be used for "compelling and scientifically sound methodological reasons." As a master of trials, Garattini comments, "It is difficult to understand what those reasons might be."[57] Garattini, Bertele', and others have been working with the European Clinical Research Infrastructures Network (ECRIN) to advocate a better revision of the Declaration.[58] They point out that informed consent for trials should clearly explain to patients how the use of a placebo or a noninferiority design may negatively impact the individual and will not provide useful information about whether the drug is better than existing medicines. The full research protocol, any amendments, recruitment performance, conflicts of interest, incentives, and the raw, anonymized data should be entered on the WHO International Clinical Trials Registry Platform.[59]

Orphan Drugs—Few Known Benefits

Since 1999, a, European law that offers rich inducements for developing drugs to treat rare diseases, and its 1983 counterpart in the United States, have succeeded in persuading companies to undertake research for rare diseases, or tie in with university or other research groups that have discovered something. People treat orphan drugs with reverence. Yet if one asks for evidence that patients actually got better, little exists. Regulators, eager to approve orphan drugs as miracles for suffering patients, allow companies to carry out low-grade trials and get by with little evidence about clinical benefits or risks.

Roberta Joppi from the Mario Negri Laboratory of Drug Regulatory Policies analyzed the quality of the data submitted to the EMA for all orphan drugs approved through 2004.[60] With Bertele' and Garattini, she found a "frequent lack of dose-finding studies, of controlled studies, of active comparator where available [using placebo instead] . . . insufficient exposure to the treatment, use of surrogate end-points or weak proof of clinical benefit." Two-thirds were tested on fewer than 200 patients, even when there were 50–100 times more patients with the same rare disease in Europe.

The same team from Mario Negri updated their study in 2010 by reviewing every one of the 63 orphan (OMP) marketing authorizations granted by the EMA, for 73 indications. They found reason to be concerned that pharmaceutical companies are exploiting the public's compassion for people with rare diseases to develop drugs, or new indications for drugs already in use, for high prices and profits with little evidence that patients benefit.[61] Two-thirds of the drugs were still tested on 200 patients or less, and trials ran much too short a time to realistically assess the drugs' possible benefits or harmful side effects. The authors write, "the number of patients studied, the use of placebo as control, the type of outcome measure and the follow-up have often been inadequate . . . Joppi and her Mario Negri colleagues found reason to be concerned with how poorly toxicity is tested for the EMA, which allows a "lack of genotoxicity, carcinogenicity or reproduction toxicity studies." In plain English, the EMA approves drugs without tests to see if they do genetic damage, cause cancer, or damage pregnancies. They concluded that more stringent criteria to assess [orphan drugs'] efficacy and cost-effectiveness would improve the clinical value and the affordability of products allowed on the market." Another recent assessment concluded "Orphan drug designation predicts reimbursement [at high prices] despite poor quality of clinical evidence."[62]

Companies have learned to exploit the orphan drug acts for quicker approvals on less evidence and greater chance of reimbursement at very high prices. Often the companies' goal is to market to much larger populations than the "orphan" designation through off-label prescribing for unapproved conditions or diseases.[63] An authoritative study from Harvard University found that three of four orphan drugs were largely being used to treat "common clinical symptoms (pain and fatigue) or laboratory abnormalities," rather than the rare disease itself.[64] One might call this pattern the Orphan-Drug Scam. The Harvard authors conclude, "We should continue to monitor orphan drug use after approval to identify products that come to be widely used for non-FDA approved indications, particularly those without adequate evidence of efficacy."

While regulators approve orphan drugs with little evidence of patient benefit, health-care systems are suffering under the burden of the high prices being charged. Garattini estimates that current law allows companies to generate up to $1 billion a year in revenues per rare disease, just from European patients and despite large public subsidies for the research.[65] Worldwide, revenues would be up to $3 billion per new orphan drug. Given that patients with rare diseases take a drug for years, such high prices go too far, and Garattini calls for a ceiling on public expenditures per drug. He also thinks that the great expansion of population in the EU should change the threshold criteria for orphan drug status from 5 cases in 10,000 to 5 in 50,000–100,000. Further, if there are two or more indications (especially for cancer indications, which make up more than one-third of all "orphan drugs"), the prices should be renegotiated.

The Need for a Good-Pharma Regulator

When he arrived at the EMA in 1997, Garattini wrote in *Science* about the "discrepancy between patients' needs and the availability of new drugs."[66] Because society delegates drug development almost entirely to drug companies, who fund them by patenting and charging high prices, few studies are done on any number of other neglected needs because they are not sufficiently profitable to warrant corporate investment. For example, companies are not developing drugs to counteract resistance to antibiotics, and they are dropping research for new psychotropic drugs to treat the suffering from mental disorders. Studies of the risks and costs involved in long-term use of drugs for prevention are lacking, as are studies on why some patients with a disorder do not respond well while others do. Clinical trials that address the comparative benefits and risks of different drugs, many with expired patents, are not done outside a few places like the Mario Negri Institute. A good-pharma regulator would be given funds to commission such studies as part of its mission to promote the effective use of medicines and look out for drugs or uses that put people's health at risk. A good-pharma regulator "should be enabled to promote the preclinical studies or the clinical trials needed to complete the outstanding safety or efficacy profiles, regardless of the manufacturer's willingness to do it." Second, it should be publicly funded and empowered to acquire drugs abandoned by companies as not profitable enough yet therapeutically promising, so that their development can be completed and they could be licensed to companies willing to manufacture then as generics.[67]

Other elements of a good-pharma regulator include accepting for review only evidence from trials designed to provide scientifically valid information about a drug's comparative effectiveness and initiating tests or trials when they serve the public interest.[68] Behind these suggestions is the radical idea that society's regulator should work to improve patients' health and safety independent of whether products meet Big Pharma's high threshold of profitability in order to develop them. There is also the problem of companies creating shortages, which leave patients without needed drugs, in order to increase the price by several multiples to end a "shortage."

In 2004, Garattini joined others, including Giuseppe Remuzzi and Richard Horton, the editor of *The Lancet*, to summarize the Bergamo Symposium of experts from across Europe. They concurred with the Mario Negri leaders about biased trials, trials with inappropriate dosages or sample sizes or end points or duration, still more biased articles making up medical science, institutionally corrupted academics, and medical journals under siege from systematically corrupted articles. These European leaders of good pharma expressed a "pressing need for independent comparative trials" because "there are so many clinical problems that only independent research (i.e., driven by public-health interests and not merely by profit) can address." They called for "a new European funding agency, with no commercial interests . . . in a framework of a non-profit, public-health-oriented funding system."[69] "Freed of the shackles of direct commercial interests, drug development could focus on clinical conditions dictated by the global burden of disease while also taking account of areas that tend to be neglected."

Funding for this new, independent agency should come from taxes and "enable the agency to do its own investigations on the data reported by industry [and] . . . cover other activities of fundamental public health importance . . . [such as] to contract independent research to third parties . . . to effectively deal the pharmaco-vigilance, to review drug use, and to make proactive investigations on the real benefits of drugs already introduced in the market."[70] Public funding would also replace the vicious circle of researchers having to please their corporate paymasters by making drugs look more effective than they are in practice, with the virtuous circle of researchers using their best scientific judgment to improve the public's health through good pharma.

The Price of Moral Integrity

A recent, courageous stand taken by the Mario Negri Institute against unethical behavior by Big Pharma occurred when GSK (GlaxoSmithKline) betrayed its commitment to transparency in 2013. The Innovative Medicines Initiative (IMI) is "a joint undertaking between the European Union and the pharmaceutical industry . . . to speed up the development of better and safer medicines for patients. IMI supports collaborative research projects and builds networks of industrial and academic experts in order to boost pharmaceutical innovation in Europe."[71] IMI aims to foster close research collaboration between public, corporate, and nonprofit research centers like the Mario Negri Institute. However, when as a member, the Mario Negri Institute sought discussions with GSK about their methodological choices in a collaborative research project, the Institute discovered that GSK ruled these choices as "not open for discussion."[72]

Although Andrew Witty, the chief executive of GSK, has formally embraced full transparency, GSK attached to the study's protocol "dozens of pages of rules and conditions" that gave it total control and even meant that the Mario Negri would have to ask permission for access to its own data from its own trial! Further, GSK rules gave it the right to block publication of Mario Negri's analysis of those data at any time after the study was completed. Yet public EU funding and independent research institutes are contributing to the project. What is promoted to the public as a grand coalition between Big Pharma, academia, government, and independent research institutes in order to develop better medicines for patients in need has in fact a subterranean tangle of controls by company lawyers that undermine transparency and open, collaborative science.

The Mario Negri protested, appealed, but other members of the IMI did not join in; so the Institute decided the only ethical thing to do was to resign from a coalition that allows violations of its own principles of open collaboration and transparency. This will cost the Institute dearly, because coalition members qualify for millions in IMI funding. Moral integrity can exact a high price, but the 50-year history in the last chapter and this one shows how the price of living out a simple ethic of applying open, independent science to develop good medicines for patients is still far from accepted.

Good Science for Good Pharma—A Public-Health Model

It's worse than you think but could be much better than you imagine. In the Introduction, we described and documented the ways in which patent-driven research and prices set at 50–100 times manufacturing costs, have corrupted the research process, the products of pharmaceutical research, medical knowledge, the way drugs are approved, and the prescribing choices physicians make. Drug companies distort each of these steps to maximize profits, usually with little benefit to patients. Risks of serious adverse reactions from new drugs are one in five.[1] While patenting may work out better in other areas of industrial research like software development, funding research to find better medicines through patent-protected high prices and monopolistic submarkets has inverted or corrupted biomedical research, especially in rich countries.

In the United States, if one takes the number of real clinical advances since the Bayh-Dole Act was passed in 1980, together with the thousands of clinically minor "innovations" and millions of patients who were hospitalized or died from 34 years of adverse reactions, and compares it to the number of clinically superior drugs discovered and developed in the 34 years *before* the Bayh-Dole Act commercialized the minds and strategies of researchers, one would find fewer clinically important new drugs since Bayh-Dole than before.[2] In the past 15 years, pharmaceutical innovation has continued to stay stagnant or decline, while prices and profits have soared.[3] The drive for more patents and profits from drugs with few new benefits and substantial risks of serious harm is the opposite of what people want.

Accelerating approvals or relaxing rules of evidence simply reward companies to develop still more minor variations, not more "life-saving" new drugs. And strong, long protections reduce incentives to develop clinically better drugs as they increase incentives to defend and extend patent protections on existing drugs through a variety of legal, quasi-legal, and illegal tactics.[4] Why do the EMA and FDA not realize they are largely rewarding more minor variations as rational, economic responses to lower and looser evidence of safety and efficacy? Perhaps because they and the politicians supporting these developments are being co-opted by the drug companies that also fund the regulators as the protectors of public safety. Advocating quicker reviews with less evidence, however, serves the interests of regulators by generating more fees.

Getting doctors to prescribe all these minor innovations has led to techniques underlying The Inverse Benefit Law: the more widely drugs are marketed, the more diluted become their benefits but the more widespread become their risks of harm.[5] Techniques include putting lead clinicians on retainers and having them serve on expert committees that lower the thresholds for prescribing drugs to healthier patients.[6] This adds tens of millions of people who were not "sick" before.[7] Creating or medicalizing new illnesses or risks adds tens of millions more, without valid clinical evidence that patients get healthier, and without counting adverse side effects. Another tactic to generate inverse benefits from more marketing is overstating the safety and efficacy of the drugs, based on clinical trials designed to produce this evidence. Testing against surrogate end points and not comparing new drugs to existing ones allows the Inverse Benefit Law to manifest itself in the absence of clear, clinical evidence, a kind of institutionally induced ignorance.[8] What a contrast are these tactics to the moral integrity and full-disclosure of the public health Mario Negri model of patient-based research that tests for real clinical advances.

An extensive body of research studies has detailed how the pursuit of high gross profits from government-protected prices and markets has corrupted nearly every part of drug discovery and development. In *Bad Pharma*, Ben Goldacre focuses particularly on the hiding, lying, and distorting of randomized clinical trials as "the gold standard" of medical science. Each of his examples stems from making new drugs look safer and more effective than they are in order to exploit high prices protected by intellectual property (IP) rights. These distortions of medical knowledge then become "evidence-based" medicine, a great advance now undermined by the substance and techniques of patent-driven research.[9]

The costs to nations and health-care systems are huge: About 80 percent of increased expenditures are wasted on new drugs with few or no clinical advantages to offset their risks of harm, which harms patients and society.[10] This is not counting the huge waste of taxpayers' money through pharmaceutical tax breaks and tax credits, plus data exclusivity provisions and so-called patent restoration clauses that do not return very many clinically superior drugs compared to the mass of minor variations and me-too drugs. Then governments pay twice when they buy the clinically minor new drugs. By contrast, the Mario Negri ethos and practices led Garattini, Tognoni, and others to remove or reclassify many of these drugs in the 1970s and again in the 1990s, saving 30 percent of the national drugs budget (see Chapter 7).

Two new books provide insights and evidence on the damage that the patent paradigm of pharmaceutical innovation is causing societies and patients. Courtney Davis and John Abraham, who between them have produced an authoritative body of policy research on drug regulation and its implications for society, have written a major book on "promissory science" and the myths of new drug regulation to get "life-saving" drugs to patients faster so they can be healthier.[11] They write "laboratory scientists make promissory claims about the social/health value of new technology/drugs, which create powerful expectations about (and hence demand for) that technology within the wider society, including patients." Promissory science is the principal way in which patent-driven pharmaceutical research diverts attention away from the hidden business model that produces scores of new products each year with few or no new benefits to offset their little-known risks of serious adverse reactions.

Based on the rhetoric of promissory science, heavy lobbying by a congress of lobbyists more than twice the size of the US Congress, and hundreds of millions in political payments, the industry has persuaded Congressmen and government officials to institute a new era of quicker reviews requiring less evidence of safety or benefit before approval. Approval has morphed from a binary decision of approve/reject to a semi-continuous variable of provisional and contingent forms of approval. Because patent-holding companies immediately start mass-marketing to maximize profits before their patents run out and free-market competition commences, conditional approvals work like complete approvals but with less evidence of safety or clinical effectiveness.

Davis and Abraham show that the dilution and speed-up of review was not driven by patient demand, as companies and regulators claim, but rather by neoliberal beliefs that less regulation fosters greater innovation, facts to the contrary conveniently ignored. Careful analyses of the consequences by top, independent researchers have found that faster reviews lead to more serious warnings of risk, hospitalizations, or deaths.[12]

No one has told the public. No one told politicians or patients or doctors that faster approvals put through in the 1990s, in response to pressures from the companies that fund the public regulator as the public defender against harmful drugs, significantly increased patients hospitalized and killed.[13] The EMA has used the same rhetoric, contrary to evidence that speed-up approvals reduce evidence that new drugs are either clinically safe or better for patients. Davis and Abraham also detail, as they famously have before, how industry funding and influence undermine the regulator's own evaluation of new drugs.

The new, neoliberal approach is to get drugs faster into patients' bloodstreams and then use "risk management" to protect them from harm. But Davis and Abraham point out that this claim "is not supported by our investigations, which indicate that risk management was used as a means to maintain on the market drugs with known risks."[14] Davis and Abraham conclude that "since the mid- to late-2000s, the EU regulatory states appear to be following the US approach . . . as a means of maintaining unsafe drugs on the market."[15]

Unauthorized or "off-label" uses not approved by regulators proliferate use and sales. Between 20 and 60 percent of sales in a disease area are for unauthorized uses with little or no evidence of benefit.[16] Thus the regulatory mandate to protect the public from ineffective and harmful drugs is weakened, and off-label promotion undermines the whole purpose of testing drugs as "safe and effective" in the first place.

What a contrast to the Mario Negri paradigm (Chapter 8) of publicly funded regulators and independent advisory groups who require evidence from externally funded trials for which trial teams compete based on the quality of their trial design and track record for scientific integrity, that a new drug is superior to existing drugs based on patient-oriented outcomes.

In a second book, Peter Gøtzsche, a physician, former drug salesman and product manager who has become one of the most authoritative experts on drug evaluation and evidence, provides lively detail to show that drug companies have become like organized crime.[17] They are certainly organized, and their premeditated criminal actions have been rising sharply.[18] Extortion, fraud, drug offenses, obstruction of justice and law enforcement, legal and illegal bribery, collusion, witness tampering, intimidation of critical academics, and political corruption—all are documented corporate tactics used to keep the public ignorant of the real efficacy and safety of new drugs[19] and to fend off actions that threaten patent-protected profits.

In making his case, Gøtzsche is building on *Corporate Crime in the Pharmaceutical Industry* by John Braithwaite, a 1984 classic that is being updated.[20] Recently, Braithwaite told a reporter, "In the area of research fraud, things are again worse than 30 years ago."[21] Richard Smith, the distinguished editor-in-chief of *BMJ* from 1991 to 2004, writes, "Many people are killed by the industry, many more than are killed by the mob. Indeed, hundreds of thousands are killed every year by prescription drugs."[22]

Gøtzsche estimates that prescription drugs have become the third leading cause of death after heart disease and cancers, substantially more than our own estimate of medicines being the fourth leading cause.[23] About 330,000 patients die each year in just the United States and Europe from prescription drugs, 200,000 in Europe and 130,000 in the United States.[24] In short, the patent-based paradigm of pharmaceutical innovation has become a deadly distortion of good medicine. He exposes such myths as "prediabetes" and "prefracture," or osteopenia, a disorder created whole-cloth by Merck that even involved getting the US Congress to change the law so that Medicare would pay for a nonscientific test that "detects" a health problem that is not supported by independent clinical evidence.[25]

Gøtzsche discredits the myth that drugs are expensive because company research costs are so high and that if we don't pay high prices, innovation will dry up. He documents how most of the key research for breakthrough drugs came from publicly funded labs or grants, before drug companies take them over for final testing and marketing. He describes how GSK has lied and suppressed information about harms to patients; how Roche has grown from early, illegal sales of heroin to making far more by misleading governments about Tamiflu; how Pfizer keeps breaking the law and even the Corporate Integrity Agreements imposed to make it go straight, like a repeat offender;

and how Merck "lied to the FDA and Congress about what and when the company knew that Vioxx is deadly . . . [as it] killed about 120,000 people."

Isn't it time for a revolution in how pharmaceutical research is done? Don't we want honest researchers to work together, not separately in high-security labs, and to learn from each other's failures as well as successes while trying any active ingredient that might work, regardless of its patentability? Isn't it time to redirect pharmacological research to improving the public's health, using the methods of the Mario Negri Institute?

Gøtzsche writes that "general system failure calls for a revolution." First, developing drugs based on patents and profits is the wrong model. Instead, research should be funded through large prizes in proportion to health improvement and then drugs could be licensed to multiple firms for free-market competition. Formal European bodies have called for such a revolution. Gøtzsche calls for prescribing far fewer medicines to patients and decommercializing health care.

Second, as an authority on trials run by drug companies, Gøtzsche writes, "We cannot trust industry trials at all" and should fund independent trials that fully report·adverse events as well as benefits. This is exactly what the Mario Negri has been doing for years and is a living model of success.

Third, funding of regulatory agencies by the companies they are supposed to be watchdogging must be replaced with public funding to become independent. They should no longer allow surrogate end points, or random samples on biased populations, or misleading comparators, or small, short trials when long, large ones are required to protect the public from the epidemic of harm. This is just what the Mario Negri Institute has been advocating for years as the alternate paradigm for how regulators should review new drugs, and just the kind of trials it actually does: large, long trials based on the full practice population to test for superiority based on real clinical end points. (See Chapters 6 and 8.)

Fourth, drug marketing is not needed because word gets around about clinically superior drugs. Nor is corrupting physicians and patient associations needed to serve as seemingly independent but drug-dependent marketing arms of companies to promote the wider uses of usually ineffective and risky new products. These associations often receive "unrestricted educational grants" that are, in fact, restricted, uneducational grants.

Finally, the dependence of medical journals on revenues from pharmaceutical companies needs to be addressed, because it may affect what they publish that becomes medical knowledge on which everyone depends. It is estimated that advertising revenues could be just as great if medical journals turned their rule that ads be relevant to medicine on its head, by mandating that ads must *not* be about medicine. With their concentrated, affluent audience, medical journals could charge as much or more per column inch for ads about great condos, cars, travel, fashions, and other luxury goods, so that their ads would look like those in *The New Yorker*. Huge profits from reprint sales should stop. No one need glossy reprints anymore, and making journals drug-dependent rewards them for publishing articles with positive results on patented drugs.

The state of affairs in Big Pharmaland is nicely captured by a 2014 *New York Times* overview of merger activity.[26] "Instead of spending money researching new products that may yield little success, several companies are instead looking to buy likely winners." Why undertake the high risks of failure in real research to find better medicines when you can buy in later at low risk? Instead of looking for products that have real clinical impact, companies are looking for "products that have strong pricing power." More profits, and more costs for everyone else, with no mention of improved health or addressing unmet needs.

The No-Patent Research Model

The practices, rules, and achievements of the Mario Negri Institute show that the case for patient-based, no-patent research is much deeper that even incisive critics like Peter Gøtzsche, Marcia Angell, or Merrill Goozner indicate.[27] Patents may work in other realms of innovation and technology; but in medicine they have not. Morally, societies exempted medicines from patents for decades because they were regarded as a social, not a commercial, good.[28] Medically, patenting distorts every step of the research process as well as testing, publishing, marketing, and finally prescribing. Making drugs subject to patents has led to the current proliferation of pseudoinnovation and serious risks we have discussed. But the Mario Negri Institute, as an oasis of classic science—independent, transparent, and funded for just the costs of research—represents a classic, alternate model for how to do good science to develop good medicines without any of these distortions.

Consider Figure 9.1 and ask how would we like researchers to choose what to research and how to develop new drugs for our loved ones and for the world? Would we rather have researchers allowed to decide for themselves which promising scientific strategies to pursue to find an effective medicine, with no financial interest beyond their salary and grants (Column 2)? Or be directed by executives concerned about which areas and strategies are most likely to generate profitable patents (Column 1)? Would we rather have the research be subjected to transparent, independent review by peers for funding and publication, or be subjected to a corporate director of research whose compensation depends on how his or her thousands of stock options perform?

Would we rather have researchers in a disease area be free to draw on any promising drug developed, past or present, regardless of its patent status, and draw on unpatentable but promising agents (Column 2), or only on active ingredients that are patentable (Column 1)?

Would we prefer that researchers in a disease area feel free to share and brainstorm about better methods and research strategies to find a solution (Column 2), or work under strict rules of secrecy within a corporate group (Column 1)? Do we think that patients who volunteer to participate in

Pharmaceutical Research to Maximize Patents & Profits *The Big Pharma Model*	*Pharmacological* Research to Maximize Health of Individuals and Populations *The Mario Negri Institute Model*
Goal it to maximize number of new patented products and profits from them in govt-protected markets. Clinical benefits to patients or populations secondary	Goal is to develop clinically beneficial new ways to address health problems of patients or populations without considering their profitability.
Diseases of the poor and other unprofitable diseases are not studied. Health inequities are reinforced.	All diseases, regardless of patents and profits, are considered, based on need and funding.
Research driven by executives and high-profit goals. Less profitable projects or teams or whole disease areas not funded, or abandon them when profit projections fall. Priorities shift as markets or priorities shift.	Research self-directed by researchers, supported by brainstorming witth colleagues
Reaseach funded out of high profits from protected prices as an investment in future profits. Priorities driven by marketing.	Research paid in classic ways - grants, contracts, budgets - by a range of public & private funders. No patenting to seek additional profits because distorts priorities, pathways, product development. Or, long arms-length patenting by host institution.
Short-term research for profitable results. Earlier long-term research less and less supported	Relentless pursuit for years ir decades to figure out how to help patients with a difficult problem.
"innovation" measured by new molecules, best in class, or first in class, even if clinically no better or worse.	"Innovation" measured by improved clinical or population health status or reduced suffering.
Closed-science secrecy. Guard info on projects, progress, failures, success, budgets, patenting startegies, to ward off competitors and poachers. Closely manage disclosures. Sculpt research findings.	Open-science transparency, sharing, network-building. Publish all results and learn from failures. Share new solutions, methods, strategies to find effective intervetions.
Ghose management or ghost writing of publications. The corporate distortion of medical knowledge.	Researchers write their own papers and publications.
Develop slightly different new drugs for large-profit conditions already treated. Occasional superior meds occur.	Focus on finding clinically superior drugs for serious, often untreated medical conditions.
Consider no promising medicines, past breakthroughts, ingredients in nature, or traditional cure that can't be patented. Minimum or no comparing or sharing.	Consider all possibly helpful medicines, past breakthroughts, ingredients in nature, traditional cures, regardless of patents. Can compare & share across companies and patent status.
Trials designed to minimize evidence of harms & maximize evidence of benefits in artifical populations that exclude those who might experience adverse reactions and include those likely to have a positive reaction. Often exclude the elderly, women, people with co-morbidities.	Trials designed to test clinical outcomes on populations that will take the medicine. Test for superiority over current treatments, regardless of patents staus. Include the natural diversity of the practice population.
Trials undertaken whenever better market information seems possible or prescribing doctors can be signed up. Very costly, measure everything to find something.	Trails undertaken only after careful review of what is known and careful work to identify a strong end point. Clean, simple & cheap, about $1/10$th the cost per patient.
Trials pay doctors and patients so well that doing or being in them is a profit stream. Distorts design, data, and results.	Patients volunteer for no pay, doctors for no or modest pay for their time. Trials part of practice and communal.
Goal to maximize the number of people on as many patented drugs as possible, with few benefits to affset risks of harm. Costs taxpayers & others about $1 trillion	Goal to maximize the number of superior drugs, at low prices, while minimizing drug consumption. Would cost taxpayers & others $1/5$th as much.

Figure 9.1   Big Pharma versus Mario Negri Institute

trials should be given a full account of the design, methods, and outcomes (Column 2), or is that the company's business (Column 1)? Do we want patients, their doctors, and health-care administrators to be given a full account of benefit and the risks of harm in new drugs (Column 2), or be given a selection that hides serious risks?[29]

Do we want trials designed so that they produce valid information about a significant clinical question and help doctors choose how or when to use a drug (Column 2)? Or do we want trials designed to produce marketing information to persuade doctors and patients to use a new drug, even though independent clinicians and pharmacists conclude it has few or no advantages over existing drugs whose risks are much better known (Column 1)? The incentives and logic of patent-based medical research lead to the former. In our Introduction, we outlined the features of a Mario Negri Trial. They essentially reflect well-established standards for objective, scientifically valid, and socially beneficial trials.

Do we trust more articles written by the researchers themselves (Column 2), or by teams of writers and statisticians on retainer with a company, who do not include negative trial results and alter end points and statistical analyses of those included to make a drug look safer and more effective than it is (Column 1)? An important study funded by the Edmond J. Safra Center for Ethics at Harvard University found that doctors do not trust the results about prescribing from trials funded by industry as much as independently funded trials.[30] The editor-in-chief of the *New England Journal of Medicine*, who used to work for several pharmaceutical companies and who keeps favoring proindustry articles, dismissed this important study by likening the self-interest of pharmaceutical executives to the self-interest of young researchers.[31] Do you agree? We did not.[32]

Patent-based research for better drugs is widely hailed as the strongest, most successful case for why patents are indispensable. Richard Posner believes that "pharmaceuticals are the poster child for the patent system."[33] But he seems not to have considered the evidence here that pharmaceutical companies have corrupted patenting and the patent system away from rewarding clinically superior drugs and toward pseudoinnovation. Does Posner believe that government-protected prices in an unfree market should make people pay very high prices for molecular manipulations that have few or no new benefits? In the past 30 years, patent proliferation, patent thickets, patent evergreening, patent stonewalling, and patent-driven mergers are far more prevalent than important clinical advances for patients. Alessandro Liberati described the corrupting effects on researchers shortly before his death:

> Pharmaceutical companies avoid research that might show that new and expensive drugs are no better than another comparator already on the market . . . Researchers are trapped by their own internal competing interests—professional and academic—which lead them to compete for pharmaceutical industry funding.[34]

Champions of patents do not even mention their deleterious effects on the quality of medical science that have been so carefully documented, or the central role of corporate actions that harm patients through overuse and misleading activities designed to make their so-called innovations look better than they are, in order to sell millions more doses before the patents run out.[35]

US Examples of No-Patent Research

What would no-patent research actually look like? It's beyond many people's imagination. Yet no-patent research is what the researchers at the large, multi-campus Mario Negri Institute have been doing every day for the past 50 years, and it is the foundation of great public research programs or organizations like the National Institutes of Health.

NIH has never been "the National Institutes of Patented Health Research," though recent changes may be taking it in that unfortunate direction. NIH is founded on having society pay for the very high risks and costs of basic research so that their discoveries are available to all. But then companies can patent the fruits of this research for society and sell them for very high prices without having to pay back society or taxpayers for bearing the high risks and costs of research. Within the NIH, we have found two vertically integrated, bench-to-bedside research units that resemble the Mario Negri model except that they are entirely funded by government.

No-Patent Research for Cancer

More interesting is the extent to which the National Institutes of Health (NIH) and other national programs of government-funded research are carrying out no-patent research. For example, the Cancer Therapy Evaluation Program (CTEP) at the National Cancer Institute (NCI) has a hand-picked integrated research staff of about 50 from disciplines needed to investigate new ways to develop drugs for cancers, then develop them in vitro and in vivo through small animal trials, and finally organize larger animal trials and human trials. They work full-time on salaries, and do not think about or apply for patents. "We follow the science," said James Zweibel, the chief. "We are not constrained by commercial issues." All scientific articles are written personally by the researchers, without ghost management or ghostwriting.

Besides CTEP doing its own research and developing its own discoveries, companies can bring a promising idea or discovery to CTEP and ask the team there to use its independent research methods to take over its development, not unlike pharmaceutical companies bringing a promising idea to the Mario Negri for development, only the funding differs. These are called "Collaborative Agreements" and the language emphasizes "joint," "shared," and "cooperative." But outside experts we have talked with, like senior oncologists who work with venture capital firms, emphasize how the CTEP research team requires that it control the research design.

As at the Mario Negri, Dr. Zweibel described how the staff respond to a request by putting together a research design that specifies end points, sampling for trials, trial sites, and other details. The company comments and then signs a Collaborative Agreement. Thus like Mario Negri, CTEP controls the science and development. This takes CTEP, like the Mario Negri, down unanticipated paths as it "follows the science." "We can address scientific questions they cannot afford or can't take the time to address," said Zwiebel. "We're not in the great rush the companies are." CTEP sets its own criteria and deadlines as a way to focus on leads that are working out and drop ones that are not.

Besides addressing leads and questions that the team thinks are valuable, CTEP has the same important advantage as the Mario Negri Institute of being able to combine drugs from different companies if research indicates they would be more effective—a sort of cancer research commons. For example, some drugs have short-term effects on tumors and can be combined with another drug that prolongs the effect. CTEP also can draw on a national clinical trials network, based at academic research centers that can mount trials more quickly and control their quality. It "provides a unified clinical and translational infrastructure," which can draw on nationally integrated tissue resources and test less common malignancies better. It can also draw on closely related groups, like the Cancer Image Program and the Cancer Diagnostic Biomarker Group. CTEP applies to the FDA for approval of its trials and takes promising drugs up through at least phase-2 trials. Regardless of when its work ends, it turns the drug over to a company after most of the risk and cost of development are paid for and completed. The company locks in patent rights and then charges $100,000 a year or more for a patient to benefit.

Based on this preliminary information, CTEP also seems like a model of no-patent research integrity, free of the dependency corruption that has been found to bias the work of commercial researchers and trialists as they develop the most marketable products and measure benefits by surrogate or substitute end points rather than hard evidence of patient improvement, while minimizing evidence of harmful side effects. It could be replicated in other major disease areas so that researchers could focus on drugs that measurably improve patients' health and survival, uncorrupted by conflicts of interest.

Research without Patenting

The Vaccine Research Center (VRC) is a second NIH unit that is widely admired as a fully integrated, independent research organization that can take an idea or molecule from basic research to final clinical trials. It focuses on diseases that most need vaccines, not the ones that most make profits. It patents none of its discoveries, seeks no revenues from its products, and makes all its work fully available. In this difficult field, it has created 37 vaccine products over the first ten years, nearly all of which are in development or testing.

Its 211 staff have published 670 scientific articles, all written by the research-ers themselves.[36] As an intramural NIH center, VRC is fully funded by the National Institute of Allergy and Infectious Diseases (NIAID), and its staff is on full-time salaries. Like CTEP, it is a multidisciplinary institute dedicated to discovering and developing better medicines for unmet needs everywhere.

VRC is regarded by some of its principal investigators as a model of inte-grated pharmacological science that could also be emulated elsewhere, with modifications. It has its own virology lab, immunology lab, and clinical tri-als core lab, as well as an animal lab. It even has its own small manufacturing facility to make batches for trials. For advanced trials, it draws on the HIV Vaccine Trials Network (HVTN), an international collaboration of scien-tists and physicians who can conduct all phases of clinical trials through a network of sites. "Protocols are developed by HVTN investigators and include partnerships between vaccine developers, clinical experts, and bio-statisticians [who] work closely with NIH staff in initiating, conducting, funding, and coordinating all . . . processes." One principal investigator called it "the Manhattan Project of vaccine research. It could be used for developing drugs too." However, under current arrangements a company patents the fruit of all this publicly paid research and testing to charge the public a high price. The public health model is destroyed by patenting for high prices.

On the wider stage beyond these two centers, NIH has created a new, large division dedicated to translational research in order to develop more leads from basic research into safe and effective drugs. Big Pharma can hardly believe its luck—still more research development and risks borne by taxpayers and then handed over to them for monopoly patenting and high prices, espe-cially for the most profitable and expanding area known as specialty drugs, for severe conditions and rare diseases. No one seems to be talking about the obvious: If the public is paying for basic, applied, and translational research, and if the public also pays for most of the doses, why not exempt these new drugs and vaccines from patenting as societal goods, or have NIH take out the patents in order to issue licenses to manufacturers so there can be free-market competition and lower prices? Then world-class, patient-oriented discoveries could be available to everyone at low prices, and the royalties could replenish part of the NIH budget.

Beyond these two successful, American models of no-patent research integrity, Big Pharma itself has been rapidly moving toward open-science, collaborating, brainstorming models of research. The world of innovation and pharmacological research is rapidly shifting toward Internet-based consortia of brainstorming researchers who love the challenge of a problem, especially an unsolved problem that could help the needy and suffering. Bernard Munos is a leader of pharmacological innovation who gives more than a dozen exam-ples of open-science networks that have developed new medicines for one-tenth the cost of Big Pharma or less. They are not trying to get rich.[37] Munos points out that mid-sized and large drug companies do research in much more costly and distorting ways, largely to charge high prices.

Profiles of Research without Patenting at the Mario Negri

In order to provide specific examples beyond those in other chapters of the book, we offer profiles of current research at the Mario Negri.

An Unpatentable Treatment for Breast Cancer

As he tried to explain to sociologists unschooled in molecular biology the exciting work he is pursuing, the soft-spoken, self-effacing physician Enrico Garattini told us that he has been on the trail of a cure for certain breast cancers for 25 years. And the key letter is "s." "Breast cancer is a misleading term," he said. "Women have breast cancers, with six major types and many subtypes."

Behind this systematic molecular research to find how a certain cancer works and how it can be "killed" or differentiated into an innocuous form is funding from some of the great Italian charities, like AIRC (http://www.airc.it) and Foundation Monzino. Each grant cycle is highly competitive, but they have repeatedly judged the Mario Negri research project as among the best. Still, the search for research support is difficult.

Enrico, the eldest son of Silvio, believes that retinoic acid—a major form of vitamin A long used in traditional Chinese medicine against tumors and currently employed in the treatment of acute promyelocytic leukemia (APL)—has great promise against a subtype of HER-plus, or HER+ breast cancer. Recently he and his group demonstrated that 25 percent of all HER 2+ breast cancers are sensitive to retinoic acid because of an amplification of the gene coding for the major retinoic acid receptor. The finding indicates that an identifiable subgroup of breast cancer patients may benefit from retinoic acid–based therapeutic strategies.

Up to 20 years ago, APL was treated with cycles of chemotherapy and had remission rates of about 25 percent. But after the introduction of all-trans-retinoic acid into the standard therapeutic regimens, remission rates shot up to 85–90 percent and patients stayed free of leukemia for 5 years or longer.

The leukemic cells are "killed" in a novel way, by differentiating them into healthy cells with a half-life of 24 hours so they die a natural, innocuous death and exit the body—a neat trick. Enrico contributed to the understanding of the mechanisms underlying the antileukemia action of retinoic acid, and some of his work has appeared in *Blood* since 1993. After persistent research for 20 years into the promise of this traditional Chinese medicine, Enrico is now setting up a phase-2 clinical trial to scientifically assess its value as a cancer drug.

Pharmaceutical companies have shown only marginal interest in this research because retinoic acid is natural, produced by our bodies every day, and therefore is not patentable. This long-term research, like several others at the Mario Negri Institute, is wholly dependent on donations and grants from charitable organizations, as are several other investigations into how nonpatentable new uses for serious illnesses can be developed. Enrico said, "At Mario Negri we are focused on the patient, and that is very different from being focused on patenting. *Patenting does not work in the service of the patient.* Within our Institute, we cover all phases of research using interdisciplinary teams that can take a promising idea from the bench to the bedside. And then it's important to loop back from what you learn in phase-3 trials back to the bench, to investigate certain puzzles or side effects."

Not Giving Up, When Even NCI Does

In 1991, PharmaMar, a biotech company set up by a wealthy Spanish family to find new drugs in the sea discovered several new compounds with completely new chemical structures potentially able to inhibit cell proliferation. Maurizio D'Incalci, head of oncology at the Mario Negri Institute, learned about this initiative, and started to collaborate with them. His laboratory found that one compound, ET743 now known as trabectedin (Yondelis) was particularly promising, because of its ability to kill cancer cells that were resistant to the available chemotherapeutic drugs and its novel mechanisms of action, certainly different from those of other known anticancer drugs. He collaborated with several scientists at the National Cancer Institute (NCI), confirming that the properties of this drug were unique, thus suggesting it was worthwhile testing it for the therapy of human cancer.

At that time, D'Incalci was the chairman of the Research Division of the European Organization for Research and Treatment of Cancer (EORTC), and also chair of the committee that was selecting new anticancer drugs to be developed by it in collaboration with the NCI. Considering the findings in preclinical tumors in mice, obtained mainly at Mario Negri Institute, both EORTC and the NCI agreed to start a program to develop the drug in the clinic. NCI invested significant resources to formulate the compound and to study its toxicological properties in different animal species—required by regulatory authorities like FDA to start any clinical investigation.

Trabectedin, however, was so toxic on the liver that the NCI toxicologists ended the project. But the EORTC committee chaired by D'Incalci decided to continue the research because in mice the drug was effective in sarcomas, a type of tumor very difficult to treat and for which no new drugs had been discovered for more than 30 years. D'Incalci turned to addressing the severe toxicity of this effective drug that even NCI toxicologists had abandoned. In order to address this problem, he teamed up with Andreas Gescher, an international expert on toxicology at the University of Leicester who spent a year at the Mario Negri, to test each part of the complex mechanisms by which the compound was toxic on the liver. They could not find out how it worked until they tried a whole-mouse approach, where they could see the whole interaction. By understanding that the mechanisms of toxicity were related to inflammation of the biliary ducts, they designed experiments to inhibit toxicity by using anti-inflammatory agents, such as corticosteroids, before trabectedin treatment.

The results were astonishing. Toxicity almost disappeared in rodents, and this finding was then confirmed in patients with sarcoma at the National Cancer Institute in Milan. The discovery was essential for the further development of the drug that was then approved in Europe in 2007 for patients with soft-tissue sarcoma. More than 100 different cancers make up what is called "soft-tissue sarcoma," and the studies at the Mario Negri Institute were essential to establish that in one particular subtype named myxoid liposarcoma, trabectedin has a high specific activity, much better than any other drug. This, however, is a very rare disease and there is a very limited commercial interest in developing drugs for it. Once again, a major Italian Cancer Charity, the Italian Association for Cancer Research, funded the studies done on this rare tumor at the Mario Negri Institute.

An additional important finding from the laboratory of the Department of Oncology at Mario Negri was that trabectedin was also very effective in animal models of ovarian cancer. These data convinced PharmaMar to sponsor a phase II study that was coordinated by the Institute and conducted in Italy, on patients with advanced ovarian cancer who had relapsed after several previous chemotherapies. Approximately 40 percent of patients responded to treatment, an impressive outcome.

Because of these data, Johnson & Johnson agreed to fund a critical phase-3 trial in return for the patent and intellectual property rights, but only for ovarian cancer because J&J only had interest in the larger market for ovarian cancer. This upset many oncologists because it meant the promise of a new, effective drug against other sarcomas would not be tested. "This is a good example of why public funding is needed for clinical trials," said D'Incalci, "so that promising drugs will be tested regardless of market size and profit potential."

The phase-3 trial was successful and in 2009, after 15 years of persistent efforts by the Mario Negri Laboratory in Oncological Research, trabectedin was approved. It added 6 months of overall survival for women with ovarian cancer who had relapsed after 6 months from the previous therapy. Only because the Mario Negri research team kept looking at the science for solutions for patients at risk and in need, without regard to patents and profit potential, was a way found to use trabectedin against cancer. The methods and research strategies developed at the Mario Negri Lab, mainly based on deep preclinical assessments using reliable experimental animal models, can now be applied to many other cancers in order to find effective compounds against them.

Getting Cancer Drugs to Penetrate Tumors

About 25 years ago, Mario Negri researchers figured out why so many cancer drugs are not as effective as they seem to be in the lab. They developed new methods including imaging mass spectrometry and a series of advances in measurement that date back to Garattini's emphasis in the 1960s on seeking better ways to measure an active agent in all parts of an organ. What they discovered was that many cancer drugs do not penetrate into a tumor but rather stay around the outer edges. Researchers had missed this crucial observation because they tested a drug's presence in the blood. However, in tumors that lack many blood vessels, an effective drug cannot penetrate into its interior.

Maurizio D'Incalci and his team are revisiting this work because now they may have a new way to transport anticancer drugs deep into tumors. Nanotechnologies developed with chemical engineers on the Mario Negri multispecialty team might be used to transport cancer drugs inside poorly vascularized tumors. They are starting up a number of projects using these new methods and seek funders to support the work.

Turning Epilepsy on Its Head

Annamaria Vezzani has been rethinking what epilepsy is. We think of an epileptic seizure as just that, a seizing or sudden forcible grasping that can range from a small, short seizing of the body to full-blown convulsions and loss of consciousness. People who have recurrent seizures are said to have epilepsy. About 1 percent, or 60 million people have epilepsy in the world, three million in the United States, and half a million in Italy. This is not a "disease" in the usual sense, with a pathogen and course of illness, and Vezzani explained to us that epilepsy was not considered a disease until recently.

The first anticonvulsive drug was bromide discovered by chance in 1857 by Locock. Subsequently, in the early 1900s phenobarbital was discovered to have anticonvulsive effects. Other, currently used drugs for the symptomatic control of seizures were developed in the 1950s.

While effective in about three quarters of cases, these drugs do not help the other quarter. They represent the patient population for which new drugs are required.

One advantage of research at a nonprofit, independent institute like the Mario Negri is that one can get close to and live with a disease and try to imagine how it really works, like Barbara McClintock's famous account in *A Feeling for the Organism* of how she won the Nobel Prize by living with corn, and getting to know each ear. Vezzani began to wonder, suppose we turn the concept of a "seizure" inside out. Suppose we all have electrical charges firing in the brain, but some kind of mechanism keeps neuron excitability within the homeostatic range and prevents it from breaking through, except for the 1 percent who experience seizures. If that model is accurate (and nearly all medical research is based on models that imagine how things work), then attention shifts from the convulsions themselves to what causes convulsive-like action to exceed its normal threshold in the 1 percent who experience epileptic seizures. The question then becomes how to prevent that threshold of normal excitability from being exceeded.

In Vezzani's new model, the threshold for convulsions is lowered by inflammation developing in the brain, which comprises certain molecules that make neurons more excitable. The question became, which of these molecules plays a key role? Working with mice, Vezzani and her team discovered an inflammatory pathway with proconvulsive activity involving High Mobility Group Box1 (HMGB1) and Interleukin-1 (IL-1β) proteins and their interaction with Toll-like receptor (TLR4) and IL-1 receptor type 1 (IL-1R1), respectively. Experimental data gathered so far "suggest a role for the HMGB1-TLR4 and IL-1β-IL-1R1 axis in human epilepsy."[38] Perhaps an anti-inflammatory therapy would be effective in the 15 million who do not respond to the classical anticonvulsive drugs.

The clinical development of a compound that blocks the biosynthesis of IL-1β by inhibiting interleukin converting enzyme represents an example of a more advanced therapeutic approach, whereby an anti-inflammatory drug has been tested with encouraging results in a small cohort of patients recruited in phase-2 clinical studies for the treatment of pharmaco-resistant epilepsy.

This long-term search for new, more effective medicines to control epilepsy is funded by charities in the United States, including the Epilepsy Therapy Project (http://www.epilepsy.com) and CURE (http://www.cureepilepsy .org), where Susan Axelrod is dedicated to promoting the search for the new treatments with no side effects. In the EU, funding comes from the European Commission Framework Programme and other charities. What makes working at the Mario Negri different, Vezzani said, was "how free we are to develop our own ideas. Not only can one concentrate mainly on one's research with few time-consuming obligations, but the department may also support your work for periods of time if you don't find full external funding."

A Rising Star Leaves America for the Mario Negri

Before Giuseppe Ristagno left a fine position at the Weil Institute of Critical Care Medicine in California to accept an offer from the Mario Negri, he had earned a degree in medicine and surgery at the University of Palermo with a score of 110 out of 110, plus honors. Soon after he finished medical school, Ristagno won a substantial three-year grant from the American Heart Association (AHA) on how to reduce permanent damage from cardiac arrest and how to do cardiopulmonary resuscitation (CPR) better. He then entered residency in anesthesia and intensive care at the University of Trieste and graduated with a perfect score of 50 out of 50 and honors again.

At a conference, he met Max Weil, the "father" of critical care and cofounder of the Weil Institute of Critical Care Medicine in Rancho Mirage, California. By the end of the conversation, Dr. Weil had decided to offer him the research fellowship in cardiac arrest and CPR. At the Weil Institute, Ristagno was soon given responsibility for all the projects and slated for promotion. But he missed Italy and his family and so he accepted a position at the Mario Negri in 2009. While working full-time on his grants, he entered the PhD program that the Mario Negri has with the Open University and completed his PhD in

November 2013. The next month, Mario Negri senior staff promoted him to the ranks of those with life tenure.

Ristagno then won a larger grant from the European Commission and another from the Italian Ministry of Health to evaluate the effectiveness of different drug combinations and pharmacological approaches in order to find out which work better—something companies are not interested in because they cannot patent or profit from it. Ristagno is also doing clinical studies in an emergency room on how to decide when to defibrillate and use drugs more effectively. He holds faculty positions at the Weil Institute and the University of Palermo.

We asked how the Mario Negri is different, and he said it's so multidisciplinary, with many possibilities to collaborate with experts in different fields, but in a culture of cooperation, not competition. When he left the Weil Institute for the Mario Negri, his friends said, "You're crazy. You won't be able to fund your own work." But funding has been easier at the Mario Negri, he told us, because it encourages each investigator to pursue his or her ideas, with full technical support. The Weil Institute has made generous offers to get Dr. Ristagno back, but he's happy at the Mario Negri and sees a bright future, saving lives by changing drug use and practices in cardiac arrest and CPR around the globe.

Cognitive Decline in the Oldest Old

For 12 years now, Ugo Lucca and his colleagues have been running "probably the largest prospective study specifically designed to investigate dementia and cognitive decline in a very large and representative population of the oldest old (some 2,500 persons 80 years and older), including a considerable number of individuals in the extreme age groups (more than 250 95–99 year olds and more than 250 centenarians)."[39] Of all residents over 80, a remarkable 89 percent agreed to participate. All lived in neighboring towns in the province of Varese, and before most of them died, all were visited in their place of residence, whether home or institution, by a skilled psychologist who administered a series of well-established questionnaires and scales, including with cognitive tests, about every aspect of their current and past lives. A proxy informant was interviewed as well. Blood, urine, and neurological examinations followed for those who agreed or were suspected of having dementia.

The study has found that among those over 80, about 28 percent of the women and 18 percent of the men suffered from dementia. One major finding is that after the age of 85, the prevalence of dementia is not doubling exponentially every five years, as many fear from the increase in earlier years. Rather dementia increases at a slower, linear rate, without leveling off in the extreme ages. The research finds that people with dementia have a 70 percent greater chance of dying, after controlling for possible confounders.

The only drugs that physicians have to treat patients with mild to moderate Alzheimer's disease are the cholinesterase inhibitors; but the patients

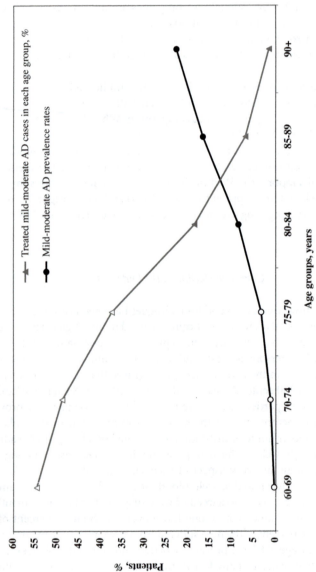

Figure 9.2 Percentage treated for Alzheimer's disease declines as prevalence increases

actually treated are a small proportion of those affected. This proportion decreases as the percentage of the patients with mild-moderate Alzheimer's increases with age. While 54.7 percent of people aged 60–69 are put on them, only 18.6 percent receive them in their 80s and just 1.6 percent in their 90s.[40] (See Figure 9.2). This may reflect difficulties in diagnosing different types of dementia, or the presence of other abnormalities, a fatalistic acceptance of the condition, or the frequency of adverse drug reactions, or the diminished effectiveness of the drugs in older patients.

No pharmaceutical company, bent on patenting and profiting, would fund a long-term, observational study like this one, and pharmaceutical companies rarely fund epidemiologic surveys, though we saw exceptions in Chapters 3 and 6. Companies exclude the old from nearly all their trials across all disease areas, including trials on drugs for Alzheimer's disease. Thus, despite huge sums spent on testing drugs, we have little data on how they affect the very old, even as their numbers grow rapidly.

The Monzino Foundation is to be commended for funding this important, prospective study. Equally significant are the dozens of survey experts, psychologists, neurologists, physicians, nurses, town counselors, laboratories, residential homes, and voluntary associations who are making the survey a success. Their names fill nearly a page in fine type, very much a Mario Negri signature as we saw in Chapters 3 and 6. They keep cash outlays low by turning Mario Negri surveys and clinical trials into a shared undertaking. The reported costs of commercial clinical trials are rising like a plane taking off because each aspect of running a trial or doing an observational study has been corporatized, and profits are fat. Even the Institutional Review Boards, originally set up as voluntary bodies by bioethicists concerned about the rights of participants, have become investor-owned giants and charge so much that hedge funds are buying into them. The Mario Negri Institute offers another paradigm—participatory but rigorous studies without the distorting effects of payoffs for everyone involved.

Managing Polypharmacy in the Elderly

Unlike most nonprofit, academic pharmacological research institutes in the world and commercial pharmaceutical ones as well, the Mario Negri has been committed to and taken responsibility for how drugs are actually used—or misused—in the community. As we read in Chapter 4, the Institute launched several initiatives to provide guidance for doctors and patients and to oppose false cures. Chapter 7 describes several initiatives of international significance by the Mario Negri to minimize use of ineffective and unsafe drugs. This is a model that other nations might want to emulate to stop wasting so much money on these drugs.

Polypharmacy in the elderly is a formidable problem, because so many older adults take potentially inappropriate medications, which puts them at an increased risk of adverse reactions and leads to multiple visits to the emergency room, hospital admissions, readmissions, and deaths. Within the Department of Neuroscience, the Mario Negri Institute has organized a Laboratory for Quality Assessment of Geriatric Therapies and Services. One initiative, led by Alessandro Nobili, establishes a registry for elderly in hospitalized medical wards known at REPOSI (http://www.reposi2013.org).[41] This research-in-action serves several functions. First, it creates a continuing record of morbidities and drugs among those over 65. Second, it provides the doctors who care for these patients with an ongoing comparative tool for looking at their practice and experience. Third, the registry provides the basis for research studies. Having a single-payer national health service greatly facilitates this kind of tracking patients and minimizing adverse events.

Other data in the registry include cognitive function, disability, and basic demographic information. About 45 percent of the participants are over 75 and 25 percent are over 85 years old. Patients average 5.6 diagnoses and are taking an average of 5.4 medicines. This overall average rises with age. A quarter of the elderly have severe drug-drug interactions—a deep worry since all the drugs were prescribed to help the patients get better. Complementing REPOSI is a Web-based program for physicians to teach how to do a comprehensive geriatric assessment, medication reconciliation, and medication review to improve the quality of prescribing. Mario Negri is running the registry in collaboration with the Society of Internal Medicine and the IRCCS Cà Granda Maggiore Policlinico Hospital Foundation of Milan.

A crucial aspect of appropriate drug prescribing is the need to implement a patient-centered approach. Patient centeredness implies the engagement of older people, their relatives and caregivers about options and the value of different treatments. Patients' feelings and beliefs about their health, their medical conditions and treatment options are key determinants of whether or not they will carry out recommended treatments. A free telephone service for drug and clinical information is available for physicians and the elderly.

A related initiative is to identify the possible misuse of drugs, or "potentially inappropriate medications" (PIMs) and deal with them using CPSS, the Computerized Prescription Support System. In a one-year study, this tool enabled clinicians to reduce PIMs by three-quarters.[42] If these methods were used across Europe, the United States, and elsewhere, far fewer elderly would be hospitalized or die from adverse interactions from the drugs they are being given to be healthier.

Good Pharma for Healthier Patients

These are only eight out of dozens of equally important research projects being carried out under the Mario Negri public health model of no-patent research, and they indicate how many critical needs and problems are neglected by patent-driven researchers. If people think that these kinds of unmet needs should be researched to find effective treatments and minimize adverse reactions, then they should consider the Mario Negri model and think about exempting medicines from patents once again, or instituting a model of patenting with compulsory licensing to maximize low prices and access.

From these examples and those in the rest of the book, readers can see that the Mario Negri's patient-centered outcomes research leads not only to developing clinically better medicines but also to addressing harmful practices that put patients at risk. These include biased and unethical trial designs, approving drugs by industry-funded regulators that do not require evidence based on representative populations that drug-candidates improve health, and prescribing more medicines at higher doses than are necessary. The Mario Negri Institute as a public health model attends to research on diseases and health problems that companies consider too unprofitable or unpatentable to support. The breakthrough work on arresting renal failure in Chapter 3, for example, did not come from discovering a breakthrough drug but on developing new therapeutic uses of existing drugs at low cost and by investigating in depth the mechanisms of action that can lead to more effective therapies.

Nations and universities everywhere have spawned a proliferation of patents to generate income through technological advances. But when it comes to medicines, the apparent success is largely illusory, because the number of *clinically* superior drugs pales before the flood of minor variations with substantial risks of serious harm, all heavily marketed at high prices as "better."[43] These new drugs may make patients worse.[44] With exceptions, net income to universities after the high costs of technology transfer is usually small, while the compromises to open, independent research are great.[45] Promising, unpatentable interventions are not even considered. Meantime, the paradigm of patenting medical research for profits is bankrupting entire health-care systems.[46]

It is time for a paradigm shift to research measured by how much products improve patient health, funded by foundations, charities, and governments, and uncorrupted by commercial pursuits. For over 50 years, the Mario Negri Institute has worked out ways to do first-class research in a collegial, open-science culture, where its dozens of research teams control the design, data, analysis, and publication of all results, independent of commercial or political pressures. It offers societal and institutional solutions to the pathologies of commercialized pharmaceutical research.

Appendix 1

Psychotropic Drugs: An Example of Mario Negri Research in the 1960s

This Appendix was prompted by the *New York Times* quoting Dr. Richard A. Friedman, professor and director of the Psychopharmacology Clinic at Weill Cornell Medical College, on Aug 19, 2013, as saying "With rare exceptions, it is hard to think of a single truly novel psychotropic drug that has emerged in the last 30 years . . . So why has the pharmaceutical industry churned out so many copycat drugs? The simple answer is that we don't yet understand the fundamental cause of most psychiatric disorders." This view is shared by researchers at the Mario Negri Institute for Pharmacological Research, who made several contributions more than 30 years ago to antidepressants, antipsychotics, and related drugs, and who have continued on the search for ways to relieve the great suffering caused by depression and schizophrenia.

An early illustration of pharmacological research by Garattini and his team was their investigations into what was happening physiologically and biochemically when people become seriously depressed or schizophrenic. This summary is based on Garattini's account in 1995.[1]

The international conference that Garatttini organized in May 1957 brought together many clinicians and scientists involved in psychopharmacology from all around the world. At that time, chlorpromazine (Thorazine), reserpine (Reserpine), meprobamate (Miltown, Equanil), iproniazid (Euphozid, Iprazid, Ipronid, Ipronin, Marsilid, Rivivol), and the amphetamines ("speed") had been developed and were all being used.

At the 1957 conference, Garattini recalled, "one could sense from the presentations the direction psychopharmacology was taking and the tremendous amount of work that still needed to be done to understand brain function. I see psychotropic drugs as tools to understand how the brain is functioning, to generate knowledge that could provide ideas to open new avenues for developing new drugs, more than just treatments. Actually only a few psychotropic drugs proved important in treatment . . . The brain is so complicated that probably there were few other ways but using drugs for learning about its functioning."

Research at the Institute was not restricted to psychopharmacology but also included neuroendocrinology and neuroimmunology, newly emerging research areas. The research ranged from basic molecular biology to clinical work in psychiatry that researchers did in collaboration with others because the Institute had no clinical arm. They did research with drugs in biochemistry, neurophysiology, behavioral pharmacology, endocrinology, and immunology. They also did research on psychiatric epidemiology and the evaluation of psychiatric services.

During the 1960s, most people bet that the most important neurotransmitter in depression was norepinephrine (also known as noradrenaline), and interest in serotonin was kept alive mainly in Europe. But then serotonin gained more attention, especially with the new class of selective serotonin reuptake inhibitors (SSRI drugs). Garattini and his team knew there was an interaction between serotonin and norepinephrine, and also between these and some of the other transmitters. "If you touch one neurotransmitter you induce a lot of interactions," he said. They also studied interactions with receptors, receptor subtypes, and transport mechanisms. In time, with microdialysis, they could measure the serotonin that was free and acting on receptors or various other targets, such as causing changes at pre- or postsynaptic receptors.

"We were probably the first to show the antagonistic effect between serotonin and chlorpromazine but we didn't get any recognition for it because we were obliged by the university to publish in Italian," Garattini said, a frustrating experience that reinforced his determination to publish only in English at the new Institute.

> We were doing experiments at the time with serotonin in isolated organs . . . and tried chlorpromazine, among many other substances. We were surprised to see the great antagonism between chlorpromazine and serotonin. We did our experiments in several isolated organs and also did some studies *in vivo*.
>
> There is really no difference between chlorpromazine and the new atypical antipsychotics except that chlorpromazine is also very active on norepinephrine. If we look back at the last 40 years we have not developed any antipsychotics that are clinically more effective than chlorpromazine. In the anxiolytic field we have added benzodiazepines (Xanax, Lexotan, other brands) and buspirone (Buspar) to meprobamate (Miltown, Equanil), but they don't offer major advances. None of the new antidepressants is superior to imipramine. The selective serotonin uptake inhibitors might have a different side-effect profile from tricyclic antidepressants, although even on looking carefully though the literature that is not completely clear. In any case, what we have in new drug development is still disappointing.
>
> Since what people and clinicians call depression has no clear biomarkers and cannot be induced as a disease, how can one know that antidepressive drugs relieve it?
>
> We were also the first to show the antagonism between reserpine and imipramine (Tofranil), the first tricyclic antidepressant. Imipramine was considered

to be a chlorpromazine-like drug. There was some skepticism in those years about whether a drug could have antidepressant effects. There was no animal model for depression we could use to show antidepressant activity. So since some clinical experience indicated that reserpine might have caused depression in some patients treated for hypertension, we used some of the behavioral effects of reserpine as a model for depression. We induced changes like hypothermia and ptosis with reserpine in the animal and tried to see whether imipramine antagonized these changes. It worked, and reserpine reversal became an important pharmacological test for screening and developing new antidepressants . . . It was interesting to see that imipramine was an antagonist of reserpine and chlorpromazine was not. So I think the development of an animal model of depression that could be used in screening for antidepressants was also an important contribution we made.

These methods, however, have a circular, self-referent character that raises fundamental issues discussed below. Tognoni and Garattini were among the first to find that *increasing the dosage of antidepressants did not reduce symptoms of depression but did increase the risks of toxic side effects.* "Psychiatrists began prescribing tricyclic anti-depressants in the early 60s and believed the higher the dose, the more effective the drug," Garattini said. "Our findings showed that higher doses increased the risk of side effects, such as cardiac complications, constipation, and bronchoconstriction with no increased benefit. On the whole, however, psychiatrists ignored this important finding and did not lower doses—they had no motive to." Through the international network of medical writers and sponsored journals, pharmaceutical companies kept important, independent work like this away from the attention of practitioners.[2]

"In the late 1950s we [also] studied the effects of electroshock and showed that it produced changes in serotonin. Later on this was also shown by others, using more sophisticated techniques. We made contributions to understanding of the mechanism of action of benzodiazepines too . . . We also did a lot of research on benzodiazepine pharmacokinetics at the time and published the first reports on these."

Garattini raised a radical question about the role of serotonin in depression by relating it to research on the diet drug, fenfluramine. "We invested a lot of research in the area of anorectic agents, like fenfluramine and the active metabolite of fenfluramine . . . We found that the metabolite of fenfluramine accumulates in the body differently from the parent substance, and with high doses can lead to a long-lasting decrease of serotonin." There are probably hundreds of thousands of people taking fenfluramine, and if they don't experience any effect from decreased serotonin, "*it makes one wonder about the role of serotonin in brain function.*"

"At the time of the Milan symposium, when I started my research with serotonin, it looked as if we would progress rapidly in understanding how the brain functions and develop drugs to take care of all psychiatric diseases. After almost 30 years, though, I must say these expectations have not been fulfilled."

"One of the problems is that we used the drugs as tools to find out what they do, and then we used that understanding to pick up new compounds. [a self-referring circularity] *If one picks compounds this way, they are bound to have actions similar to what we started with.*" But now that we are accessing postreceptor mechanisms all the way down the chain of events [in 1995], we should find new points in the system that drugs might attack. "Some time ago I organized a meeting in Milan on new tests for new drugs, because if we continue with the same tests as today we will just have more chemical entities of the same type. *Maybe all the drugs we have are similar because they have been detected by the same tests.* [No major advances have been made in developing novel animal models.] We should probably work to develop drugs that are selectively effective for one or more subpopulations of patients."

"In other words, we might develop drugs for a certain type of depression but not for all depressions. But to do that will require changes in our approach to drug development, because industry will not be interested in developing drugs without a sufficiently large market to get back their investment. This is a problem that needs to be solved. In order to progress we need to find a way to dissociate the development of the drug from the question of profit. There is a conflict between our needs and what companies are developing that will have to be overcome."

"I think we shall have to find a way in the future to bring together the know-how of industry with the know-how of independent research institutions and reconcile their interests with the interests of the public . . . It is time to think in a different way about how to develop psychotropic drugs. Take as an example the field of anti-hypertensives. We have so many anti-hypertensives that work through different mechanisms and they may be effective on different subpopulations. But we don't take advantage of that to prescribe the specific anti-hypertensive agent for each [specific] group of patients." Funding for such trials of postpatent drugs is not available.

"This is more or less what is happening in psychopharmacology [in 1995], when we talk about the use of neuroleptics in schizophrenic or other psychotic patients. We have many neuroleptics, and one or another of these may be more selectively effective in one subpopulation of patients or another [what is now called "personalized medicine"]. *But testing and evaluation need to be independent of profit* (for example, trials run through NIH in the U.S. and similar institutions in other countries) in order the find out which one works best on which type of patient."

Appendix 2

Published Trials by the Mario Negri Institute since 2000

1. Effectiveness of nebulized beclomethasone in preventing viral wheezing: An RCT. Clavenna A. Sequi M. Cartabia M. Fortinguerra F. Borghi M. Bonati M. Pediatrics (2014) 133:3 (e505–e512). Date of Publication: 2014
2. Differences in the acute effects of aerobic and resistance exercise in subjects with type 2 diabetes: Results from the RAED2 randomized trial. Bacchi E. Negri C. Trombetta M. Zanolin M.E. Lanza M. Bonora E. Moghetti P. Diabetes Technology and Therapeutics (2014) 16: SUPPL. 1 (S94–S95). Date of Publication: 2014
3. Efficacy of coupled plasma filtration adsorption (CPFA) in patients with septic shock: A multicenter randomised controlled clinical trial. Livigni S. Bertolini G. Rossi C. Ferrari F. Giardino M. Pozzato M. Remuzzi G. BMJ Open (2014) 4:1 Article Number: e003536. Date of Publication: 2014
4. Doxycycline in Creutzfeldt-Jakob disease: A phase 2, randomised, double-blind, placebo-controlled trial. Haik S. Marcon G. Mallet A. Tettamanti M. Welaratne A. Giaccone G. Azimi S. Pietrini V. Fabreguettes J.-R. Imperiale D. Cesaro P. Buffa C. Aucan C. Lucca U. Peckeu L. Suardi S. Tranchant C. Zerr I. Houillier C. Redaelli V. Vespignani H. Campanella A. Sellal F. Krasnianski A. Seilhean D. Heinemann U. Sedel F. Canovi M. Gobbi M. Di Fede G. Laplanche J.-L. Pocchiari M. Salmona M. Forloni G. Brandel J.-P. Tagliavini F. The Lancet Neurology (2014) 13:2 (150–158). Date of Publication: February 2014
5. Perinatal factors and the risk of atopic dermatitis: A cohort study. Parazzini F. Cipriani S. Zinetti C. Chatenoud L. Frigerio L. Amuso G. Ciammella M. Di Landro A. Naldi L. Pediatric Allergy and Immunology (2014) 25:1 (43–50). Date of Publication: February 2014
6. Sorafenib does not improve efficacy of chemotherapy in advanced pancreatic cancer: A GISCAD randomized phase II study. Cascinu S. Berardi R. Sobrero A. Bidoli P. Labianca R. Siena S. Ferrari D. Barni S. Aitini E. Zagonel V. Caprioni F. Villa F. Mosconi S. Faloppi L. Tonini G. Boni C. Conte P. Di Costanzo F. Cinquini M. Digestive and Liver Disease (2014) 46:2 (182–186). Date of Publication: February 2014
7. Bardoxolone methyl in type 2 diabetes and stage 4 chronic kidney disease. De Zeeuw D. Akizawa T. Audhya P. Bakris G.L. Chin M. Christ-Schmidt H. Goldsberry A. Houser M. Krauth M. Lambers Heerspink H.J. McMurray J.J. Meyer C.J. Parving H.-H. Remuzzi G. Toto R.D. Vaziri N.D. Wanner C. Wittes

J. Wrolstad D. Chertow G.M. New England Journal of Medicine (2013) 369:26 (2492–2503). Date of Publication: 2013

8. Twenty-four hour efficacy with preservative free tafluprost compared with latanoprost in patients with primary open angle glaucoma or ocular hypertension. Konstas A.G.P. Quaranta L. Katsanos A. Riva I. Tsai J.C. Giannopoulos T. Voudouragkaki I.C. Paschalinou E. Floriani I. Haidich A.-B. British Journal of Ophthalmology (2013) 97:12 (1510–1515). Date of Publication: December 2013

9. Effect of longacting somatostatin analogue on kidney and cyst growth in autosomal dominant polycystic kidney disease (ALADIN): A randomised, placebo-controlled, multicentre trial. Caroli A. Perico N. Perna A. Antiga L. Brambilla P. Pisani A. Visciano B. Imbriaco M. Messa P. Cerutti R. Dugo M. Cancian L. Buongiorno E. De Pascalis A. Gaspari F. Carrara F. Rubis N. Prandini S. Remuzzi A. Remuzzi G. Ruggenenti P. The Lancet (2013) 382:9903 (1485–1495). Date of Publication: 2013

10. Thymidylate synthase, topoisomerase-1 and microsatellite instability: Relationship with outcome in mucinous colorectal cancer treated with fluorouracil. Negri F.V. Azzoni C. Bottarelli L. Campanini N. Mandolesi A. Wotherspoon A. Cunningham D. Scartozzi M. Cascinu S. Tinelli C. Silini E.M. Ardizzoni A. Anticancer Research (2013) 33:10 (4611–4617). Date of Publication: October 2013

11. Both resistance training and aerobic training reduce hepatic fat content in type 2 diabetic subjects with nonalcoholic fatty liver disease (the RAED2 randomized trial). Bacchi E. Negri C. Targher G. Faccioli N. Lanza M. Zoppini G. Zanolin E. Schena F. Bonora E. Moghetti P. Hepatology (2013) 58:4 (1287–1295). Date of Publication: October 2013

12. Comparative pharmacokinetic and pharmacodynamic evaluation of branded and generic formulations of meloxicam in healthy male volunteers. Del Tacca M. Pasqualetti G. Gori G. Pepe P. Di Paolo A. Lastella M. De Negri F. Blandizzi C. Therapeutics and Clinical Risk Management (2013) 9:1 (303–311). Date of Publication: 2013

13. In kidney transplant patients, alemtuzumab but not basiliximab/low-dose rabbit anti-thymocyte globulin induces B cell depletion and regeneration, which associates with a high incidence of de novo donor-specific anti-HLA antibody development. Todeschini M. Cortinovis M. Perico N. Poli F. Innocente A. Cavinato R.A. Gotti E. Ruggenenti P. Gaspari F. Noris M. Remuzzi G. Casiraghi F. Journal of Immunology (2013) 191:5 (2818–2828). Date of Publication: 1 Sep 2013

14. Effect on blood pressure of combined inhibition of endothelin-converting enzyme and neutral endopeptidase with daglutril in patients with type 2 diabetes who have albuminuria: A randomised, crossover, double-blind, placebo-controlled trial. Parvanova A. van der Meer I.M. Iliev I. Perna A. Gaspari F. Trevisan R. Bossi A. Remuzzi G. Benigni A. Ruggenenti P. The Lancet Diabetes and Endocrinology (2013) 1:1 (19–27). Date of Publication: September 2013

15. Erlotinib versus docetaxel as second-line treatment of patients with advanced non-small-cell lung cancer and wild-type EGFR tumours (TAILOR): A randomised controlled trial. Garassino M.C. Martelli O. Broggini M. Farina G. Veronese S. Rulli E. Bianchi F. Bettini A. Longo F. Moscetti L. Tomirotti M. Marabese M. Ganzinelli M. Lauricella C. Labianca R. Floriani I. Giaccone G. Torri V. Scanni A. Marsoni S. The Lancet Oncology (2013) 14:10 (981–988). Date of Publication: September 2013

16. Randomized double-blind placebo-controlled trial of acetyl-L-carnitine for ALS. Beghi E. Pupillo E. Bonito V. Buzzi P. Caponnetto C. Chio A. Corbo M. Giannini

F. Inghilleri M. Bella V.L. Logroscino G. Lorusso L. Lunetta C. Mazzini L. Messina P. Mora G. Perini M. Quadrelli M.L. Silani V. Simone I.L. Tremolizzo L. Samarelli V. Tortelli R. D'Errico E. Merello M. Tavernelli F. Mancardi G.L. Mascolo M. Bendotti C. Buratti M. Floriani I. Giordano L. Giussani G. Maderna L. Maestri E. Marinou K. Mennini T. Messina S. Morelli C. Papetti L. Rizzo A. Ticozzi N. Verde F. Ferrarese C. Marzorati L. Testa L. Valentino F. Frasca V. Giacomelli E. Casa S. Malentacchi M. Calvo A. Cammarosano S. Moglia C. Cavallo E. Fuda G. Amyotrophic Lateral Sclerosis and Frontotemporal Degeneration (2013) 14:5–6 (397–405). Date of Publication: September 2013

17. The long-term multicenter observational study of dabigatran treatment in patients with atrial fibrillation (RELY-ABLE) study. Connolly S.J. Wallentin L. Ezekowitz M.D. Eikelboom J. Oldgren J. Reilly P.A. Brueckmann M. Pogue J. Alings M. Amerena J.V. Avezum A. Baumgartner I. Budaj A.J. Chen J.-H. Dans A.L. Darius H. Di Pasquale G. Ferreira J. Flaker G.C. Flather M.D. Franzosi M.G. Golitsyn S.P. Halon D.A. Heidbuchel H. Hohnloser S.H. Huber K. Jansky P. Kamensky G. Keltai M. Kim S.S. Lau C.-P. Le Heuzey J.-Y. Lewis B.S. Liu L. Nanas J. Omar R. Pais P. Pedersen K.E. Piegas L.S. Raev D. Smith P.J. Talajic M. Tan R.S. Tanomsup S. Toivonen L. Vinereanu D. Xavier D. Zhu J. Wang S.Q. Duffy C.O. Themeles E. Yusuf S. Circulation (2013) 128:3 (237–243). Date of Publication: 16 Jul 2013

18. Impact of vitamin D administration on immunogenicity of trivalent inactivated influenza vaccine in previously unvaccinated children. Principi N. Marchisio P. Terranova L. Zampiero A. Baggi E. Daleno C. Tirelli S. Pelucchi C. Esposito S. Human Vaccines and Immunotherapeutics (2013) 9:5 (969–974). Date of Publication: May 2013

19. Randomised Phase II Trial (NCT00637975) Evaluating Activity and Toxicity of Two Different Escalating Strategies for Pregabalin and Oxycodone Combination Therapy for Neuropathic Pain in Cancer Patients. Garassino M.C. Piva S. la Verde N. Spagnoletti I. Iorno V. Carbone C. Febbraro A. Bianchi A. Bramati A. Moretti A. Ganzinelli M. Marabese M. Gentili M. Torri V. Farina G. PLoS ONE (2013) 8:4 Article Number: e59981. Date of Publication: 5 Apr 2013

20. Rationale and trial design of bardoxolone methyl evaluation in patients with chronic kidney disease and type 2 diabetes: The Occurrence of Renal Events (BEACON). De Zeeuw D. Akizawa T. Agarwal R. Audhya P. Bakris G.L. Chin M. Krauth M. Lambers Heerspink H.J. Meyer C.J. McMurray J.J. Parving H.-H. Pergola P.E. Remuzzi G. Toto R.D. Vaziri N.D. Wanner C. Warnock D.G. Wittes J. Chertow G.M. American Journal of Nephrology (2013) 37:3 (212–222). Date of Publication: April 2013

21. Could interferon still play a role in metastatic renal cell carcinoma? A randomized study of two schedules of sorafenib plus interferon-alpha 2a (RAPSODY). Bracarda S. Porta C. Boni C. Santoro A. Mucciarini C. Pazzola A. Cortesi E. Gasparro D. Labianca R. Di Costanzo F. Falcone A. Cinquini M. Caserta C. Paglino C. De Angelis V. European Urology (2013) 63:2 (254–261). Date of Publication: February 2013

22. Hemoglobin stability in patients with anemia, CKD, and type 2 diabetes: An analysis of the TREAT (trial to reduce cardiovascular events with aranesp therapy) placebo arm. Skali H. Lin J. Pfeffer M.A. Chen C.-Y. Cooper M.E. McMurray J.J.V. Nissenson A.R. Remuzzi G. Rossert J. Parfrey P.S. Scott-Douglas N.W. Singh A.K. Toto R. Uno H. Ivanovich P. American Journal of Kidney Diseases (2013) 61:2 (238–246). Date of Publication: February 2013

23. Differences in the Acute Effects of Aerobic and Resistance Exercise in Subjects with Type 2 Diabetes: Results from the RAED2 Randomized Trial. Bacchi E. Negri C. Trombetta M. Zanolin M.E. Lanza M. Bonora E. Moghetti P. PLoS ONE (2012) 7:12 Article Number: e49937. Date of Publication: 5 Dec 2012

24. The postoperative analgesic efficacy of preperitoneal continuous wound infusion compared to epidural continuous infusion with local anesthetics after colorectal cancer surgery: A randomized controlled multicenter study. Bertoglio S. Fabiani F. De Negri P. Corcione A. Merlo D.F. Cafiero F. Esposito C. Belluco C. Pertile D. Amodio R. Mannucci M. Fontana V. De Cicco M. Zappi L. Anesthesia and Analgesia (2012) 115:6 (1442–1450). Date of Publication: December 2012

25. Comparison between the AA/EPA ratio in depressed and non depressed elderly females: Omega-3 fatty acid supplementation correlates with improved symptoms but does not change immunological parameters. Rizzo A.M. Corsetto P.A. Montorfano G. Opizzi A. Faliva M. Giacosa A. Ricevuti G. Pelucchi C. Berra B. Rondanelli M. Nutrition Journal (2012) 11:1 Article Number: 82. Date of Publication: 2012

26. Circadian intraocular pressure and blood pressure reduction with timolol 0.5% solution and timogel 0.1% in patients with primary open-angle glaucoma. Quaranta L. Katsanos A. Floriani I. Riva I. Russo A. Konstas A.G.P. Journal of Clinical Pharmacology (2012) 52:10 (1552–1557). Date of Publication: October 2012

27. Reply to FOLFIRI plus cetuximab versus FOLFIRI plus bevacizumab as first-line treatment for patients with metastatic colorectal cancer-subgroup analysis of patients with KRAS-mutated tumours in the randomised German AIO study KRK-0306. Pietrantonio F. Garassino M.C. Torri V. De Braud F. Annals of Oncology (2012) 23:10 (2771–2772) Article Number: mds332. Date of Publication: October 2012

28. Measurable urinary albumin predicts cardiovascular risk among normoalbuminuric patients with type 2 diabetes. Ruggenenti P. Porrini E. Motterlini N. Perna A. Ilieva A.P. Iliev I.P. Dodesini A.R. Trevisan R. Bossi A. Sampietro G. Capitoni E. Gaspari F. Rubis N. Ene-Iordache B. Remuzzi G. Journal of the American Society of Nephrology (2012) 23:10 (1717–1724). Date of Publication: 28 Sep 2012

29. Immediate effects of bilateral grade III mobilization of the talocrural joint on the balance of elderly women. Pertille A. MacEdo A.B. Dibai Filho A.V. Rego E.M. Arrais L.D.D.F. Negri J.R. Teodori R.M. Journal of Manipulative and Physiological Therapeutics (2012) 35:7 (549–555). Date of Publication: September 2012

30. Carbon dioxide insufflation in open-chamber cardiac surgery: A double-blind, randomized clinical trial of neurocognitive effects. Chaudhuri K. Storey E. Lee G.A. Bailey M. Chan J. Rosenfeldt F.L. Pick A. Negri J. Gooi J. Zimmet A. Esmore D. Merry C. Rowland M. Lin E. Marasco S.F. Journal of Thoracic and Cardiovascular Surgery (2012) 144:3 (646–653.e1). Date of Publication: September 2012

31. Systematic lymphadenectomy in ovarian cancer at second-look surgery: A randomised clinical trial. Dell Anna T. Signorelli M. Benedetti-Panici P. Maggioni A. Fossati R. Fruscio R. Milani R. Bocciolone L. Buda A. Mangioni C. Scambia G. Angioli R. Campagnutta E. Grassi R. Landoni F. British Journal of Cancer (2012) 107:5 (785–792). Date of Publication: 21 Aug 2012

32. Final overall survival results of phase III GCIG CALYPSO trial of pegylated liposomal doxorubicin and carboplatin vs paclitaxel and carboplatin in platinum-sensitive ovarian cancer patients. Wagner U. Marth C. Largillier R. Kaern J. Brown C. Heywood M. Bonaventura T. Vergote I. Piccirillo M.C. Fossati R.

Gebski V. Lauraine E.P. British Journal of Cancer (2012) 107:4 (588–591). Date of Publication: 7 Aug 2012

33. A multicentre, randomised, open-label, controlled trial evaluating equivalence of inhalational and intravenous anaesthesia during elective craniotomy. Citerio G. Pesenti A. Latini R. Masson S. Barlera S. Gaspari F. Franzosi M.G. European Journal of Anaesthesiology (2012) 29:8 (371–379). Date of Publication: August 2012

34. Intravenous immunoglobulin versus intravenous methylprednisolone for chronic inflammatory demyelinating polyradiculoneuropathy: A randomised controlled trial. Nobile-Orazio E. Cocito D. Jann S. Uncini A. Beghi E. Messina P. Antonini G. Fazio R. Gallia F. Schenone A. Francia A. Pareyson D. Santoro L. Tamburin S. Macchia R. Cavaletti G. Giannini F. Sabatelli M. The Lancet Neurology (2012) 11:6 (493–502). Date of Publication: June 2012

35. Comparison of defibrillation efficacy between two pads placements in a pediatric porcine model of cardiac arrest. Ristagno G. Yu T. Quan W. Freeman G. Li Y. Resuscitation (2012) 83:6 (755–759). Date of Publication: June 2012

36. Annual or biennial CT screening versus observation in heavy smokers: 5-year results of the MILD trial. Pastorino U. Rossi M. Rosato V. Marchiano A. Sverzellati N. Morosi C. Fabbri A. Galeone C. Negri E. Sozzi G. Pelosi G. La Vecchia C. European Journal of Cancer Prevention (2012) 21:3 (308–315). Date of Publication: May 2012

37. Heparin in pregnant women with previous placenta-mediated pregnancy complications: A prospective, randomized, multicenter, controlled clinical trial. Martinelli I. Ruggenenti P. Cetin I. Pardi G. Perna A. Vergani P. Acaia B. Facchinetti F. La Sala G.B. Bozzo M. Rampello S. Marozio L. Diadei O. Gherardi G. Carminati S. Remuzzi G. Mannucci P.M. Blood (2012) 119:14 (3269–3275). Date of Publication: 5 Apr 2012

38. Increased risk of cognitive and functional decline in patients with atrial fibrillation: Results of the ONTARGET and TRANSCEND studies. Marzona I. O'Donnell M. Teo K. Gao P. Anderson C. Bosch J. Yusuf S. Canadian Medical Association Journal (2012) 184:6 (E329–E336). Date of Publication: 3 Apr 2012

39. Effects of candesartan on left ventricular function, aldosterone and BNP in chronic heart failure. Aleksova A. Masson S. Maggioni A.P. Lucci D. Urso R. Staszewsky L. Ciaffoni S. Cacciatore G. Misuraca G. Gulizia M. Mos L. Proietti G. Minneci C. Latini R. Sinagra G. Cardiovascular Drugs and Therapy (2012) 26:2 (131–143). Date of Publication: April 2012

40. Metabolic effects of aerobic training and resistance training in type 2 diabetic subjects: A randomized controlled trial (the RAED2 study). Bacchi E. Negri C. Zanolin M.E. Milanese C. Faccioli N. Trombetta M. Zoppini G. Cevese A. Bonadonna R.C. Schena F. Bonora E. Lanza M. Moghetti P. Diabetes Care (2012) 35:4 (676–682). Date of Publication: April 2012

41. A 6-month randomized controlled trial of intravenous immunoglobulins versus intravenousmethylprednisolone in chronic inflammatory demyelinating polyradiculoneuropathy (IMC study). Nobile-Orazio E. Cocito D. Jann S. Uncini A. Messina P. Antonini G. Fazio R. Gallia F. Schenone A. Francia A. Pareyson P. Santoro L. Tamburin S. Macchia R. Guarneri C. Cavaletti G. Giannini F. Sabatelli M. Beghi E. Journal of the Peripheral Nervous System (2012) 17 SUPPL. 1 (S39–S40). Date of Publication: April 2012

42. Reply to letters regarding article, "risk of bleeding with 2 doses of dabigatran compared with warfarin in older and younger patients with atrial fibrillation: An

analysis of the randomized evaluation of long-term anticoagulant therapy (RE-LY) trial." Eikelboom J.W. Connolly S.J. Healey J.S. Yang S. Yusuf S. Wallentin L. Oldgren J. Ezekowitz M. Alings M. Kaatz S. Hohnloser S.H. Diener H.-C. Franzosi M.G. Huber K. Reilly P. Varrone J. Circulation (2012) 125:3 (e293–e294). Date of Publication: 24 Jan 2012

43. Randomized phase III study of surgery alone or surgery plus preoperative cisplatin and gemcitabine in stages IB to IIIA non-small-cell lung cancer. Scagliotti G.V. Pastorino U. Vansteenkiste J.F. Spaggiari L. Facciolo F. Orlowski T.M. Maiorino L. Hetzel M. Leschinger M. Visseren-Grul C. Torri V. Journal of Clinical Oncology (2012) 30:2 (172–178). Date of Publication: 10 Jan 2012

44. Effects of manidipine and delapril in hypertensive patients with type 2 diabetes mellitus: The delapril and manidipine for nephroprotection in diabetes (DEMAND) randomized clinical trial. Ruggenenti P. Lauria G. Iliev I.P. Fassi A. Ilieva A.P. Rota S. Chiurchiu C. Barlovic D.P. Sghirlanzoni A. Lombardi R. Penza P. Cavaletti G. Piatti M.L. Frigeni B. Filipponi M. Rubis N. Noris G. Motterlini N. Ene-Iordache B. Gaspari F. Perna A. Zaletel J. Bossi A. Dodesini A.R. Trevisan R. Remuzzi G. Hypertension (2011) 58:5 (776–783). Date of Publication: November 2011

45. Phosphate may promote CKD progression and attenuate renoprotective effect of ACE inhibition. Zoccali C. Ruggenenti P. Perna A. Leonardis D. Tripepi R. Tripepi G. Mallamaci F. Remuzzi G. Journal of the American Society of Nephrology (2011) 22:10 (1923–1930). Date of Publication: October 2011

46. Antiproteinuric effect of chemokine C-C motif ligand 2 inhibition in subjects with acute proliferative lupus nephritis. Ble A. Mosca M. Di Loreto G. Guglielmotti A. Biondi G. Bombardieri S. Remuzzi G. Ruggenenti P. American Journal of Nephrology (2011) 34:4 (367–372). Date of Publication: October 2011

47. A double-blind, randomised, placebo-controlled phase III intergroup study of gefitinib in patients with advanced NSCLC, non-progressing after first line platinum-based chemotherapy (EORTC 08021/ILCP 01/03). Gaafar R.M. Surmont V.F. Scagliotti G.V. Van Klaveren R.J. Papamichael D. Welch J.J. Hasan B. Torri V. Van Meerbeeck J.P. European Journal of Cancer (2011) 47:15 (2331–2340). Date of Publication: October 2011

48. Effects of high dose aleglitazar on renal function in patients with type 2 diabetes. Herz M. Gaspari F. Perico N. Viberti G. Urbanowska T. Rabbia M. Kirk D.W. International Journal of Cardiology (2011) 151:2 (136–142). Date of Publication: 1 Sep 2011

49. Clinical characteristics of patients with asymptomatic recurrences of atrial fibrillation in the Gruppo Italiano per lo Studio della Sopravvivenza nell'Infarto Miocardico-Atrial Fibrillation (GISSI-AF) trial. Disertori M. Lombardi F. Barlera S. Maggioni A.P. Favero C. Franzosi M.G. Lucci D. Staszewsky L. Fabbri G. Quintarelli S. Bianconi L. Latini R. American Heart Journal (2011) 162:2 (382–389). Date of Publication: August 2011

50. Treatment of first tonic—Clonic seizure does not affect mortality: Long-term follow-up of a randomised clinical trial. Leone M.A. Vallalta R. Solari A. Beghi E. Journal of Neurology, Neurosurgery and Psychiatry (2011) 82:8 (924–927). Date of Publication: August 2011

51. Effect of aliskiren in patients with heart failure according to background dose of ACE inhibitor: A retrospective analysis of the aliskiren observation of heart failure treatment (ALOFT) trial. Sidik N.P. Solomon S.D. Latini R. Maggioni A.P.

Wright M. Gimpelewicz C.R. Pitt B. McMurray J.J.V. Cardiovascular Drugs and Therapy (2011) 25:4 (315–321). Date of Publication: August 2011

52. Associations of albuminuria in patients with chronic heart failure: Findings in the Aliskiren Observation of Heart Failure Treatment study. Jackson C.E. Mac-Donald M.R. Petrie M.C. Solomon S.D. Pitt B. Latini R. Maggioni A.P. Smith B.A. Prescott M.F. Lewsey J. McMurray J.J.V. European Journal of Heart Failure (2011) 13:7 (746–754). Date of Publication: July 2011

53. Neurohumoral effects of aliskiren in patients with symptomatic heart failure receiving a mineralocorticoid receptor antagonist: The Aliskiren Observation of Heart Failure Treatment study. Pitt B. Latini R. Maggioni A.P. Solomon S.D. Smith B.A. Wright M. Prescott M.F. McMurray J.J.V. European Journal of Heart Failure (2011) 13:7 (755–764). Date of Publication: July 2011

54. ACE inhibition is renoprotective among obese patients with proteinuria. Mallamaci F. Ruggenenti P. Perna A. Leonardis D. Tripepi R. Tripepi G. Remuzzi G. Zoccali C. Journal of the American Society of Nephrology (2011) 22:6 (1122–1128). Date of Publication: June 2011

55. An open-label, randomized clinical trial assessing immunogenicity, safety and tolerability of pandemic influenza A/H1N1 MF59-adjuvanted vaccine administered sequentially or simultaneously with seasonal virosomal-adjuvanted influenza vaccine to paediatric kidney transplant recipients. Esposito S. Meregalli E. Daleno C. Ghio L. Tagliabue C. Valzano A. Serra D. Galeone C. Edefonti A. Principi N. Nephrology Dialysis Transplantation (2011) 26:6 (2018–2024). Date of Publication: June 2011

56. Risk of bleeding with 2 doses of dabigatran compared with warfarin in older and younger patients with atrial fibrillation: An analysis of the randomized evaluation of long-term anticoagulant therapy (RE-LY) Trial. Eikelboom J.W. Wallentin L. Connolly S.J. Ezekowitz M. Healey J.S. Oldgren J. Yang S. Alings M. Kaatz S. Hohnloser S.H. Diener H.-C. Franzosi M.G. Huber K. Reilly P. Varrone J. Yusuf S. Circulation (2011) 123:21 (2363–2372). Date of Publication: 31 May 2011

57. Intermittent versus continuous chemotherapy in advanced colorectal cancer: A randomised 'GISCAD' trial. Labianca R. Sobrero A. Isa L. Cortesi E. Barni S. Nicolella D. Aglietta M. Lonardi S. Corsi D. Turci D. Beretta G.D. Fornarini G. Dapretto E. Floriani I. Zaniboni A. Annals of Oncology (2011) 22:5 (1236–1242). Date of Publication: 2011

58. Randomized phase III clinical trial evaluating weekly cisplatin for advanced epithelial ovarian cancer. Fruscio R. Garbi A. Parma G. Lissoni A.A. Garavaglia D. Bonazzi C.M. Dell'Anna T. Mangioni C. Milani R. Colombo N. Journal of the National Cancer Institute (2011) 103:4 (347–351). Date of Publication: 16 Feb 2011

59. Oral ondansetron versus domperidone for symptomatic treatment of vomiting during acute gastroenteritis in children: Multicentre randomized controlled trial. Marchetti F. Maestro A. Rovere F. Zanon D. Arrighini A. Bertolani P. Biban P. Da Dalt L. Di Pietro P. Renna S. Guala A. Mannelli F. Pazzaglia A. Messi G. Perri F. Reale A. Urbino A.F. Valletta E. Vitale A. Zangardi T. Tondelli M.T. Clavenna A. Bonati M. Ronfani L. BMC Pediatrics (2011) 11 Article Number: 15. Date of Publication: 10 Feb 2011

60. Effects of verapamil added-on trandolapril therapy in hypertensive type 2 diabetes patients with microalbuminuria: The BENEDICT-B randomized trial. Ruggenenti P. Fassi A. Ilieva A.P. Iliev I.P. Chiurchiu C. Rubis N. Gherardi G.

Ene-Iordache B. Gaspari F. Perna A. Cravedi P. Bossi A. Trevisan R. Motterlini N. Remuzzi G. Journal of Hypertension (2011) 29:2 (207–216). Date of Publication: February 2011

61. Circulating cardiovascular biomarkers in recurrent atrial fibrillation: Data from the GISSI-Atrial Fibrillation Trial. Latini R. Masson S. Pirelli S. Barlera S. Pulitano G. Carbonieri E. Gulizia M. Vago T. Favero C. Zdunek D. Struck J. Staszewsky L. Maggioni A.P. Franzosi M.G. Disertori M. Journal of Internal Medicine (2011) 269:2 (160–171). Date of Publication: February 2011

62. Long chain omega-3 polyunsaturated fatty acids supplementation in the treatment of elderly depression: Effects on depressive symptoms, on phospholipids fatty acids profile and on health-related quality of life. Rondanelli M. Giacosa A. Opizzi A. Pelucchi C. La Vecchia C. Montorfano G. Negroni M. Berra B. Politi P. Rizzo A.M. Journal of Nutrition, Health and Aging (2011) 15:1 (37–44). Date of Publication: January 2011

63. Effects of n-3 polyunsaturated fatty acids and of rosuvastatin on left ventricular function in chronic heart failure: A substudy of GISSI-HF trial. Ghio S. Scelsi L. Latini R. Masson S. Eleuteri E. Palvarini M. Vriz O. Pasotti M. Gorini M. Marchioli R. Maggioni A. Tavazzi L. European Journal of Heart Failure (2010) 12:12 (1345–1353). Date of Publication: December 2010

64. Selective vitamin D receptor activation with paricalcitol for reduction of albuminuria in patients with type 2 diabetes (VITAL study): A randomised controlled trial. De Zeeuw D. Agarwal R. Amdahl M. Audhya P. Coyne D. Garimella T. Parving H.-H. Pritchett Y. Remuzzi G. Ritz E. Andress D. The Lancet (2010) 376:9752 (1543–1551). Date of Publication: 6 Nov 2010

65. Effects of add-on fluvastatin therapy in patients with chronic proteinuric nephropathy on dual renin-angiotensin system blockade: The ESPLANADE trial. Ruggenenti P. Perna A. Tonelli M. Loriga G. Motterlini N. Rubis N. Ledda F. Rota Jr. S. Satta A. Granata A. Battaglia G. Cambareri F. David S. Gaspari F. Stucchi N. Carminati S. Ene-Iordache B. Cravedi P. Remuzzi G. Clinical Journal of the American Society of Nephrology (2010) 5:11 (1928–1938). Date of Publication: 1 Nov 2010

66. Supervised walking groups to increase physical activity in type 2 diabetic patients. Negri C. Bacchi E. Morgante S. Soave D. Marques A. Menghini E. Muggeo M. Bonora E. Moghetti P. Diabetes Care (2010) 33:11 (2333–2335). Date of Publication: November 2010

67. Efficacy and safety of dabigatran compared with warfarin at different levels of international normalised ratio control for stroke prevention in atrial fibrillation: An analysis of the RE-LY trial. Wallentin L. Yusuf S. Ezekowitz M.D. Alings M. Flather M. Franzosi M.G. Pais P. Dans A. Eikelboom J. Oldgren J. Pogue J. Reilly P.A. Yang S. Connolly S.J. The Lancet (2010) 376:9745 (975–983). Date of Publication: 18 Sep 2010

68. Effects of combined ezetimibe and simvastatin therapy as compared with simvastatin alone in patients with type 2 diabetes: A prospective randomized double-blind clinical trial. Ruggenenti P. Cattaneo D. Rota S. Iliev I. Parvanova A. Diadei O. Ene-Iordache B. Ferrari S. Bossi A.C. Trevisan R. Belviso A. Remuzzi G. Diabetes Care (2010) 33:9 (1954–1956). Date of Publication: September 2010

69. Lithium carbonate in amyotrophic lateral sclerosis: Lack of efficacy in a dose-finding trial. Chio A. Borghero G. Calvo A. Capasso M. Caponnetto C. Corbo M. Giannini F. Logroscino G. Mandrioli J. Marcello N. Mazzini L. Moglia C. Monsurro M.R. Mora G. Patti F. Perini M. Pietrini V. Pisano F. Pupillo E. Sabatelli M.

Salvi F. Silani V. Simone I.L. Soraru G. Tola M.R. Volanti P. Beghi E. Neurology (2010) 75:7 (619–625). Date of Publication: 17 Aug 2010

70. Sirolimus therapy to halt the progression of ADPKD. Perico N. Antiga L. Caroli A. Ruggenenti P. Fasolini G. Cafaro M. Ondei P. Rubis N. Diadei O. Gherardi G. Prandini S. Panozo A. Bravo R.F. Carminati S. De Leon F.R. Gaspari F. Cortinovis M. Motterlini N. Ene-Iordache B. Remuzzi A. Remuzzi G. Journal of the American Society of Nephrology (2010) 21:6 (1031–1040). Date of Publication: June 2010

71. New atypical antipsychotics for schizophrenia: Iloperidone. Caccia S. Pasina L. Nobili A. Drug Design, Development and Therapy (2010) 4 (33–48). Date of Publication: 2010

72. Reducing polycystic liver volume in ADPKD: Effects of somatostatin analogue octreotide. Caroli A. Antiga L. Cafaro M. Fasolini G. Remuzzi A. Remuzzi G. Ruggenenti P. Clinical Journal of the American Society of Nephrology (2010) 5:5 (783–789). Date of Publication: 1 May 2010

73. Effect of the urotensin receptor antagonist palosuran in hypertensive patients with type 2 diabetic nephropathy. Vogt L. Chiurchiu C. Chadha-Boreham H. Danaietash P. Dingemanse J. Hadjadj S. Krum H. Navis G. Neuhart E. Parvanova A.I. Ruggenenti P. Woittiez A.J. Zimlichman R. Remuzzi G. De Zeeuw D. Hypertension (2010) 55:5 (1206–1209). Date of Publication: May 2010

74. Clinical predictors of atrial fibrillation recurrence in the Gruppo Italiano per lo Studio della Sopravvivenza nell'Infarto Miocardico-Atrial Fibrillation (GISSI-AF) trial. Disertori M. Lombardi F. Barlera S. Latini R. Maggioni A.P. Zeni P. Di Pasquale G. Cosmi F. Franzosi M.G. American Heart Journal (2010) 159:5 (857–863). Date of Publication: May 2010

75. Effectiveness of a propolis and zinc solution in preventing acute otitis media in children with a history of recurrent acute otitis media. Marchisio P. Esposito S. Bianchini S. Desantis C. Galeone C. Nazzari E. Pignataro L. Principi N. International Journal of Immunopathology and Pharmacology (2010) 23:2 (567–575). Date of Publication: April-June 2010

76. Skeletonized internal thoracic artery harvesting reduces chest wall dysesthesia after coronary bypass surgery. Markman P.L. Rowland M.A. Leong J.-Y. Van Der Merwe J. Storey E. Marasco S. Negri J. Bailey M. Rosenfeldt F.L. Journal of Thoracic and Cardiovascular Surgery (2010) 139:3 (674–679). Date of Publication: March 2010

77. Impact of influenza-like illness and effectiveness of influenza vaccination in oncohematological children who have completed cancer therapy. Esposito S. Cecinati V. Scicchitano B. Delvecchio G.C. Santoro N. Amato D. Pelucchi C. Jankovic M. De Mattia D. Principi N. Vaccine (2010) 28:6 (1558–1565). Date of Publication: 10 Feb 2010

78. Effect of omega-3 fatty acids supplementation on depressive symptoms and on health-related quality of life in the treatment of elderly women with depression: A double-blind, placebo-controlled, randomized clinical trial. Rondanelli M. Giacosa A. Opizzi A. Pelucchi C. Vecchia C.L. Montorfano G. Negroni M. Berra B. Politi P. Rizzo A.M. Journal of the American College of Nutrition (2010) 29:1 (55–64). Date of Publication: February 2010

79. Double-blind placebo-controlled trial on the use of acetyl-L-carnitine for the treatment of Amyotrophic Lateral Sclerosis (ALS). Beghi E. Pupillo E. Mattana F. Millul A. Quadrelli M. Ricerca e Pratica (2010) 26:1 (19). Date of Publication: January-February 2010

80. Prospective, randomized multicentric study to compare the efficacy of myco-phenolate mofetil versus azathioprine as the only immunosuppressive treatment in preventing chronic transplant nephropathy in kidney transplant patient (ATHENA). Perico N. Ruggenenti P. Cravedi P. Marasa M. Remuzzi G. Ricerca e Pratica (2010) 26:1 (22). Date of Publication: January-February 2010

81. Prospective, randomized open-label, blinded-endpoint (PROBE) study to assess the equivalent levels of blood pressure: Combined therapy with ACE-inhibitors benazepril and angiotensin receptor antagonist valsartan more effectively reduce microalbuminuria than therapy with benazepril only or with only valsartan in hypertensive patients with type 2 diabetes and albuminuria. Ruggenenti P. Remuzzi G. Rota S. Ricerca e Pratica (2010) 26:1 (24). Date of Publication: January-February 2010

82. Prospective, randomized open-label, blinded-endpoint (PROBE) study to assess the equivalent levels of blood pressure: Combined therapy with ACE-inhibitors benazepril and angiotensin-II receptor antagonist (sartan) valsartan effectively reduce and prevent end-stage renal disease compared to treatment with benazepril or valsartan alone in patients with overt nephropathy of type 2 diabetes (VALID). Remuzzi G. Ruggenenti P. Rota S. Ricerca e Pratica (2010) 26:1 (23). Date of Publication: January-February 2010

83. Efficacy of beclomethasone versus placebo in the prophylaxis of viral wheezing in preschool age. Clavenna A. Gangemi M. Casadei G. Garattini L. Bonati M. Ricerca e Pratica (2010) 26:1 (21). Date of Publication: January-February 2010

84. Antihypertensive effects of double the maximum dose of valsartan in African-American patients with type 2 diabetes mellitus and albuminuria. Weir M.R. Hollenberg N.K. Zappe D.H. Meng X. Parving H.-H. Viberti G. Remuzzi G. Journal of Hypertension (2010) 28:1 (186–193). Date of Publication: January 2010

85. Erythropoietin in amyotrophic lateral sclerosis: A pilot, randomized, double-blind, placebo-controlled study of safety and tolerability. Lauria G. Campanella A. Filippini G. Martini A. Penza P. Maggi L. Antozzi C. Ciano C. Beretta P. Caldiroli D. Ghelma F. Ferrara G. Ghezzi P. Mantegazza R. Amyotrophic Lateral Sclerosis (2009) 10:5–6 (410–415). Date of Publication: 2009

86. Randomized, double-blind, Phase 1 trial of an alphavirus replicon vaccine for cytomegalovirus in CMV seronegative adult volunteers. Bernstein D.I. Reap E.A. Katen K. Watson A. Smith K. Norberg P. Olmsted R.A. Hoeper A. Morris J. Negri S. Maughan M.F. Chulay J.D. Vaccine (2009) 28:2 (484–493). Date of Publication: 11 Dec 2009

87. Impact of the PPAR-(gamma)2 Pro12Ala polymorphism and ACE inhibitor therapy on new-onset microalbuminuria in type 2 diabetes: Evidence from BENEDICT. De Cosmo S. Motterlini N. Prudente S. Pellegrini F. Trevisan R. Bossi A. Remuzzi G. Trischitta V. Ruggenenti P. Diabetes (2009) 58:12 (2920–2929). Date of Publication: December 2009

88. Effects of antihypertensive drugs on carotid intima-media thickness: Focus on angiotensin II receptor blockers. A review of randomized, controlled trials. Cuspidi C. Negri F. Giudici V. Capra A. Sala C. Integrated Blood Pressure Control (2009) 2 (1–8). Date of Publication: 2009

89. Modified radical hysterectomy versus extrafascial hysterectomy in the treatment of stage I endometrial cancer: Results from the ILIADE randomized study. Signorelli M. Lissoni A.A. Cormio G. Katsaros D. Pellegrino A. Selvaggi L. Ghezzi F. Scambia G. Zola P. Grassi R. Milani R. Giannice R. Caspani G. Mangioni

C. Floriani I. Rulli E. Fossati R. Annals of Surgical Oncology (2009) 16:12 (3431–3441). Date of Publication: December 2009

90. A trial of darbepoetin alfa in type 2 diabetes and chronic kidney disease. Pfeffer M.A. Burdmann E.A. Chen C.-Y. Cooper M.E. De Zeeuw D. Eckardt K.-U. Feyzi J.M. Ivanovich P. Kewalramani R. Levey A.S. Lewis E.F. McGill J.B. McMurray J.J.V. Parfrey P. Parving H.-H. Remuzzi G. Singh A.K. Solomon S.D. Toto R. New England Journal of Medicine (2009) 361:21 (2019–2032). Date of Publication: 19 Nov 2009

91. Cyclophosphamide in chronic lymphocytic leukemia first line: Final results of Chronic Lymphocytic Leukemia 8 Study. Gobbi M. Haematologica Meeting Reports (2009) 3:3 (99–102). Date of Publication: 2009

92. Motor cortex stimulation for ALS: A double blind placebo-controlled study. Di Lazzaro V. Pilato F. Profice P. Ranieri F. Musumeci G. Florio L. Beghi E. Frisullo G. Capone F. Sabatelli M. Tonali P.A. Dileone M. Neuroscience Letters (2009) 464:1 (18–21). Date of Publication: 16 Oct 2009

93. Efficacy of injectable trivalent virosomal-adjuvanted inactivated influenza vaccine in preventing acute otitis media in children with recurrent complicated or noncomplicated acute otitis media. Marchisio P. Esposito S. Bianchini S. Dusi E. Fusi M. Nazzari E. Picchi R. Galeone C. Principi N. Pediatric Infectious Disease Journal (2009) 28:10 (855–859). Date of Publication: October 2009

94. The selective vitamin d receptor activator for albuminuria lowering (VITAL) study: Study design and baseline characteristics. Lambers Heerspink H.J. Agarwal R. Coyne D.W. Parving H.-H. Ritz E. Remuzzi G. Audhya P. Amdahl M.J. Andress D.L. De Zeeuw D. American Journal of Nephrology (2009) 30:3 (280–286). Date of Publication: September 2009

95. High-grade soft-tissue sarcomas: Tumor response assessment—Pilot study to assess the correlation between radiologic and pathologic response by using RECIST and Choi criteria. Stacchiotti S. Collini P. Messina A. Morosi C. Barisella M. Bertulli R. Piovesan C. Dileo P. Torri V. Gronchi A. Casali P.G. Radiology (2009) 251:2 (447–456). Date of Publication: May 2009

96. A phase II, randomized trial of neo-adjuvant chemotherapy comparing a three-drug combination of paclitaxel, ifosfamide, and cisplatin (TIP) versus paclitaxel and cisplatin (TP) followed by radical surgery in patients with locally advanced squamous cell cervical carcinoma: The Snap-02 Italian Collaborative Study. Lissoni A.A. Colombo N. Pellegrino A. Parma G. Zola P. Katsaros D. Chiari S. Buda A. Landoni F. Peiretti M. Dell'Anna T. Fruscio R. Signorelli M. Grassi R. Floriani I. Fossati R. Torri V. Rulli E. Annals of Oncology (2009) 20:4 (660–665). Date of Publication: 2009

97. Anaesthesiological strategies in elective craniotomy: Randomized, equivalence, open trial—The NeuroMorfeo trial. Citerio G. Grazia M.G. Latini R. Masson S. Barlera S. Guzzetti S. Pesenti A. Trials (2009) 10 Article Number: 19. Date of Publication: 6 Apr 2009

98. Fondaparinux compared to enoxaparin in patients with acute coronary syndromes without ST-segment elevation: Outcomes and treatment effect across different levels of risk Joyner C.D. Peters R.J.G. Afzal R. Chrolavicius S. Mehta S.R. Fox K.A.A. Granger C.B. Franzosi M.G. Flather M. Budaj A. Bassand J.-P. Yusuf S. American Heart Journal (2009) 157:3 (502–508). Date of Publication: March 2009

99. Incidence and clinical implications of venous thromboembolism in advanced colorectal cancer patients: The 'GISCAD-alternating schedule' study findings.

Mandala M. Barni S. Floriani I. Isa L. Fornarini G. Marangolo M. Mosconi S. Corsi D. Rulli E. Frontini L. Cortesi E. Zaniboni A. Aglietta M. Labianca R. European Journal of Cancer (2009) 45:1 (65–73). Date of Publication: January 2009

100. Anti-remodelling effect of canrenone in patients with mild chronic heart failure (AREA IN-CHF study): Final results. Boccanelli A. Mureddu G.F. Cacciatore G. Clemenza F. Di Lenarda A. Gavazzi A. Porcu M. Latini R. Lucci D. Maggioni A.P. Masson S. Vanasia M. De Simone G. European Journal of Heart Failure (2009) 11:1 (68–76). Date of Publication: January 2009

101. Systematic pelvic lymphadenectomy vs no lymphadenectomy in early-stage endometrial carcinoma: Randomized clinical trial. Panici P.B. Basile S. Maneschi F. Lissoni A.A. Signorelli M. Scambia G. Angioli R. Tateo S. Mangili G. Katsaros D. Garozzo G. Campagnutta E. Donadello N. Greggi S. Melpignano M. Raspagliesi F. Ragni N. Cormio G. Grassi R. Franchi M. Giannarelli D. Fossati R. Torri V. Amoroso M. Croce C. Mangioni C. Journal of the National Cancer Institute (2008) 100:23 (1707–1716). Date of Publication: December 2008

102. TILT: A randomized controlled trial of interruption of antiretroviral therapy with or without interleukin-2 in HIV-1 infected individuals. Angus B. Lampe F. Tambussi G. Duvivier C. Katlama C. Youle M. Williams I. Clotet B. Fisher M. Post F.A. Babiker A. Phillips A. AIDS (2008) 22:6 (737–740). Date of Publication: 2008

103. Benefit of oral anticoagulant over antiplatelet therapy in atrial fibrillation depends on the quality of international normalized ratio control achieved by centers and countries as measured by time in therapeutic range. Connolly S.J. Pogue J. Eikelboom J. Flaker G. Commerford P. Franzosi M.G. Healey J.S. Yusuf S. Circulation (2008) 118:20 (2029–2037). Date of Publication: 11 Nov 2008

104. Randomized controlled trial comparing the effectiveness of 308-nm excimer laser alone or in combination with topical hydrocortisone 17-butyrate cream in the treatment of vitiligo of the face and neck. Sassi F. Cazzaniga S. Tessari G. Chatenoud L. Reseghetti A. Marchesi L. Girolomoni G. Naldi L. British Journal of Dermatology (2008) 159:5 (1186–1191). Date of Publication: November 2008

105. Effects of the timolol-dorzolamide fixed combination and latanoprost on circadian diastolic ocular perfusion pressure in glaucoma. Quaranta L. Miglior S. Floriani I. Pizzolante T. Konstas A.G.P. Investigative Ophthalmology and Visual Science (2008) 49:10 (4226–4231). Date of Publication: October 2008

106. Comparative pharmacokinetics of a single oral dose of two formulations of amlodipine: A randomized, single-blind, two-period, two-sequence, crossover study. Pico J.C. Dominguez G. Negri A.L. Caubet J.C. Terragno N.A. Arzneimittel-Forschung/Drug Research (2008) 58:7 (323–327). Date of Publication: 2008

107. Preventing left ventricular hypertrophy by ACE inhibition in hypertensive patients with type 2 diabetes: A prespecified analysis of the Bergamo Nephrologic Diabetes Complications Trial (BENEDICT). Ruggenenti P. Iliev I. Costa G.M. Parvanova A. Perna A. Giuliano G.A. Motterlini N. Ene-Iordache B. Remuzzi G. Diabetes Care (2008) 31:8 (1629–1634). Date of Publication: August 2008

108. Comparison of two humidification systems for long-term noninvasive mechanical ventilation. Nava S. Cirio S. Fanfulla F. Carlucci A. Navarra A. Negri A. Ceriana P. European Respiratory Journal (2008) 32:2 (460–464). Date of Publication: August 2008

109. Stopping a trial early in oncology: For patients or for industry? Trotta F. Apolone G. Garattini S. Tafuri G. Annals of Oncology (2008) 19:7 (1347–1353). Date of Publication: July 2008

110. Long-term outcome in patients with critical illness myopathy or neuropathy: The Italian multicentre CRIMYNE study. Guarneri B. Bertolini G. Latronico N. Journal of Neurology, Neurosurgery and Psychiatry (2008) 79:7 (838–840). Date of Publication: July 2008

111. Cost minimisation analysis of 12 or 24 weeks of peginterferon alfa-2b + ribavirin for hepatitis C virus. De Compadri P. Koleva D. Mangia A. Motterlini N. Garattini L. Journal of Medical Economics (2008) 11:1 (151–163). Date of Publication: 2008

112. ACE gene polymorphism and losartan treatment in type 2 diabetic patients with nephropathy. Parving H.-H. De Zeeuw D. Cooper M.E. Remuzzi G. Liu N. Lunceford J. Shahinfar S. Wong P.H. Lyle P.A. Rossing P. Brenner B.M. Journal of the American Society of Nephrology (2008) 19:4 (771–779). Date of Publication: April 2008

113. Adjuvant chemotherapy in completely resected gastric cancer: A randomized phase III trial conducted by GOIRC. Di Costanzo F. Gasperoni S. Manzione L. Bisagni G. Labianca R. Bravi S. Cortesi E. Carlini P. Bracci R. Tomao S. Messerini L. Arcangeli A. Torri V. Bilancia D. Floriani I. Tonato M. Journal of the National Cancer Institute (2008) 100:6 (388–398). Date of Publication: March 2008

114. TILT: A randomized controlled trial of interruption of antiretroviral therapy with or without interleukin-2 in HIV-1 infected individuals. Angus B. Lampe F. Tambussi G. Duvivier C. Katlama C. Youle M. Williams I. Clotet B. Fisher M. Post F.A. Babiker A. Phillips A. AIDS (2008) 22:6 (737–740). Date of Publication: March 2008

115. A phase II randomised clinical trial comparing cisplatin, paclitaxel and ifosfamide with cisplatin, paclitaxel and epirubicin in newly diagnosed advanced epithelial ovarian cancer: Long-term survival analysis. Fruscio R. Colombo N. Lissoni A.A. Garbi A. Fossati R. Ieda' N. Torri V. Mangioni C. British Journal of Cancer (2008) 98:4 (720–727). Date of Publication: 26 Feb 2008

116. Cetuximab plus gemcitabine and cisplatin compared with gemcitabine and cisplatin alone in patients with advanced pancreatic cancer: a randomised, multicentre, phase II trial. Cascinu S. Berardi R. Labianca R. Siena S. Falcone A. Aitini E. Barni S. Di Costanzo F. Dapretto E. Tonini G. Pierantoni C. Artale S. Rota S. Floriani I. Scartozzi M. Zaniboni A. The Lancet Oncology (2008) 9:1 (39–44). Date of Publication: January 2008

117. Combined estrogen-progestogen menopausal therapy. Anderson G.L. Autier P. Beral V. Bosland M.C. Fernandez E. Haslam S.Z. Kaufman D.G. La Vecchia C. Molinolo A.A. Newcomb P.A. Parl F.F. Peto J. Rosano G. Roy D. Stanczyk F.Z. Thomas D.B. Vatten L. Junghans T. Olin S. Shapiro S. Stafford R.S. Jameson C.W. Meyer J.U. Baan R. Berthiller J. Cogliano V.J. Dresler C. El Ghissassi F. Franceschi S. Goncalves M.-A.G. Grosse Y. Guha N. Marron M. Mitchell J. Napalkov N. Secretan B. Straif K. Ullrich A. Egraz S. Kajo B. Lezere M. Lorenzen-Augros H. IARC Monographs on the Evaluation of Carcinogenic Risks to Humans (2007) 91 (205–372). Date of Publication: 2007 Combined Estrogen-Progestogen Contraceptives and Combined Estrogen-Progestogen Menopausal Therapy, Book Series Title:

118. A double-blind, placebo-controlled, randomized trial of bupropion for smoking cessation in primary care. Fossati R. Apolone G. Negri E. Compagnoni A. La Vecchia C. Mangano S. Clivio L. Garattini S. Archives of Internal Medicine (2007) 167:16 (1791–1797). Date of Publication: 9 Oct 2007

119. Sirolimus versus cyclosporine therapy increases circulating regulatory T cells, but does not protect renal transplant patients given alemtuzumab induction

from chronic allograft injury. Ruggenenti P. Perico N. Gotti E. Cravedi P. D'Agati V. Gagliardini E. Abbate M. Gaspari F. Cattaneo D. Noris M. Casiraghi F. Todeschini M. Cugini D. Conti S. Remuzzi G. Transplantation (2007) 84:8 (956–964). Date of Publication: October 2007

120. Venous thromboembolism predicts poor prognosis in irresectable pancreatic cancer patients. Mandala M. Reni M. Cascinu S. Barni S. Floriani I. Cereda S. Berardi R. Mosconi S. Torri V. Labianca R. Annals of Oncology (2007) 18:10 (1660–1665). Date of Publication: October 2007

121. Albuminuria response to very high-dose valsartan in type 2 diabetes mellitus. Hollenberg N.K. Parving H.-H. Viberti G. Remuzzi G. Ritter S. Zelenkofske S. Kandra A. Daley W.L. Rocha R. Journal of Hypertension (2007) 25:9 (1921–1926). Date of Publication: September 2007

122. Baseline characteristics of patients recruited in the AREA IN-CHF study (Anti-remodelling Effect of Aldosterone Receptors Blockade with Canrenone in Mild Chronic Heart Failure). Boccanelli A. Cacciatore G. Mureddu G.F. De Simone G. Clemenza F. De Maria R. Di Lenarda A. Gavazzi A. Latini R. Masson S. Porcu M. Vanasia M. Gonzini L. Maggioni A.P. Journal of Cardiovascular Medicine (2007) 8:9 (683–691). Date of Publication: September 2007

123. Intercurrent Factors Associated with the Development of Open-Angle Glaucoma in the European Glaucoma Prevention Study. Miglior S. Torri V. Zeyen T. Pfeiffer N. Vaz J.C. Adamsons I. American Journal of Ophthalmology (2007) 144:2 (266–275.e1). Date of Publication: August 2007

124. Mycophenolate mofetil versus azathioprine for prevention of chronic allograft dysfunction in renal transplantation: The MYSS follow-up randomized, controlled clinical trial. Remuzzi G. Cravedi P. Costantini M. Lesti M. Ganeva M. Gherardi G. Ene-Iordache B. Gotti E. Donati D. Salvadori M. Sandrini S. Segoloni G. Federico S. Rigotti P. Sparacino V. Ruggenenti P. Journal of the American Society of Nephrology (2007) 18:6 (1973–1985). Date of Publication: June 2007

125. Albuminuria is a target for renoprotective therapy independent from blood pressure in patients with type 2 diabetic nephropathy: Post hoc analysis from the reduction of endpoints in NIDDM with the angiotensin II antagonist losartan (RENAAL) trial. Eijkelkamp W.B.A. Zhang Z. Remuzzi G. Parving H.-H. Cooper M.E. Keane W.F. Shahinfar S. Gleim G.W. Weir M.R. Brenner B.M. De Zeeuw D. Journal of the American Society of Nephrology (2007) 18:5 (1540–1546). Date of Publication: May 2007

126. Adjuvant treatment of high-risk, radically resected gastric cancer patients with 5-fluorouracil, leucovorin, cisplatin, and epidoxorubicin in a randomized controlled trial. Cascinu S. Labianca R. Barone C. Santoro A. Carnaghi C. Cassano A. Beretta G.D. Catalano V. Bertetto O. Barni S. Frontini L. Aitini E. Rota S. Torri V. Floriani I. Journal of the National Cancer Institute (2007) 99:8 (601–607). Date of Publication: 18 Apr 2007

127. Does remission of renal disease associated with antihypertensive treatement exist? Cravedi P. Ruggenenti P. Remuzzi G. Current Hypertension Reports (2007) 9:2 (160–165). Date of Publication: April 2007

128. Impact of blood pressure control and angiotensin-converting enzyme inhibitor therapy on new-onset microalbuminuria in type 2 diabetes: A post hoc analysis of the BENEDICT trial. Ruggenenti P. Perna A. Ganeva M. Ene-Iordache B. Remuzzi G. Journal of the American Society of Nephrology (2006) 17:12 (3472–3481). Date of Publication: December 2006

129. Treatment of the first tonic-clonic seizure does not affect long-term remission of epilepsy. Leone M.A. Solari A. Beghi E. Neurology (2006) 67:12 (2227–2229). Date of Publication: December 2006

130. The effectiveness of hospitalization in the treatment of paediatric idiopathic headache patients. Lanzi G. D'Arrigo S. Termine C. Rossi M. Ferrari-Ginevra O. Mongelli A. Millul A. Beghi E. Psychopathology (2007) 40:1 (1–7). Date of Publication: November 2006

131. Randomised study of systematic lymphadenectomy in patients with epithelial ovarian cancer macroscopically confined to the pelvis. Maggioni A. Panici P.B. Dell'Anna T. Landoni F. Lissoni A. Pellegrino A. Rossi R.S. Chiari S. Campagnutta E. Greggi S. Angioli R. Manci N. Calcagno M. Scambia G. Fossati R. Floriani I. Torri V. Grassi R. Mangioni C. British Journal of Cancer (2006) 95:6 (699–704). Date of Publication: 18 Sep 2006

132. Clindamycin-paclitaxel pharmacokinetic interaction in ovarian cancer patients. Fruscio R. Lissoni A.A. Frapolli R. Corso S. Mangioni C. D'Incalci M. Zucchetti M. Cancer Chemotherapy and Pharmacology (2006) 58:3 (319–325). Date of Publication: September 2006

133. Adjuvant chemotherapy vs radiotherapy in high-risk endometrial carcinoma: Results of a randomised trial. Maggi R. Lissoni A. Spina F. Melpignano M. Zola P. Favalli G. Colombo A. Fossati R. British Journal of Cancer (2006) 95:3 (266–271). Date of Publication: 7 Aug 2006

134. Cancer risk after radiotherapy for breast cancer. Levi F. Randimbison L. Te V.-C. Vecchia C.L. British Journal of Cancer (2006) 95:3 (390–392). Date of Publication: 7 Aug 2006

135. Long-term renal allograft function on a tacrolimus-based, pred-free maintenance immunosuppression comparing sirolimus vs. MMF. Gallon L. Perico N. Dimitrov B.D. Winoto J. Remuzzi G. Leventhal J. Gaspari F. Kaufman D. American Journal of Transplantation (2006) 6:7 (1617–1623). Date of Publication: July 2006

136. What blood-pressure level provides greatest renoprotection in patients with diabetic nephropathy and hypertension? Ruggenenti P. Remuzzi G. Nature Clinical Practice Nephrology (2006) 2:5 (250–251). Date of Publication: May 2006

137. Renal risk and renoprotection among ethnic groups with type 2 diabetic nephropathy: A post hoc analysis of RENAAL. De Zeeuw D. Ramjit D. Zhang Z. Ribeiro A.B. Kurokawa K. Lash J.P. Chan J. Remuzzi G. Brenner B.M. Shahinfar S. Kidney International (2006) 69:9 (1675–1682). Date of Publication: May 2006

138. The contribution of information technology: Towards a better clinical data management. Clivio L. Tinazzi A. Mangano S. Santoro E. Drug Development Research (2006) 67:3 (245–250). Date of Publication: March 2006

139. Chiropractic manipulation in the treatment of acute back pain and sciatica with disc protrusion: A randomized double-blind clinical trial of active and simulated spinal manipulations. Santilli V. Beghi E. Finucci S. Spine Journal (2006) 6:2 (131–137). Date of Publication: March/April 2006

140. Pain in cancer. An outcome research project to evaluate the epidemiology, the quality and the effects of pain treatment in cancer patients. Apolone G. Bertetto O. Caraceni A. Corli O. De Conno F. Labianca R. Maltoni M. Nicora M. Torri V. Zucco F. Health and Quality of Life Outcomes (2006) 4 Article Number: 7. Date of Publication: 2 Feb 2006

141. Epidoxorubicin versus no treatment as consolidation therapy in advanced ovarian cancer: Results from a phase II study. Bolis G. Danese S. Tateo S. Rabaiotti

E. D'Agostino G. Merisio C. Scarfone G. Polverino G. Parazzini F. International Journal of Gynecological Cancer (2006) 16: SUPPL. 1 (74–78). Date of Publication: February 2006

142. Preventing microalbuminuria in patients with diabetes: Rationale and design of the Randomised Olmesartan and Diabetes Microalbuminuria Prevention (ROAD-MAP) study. Haller H. Viberti G.C. Mimran A. Remuzzi G. Rabelink A.J. Ritz E. Rump L.C. Ruilope L.M. Katayama S. Ito S. Izzo Jr. J.L. Januszewicz A. Journal of Hypertension (2006) 24:2 (403–408). Date of Publication: February 2006

143. Circadian analysis of myocardial infarction incidence in an Argentine and Uruguayan population. D'Negri C.E. Nicola-Siri L. Vigo D.E. Girotti L.A. Cardinali D.P. BMC Cardiovascular Disorders (2006) 6 Article Number: 1. Date of Publication: 9 Jan 2006

144. Randomized trial of neoadjuvant chemotherapy comparing paclitaxel, ifosfamide, and cisplatin with ifosfamide and cisplatin followed by radical surgery in patients with locally advanced squamous cell cervical carcinoma: The SNAP01 (Studio neo-adjuvante portio) Italian collaborative study. Buda A. Fossati R. Colombo N. Fei F. Floriani I. Alletti D.G. Katsaros D. Landoni F. Lissoni A. Malzoni C. Sartori E. Scollo P. Torri V. Zola P. Mangioni C. Journal of Clinical Oncology (2005) 23:18 (4137–4145). Date of Publication: 2005

145. A randomized controlled trial of psychological interventions for postnatal depression. Milgrom J. Negri L.M. Gemmill A.W. McNeil M. Martin P.R. British Journal of Clinical Psychology (2005) 44:4 (529–542). Date of Publication: Nov 2005

146. C-reactive protein in heart failure: Prognostic value and the effect of Valsartan. Anand I.S. Latini R. Florea V.G. Kuskowski M.A. Rector T. Masson S. Signorini S. Mocarelli P. Hester A. Glazer R. Cohn J.N. Circulation (2005) 112:10 (1428–1434). Date of Publication: 6 Sep 2005

147. Usefulness of temporal changes in neurohormones as markers of ventricular remodeling and prognosis in patients with left ventricular systolic dysfunction and heart failure receiving either Candesartan or Enalapril or both. Yan R.T. White M. Yan A.T. Yusuf S. Rouleau J.L. Maggioni A.P. Hall C. Latini R. Afzal R. Floras J. Masson S. McKelvie R.S. American Journal of Cardiology (2005) 96:5 (698–704). Date of Publication: 1 Sep 2005

148. Anemia and change in hemoglobin over time related to mortality and morbidity in patients with chronic heart failure: Results from Val-HeFT. Anand I.S. Kuskowski M.A. Rector T.S. Florea V.G. Glazer R.D. Hester A. Chiang Y.T. Aknay N. Maggioni A.P. Opasich C. Latini R. Cohn J.N. Circulation (2005) 112:8 (1121–1127). Date of Publication: 23 Aug 2005

149. Mucinous histology predicts for reduced fluorouracil responsiveness and survival in advanced colorectal cancer. Negri F.V. Wotherspoon A. Cunningham D. Norman A.R. Chong G. Ross P.J. Annals of Oncology (2005) 16:8 (1305–1310). Date of Publication: August 2005

150. Safety and efficacy of long-acting somatostatin treatment in autosomal-dominant polycystic kidney disease. Ruggenenti P. Remuzzi A. Ondei P. Fasolini G. Antiga L. Ene-Iordache B. Remuzzi G. Epstein F.H. Kidney International (2005) 68:1 (206–216). Date of Publication: July 2005

151. Caudal anesthesia for minor pediatric surgery: A prospective randomized comparison of ropivacaine 0.2% vs levobupivacaine 0.2%. Ivani G. De Negri P. Lonnqvist P.A. L'Erario M. Mossetti V. Difilippo A. Rosso F. Paediatric Anaesthesia (2005) 15:6 (491–494). Date of Publication: 2005

152. A randomised controlled trial of moxibustion for breech presentation. Cardini F. Lombardo P. Regalia A.L. Regaldo G. Zanini A. Negri M.G. Panepuccia L. Todros T. BJOG: An International Journal of Obstetrics and Gynaecology (2005) 112:6 (743–747). Date of Publication: June 2005

153. Effect of valsartan on quality of life when added to usual therapy for heart failure: Results from the Valsartan Heart Failure Trial. Majani G. Giardini A. Opasich C. Glazer R. Hester A. Tognoni G. Cohn J.N. Tavazzi L. Journal of Cardiac Failure (2005) 11:4 (253–259). Date of Publication: May 2005

154. Systematic aortic and pelvic lymphadenectomy versus resection of bulky nodes only in optimally debulked advanced ovarian cancer: A randomized clinical trial. Panici P.B. Maggioni A. Hacker N. Landoni F. Ackermann S. Campagnutta E. Tamussino K. Winter R. Pellegrino A. Greggi S. Angioli R. Manci N. Scambia G. Dell'Anna T. Fossati R. Floriani I. Rossi R.S. Grassi R. Favalli G. Raspagliesi F. Giannarelli D. Martella L. Mangioni C. Journal of the National Cancer Institute (2005) 97:8 (560–566). Date of Publication: 20 Apr 2005

155. Blood-pressure control for renoprotection in patients with non-diabetic chronic renal disease (REIN-2): Multicentre, randomised controlled trial. Ruggenenti P. Perna A. Loriga G. Ganeva M. Ene-Iordache B. Turturro M. Lesti M. Perticucci E. Chakarski I.N. Leonardis D. Garini G. Sessa A. Basile C. Alpa M. Scanziani R. Sorba G. Zoccali C. Remuzzi G. Lancet (2005) 365:9463 (939–946). Date of Publication: 12 Mar 2005

156. Valsartan reduces the incidence of atrial fibrillation in patients with heart failure: Results from the Valsartan Heart Failure Trial (Val-HeFT). Maggioni A.P. Latini R. Carson P.E. Singh S.N. Barlera S. Glazer R. Masson S. Cere E. Tognoni G. Cohn J.N. American Heart Journal (2005) 149:3 (548–557). Date of Publication: March 2005

157. Starc II, a multicenter randomized placebo-controlled double-blind clinical trial of trapidil for 1-year clinical events and angiographic restenosis reduction after coronary angioplasty and stenting. Maresta A. Balducelli M. Latini R. Bernardi G. Moccetti T. Sosa C. Barlera S. Varani E. Ribeiro Da Silva E.E. Monici Preti A. Maggioni A.P. Catheterization and Cardiovascular Interventions (2005) 64:3 (375–382). Date of Publication: March 2005

158. Developmental assessment of children by means of a postal questionnaire to parents: Survival, growth, development at 18 months of life and birth-weight. Bortolus R. Chatenoud L. Restelli S. Di Cintio E. Parazzini F. Italian Journal of Gynaecology and Obstetrics (2005) 17:1 (13–23). Date of Publication: Jan 2005

159. Continuum of renoprotection with losartan at all stages of type 2 diabetic nephropathy: A post hoc analysis of the RENAAL trial results. Remuzzi G. Ruggenenti P. Perna A. Dimitrov B.D. De Zeeuw D. Hille D.A. Shahinfar S. Carides G.W. Brenner B.M. Journal of the American Society of Nephrology (2004) 15:12 (3117–3125). Date of Publication: December 2004

160. Paclitaxel 175 or 225 mg per meters squared with carboplatin in advanced ovarian cancer: A randomized trial. Bolis G. Scarfone G. Polverino G. Raspagliesi F. Tateo S. Richiardi G. Melpignano M. Franchi M. Mangili G. Presti M. Villa A. Conta E. Guarnerio P. Cipriani S. Parazzini F. Journal of Clinical Oncology (2004) 22:4 (686–690). Date of Publication: 2004

161. Follow-up for patients with colorectal cancer after curative-intent primary treatment. Johnson F.E. Virgo K.S. Fossati R. Journal of Clinical Oncology (2004) 22:8 (1363–1365). Date of Publication: 2004

162. Preventing microalbuminuria in type 2 diabetes. Ruggenenti P. Fassi A. Ilieva A.P. Bruno S. Iliev I.P. Brusegan V. Rubis N. Gherardi G. Arnoldi F. Ganeva M. Ene-Iordache B. Gaspari F. Perna A. Bossi A. Trevisan R. Dodesini A.R. Remuzzi G. New England Journal of Medicine (2004) 351:19 (1941–1951). Date of Publication: 4 Nov 2004

163. Albuminuria, a therapeutic target for cardiovascular protection in type 2 diabetic patients with nephropathy. De Zeeuw D. Remuzzi G. Parving H.-H. Keane W.F. Zhang Z. Shahinfar S. Snapinn S. Cooper M.E. Mitch W.E. Brenner B.M. Circulation (2004) 110:8 (921–927). Date of Publication: 24 Aug 2004

164. Mycophenolate mofetil versus azathioprine for prevention of acute rejection in renal transplantation (MYSS): A randomised trial. Remuzzi G. Lesti M. Gotti E. Ganeva M. Dimitrov B.D. Ene-Iordache B. Gherardi G. Donati D. Salvadori M. Sandrini S. Valente U. Segoloni G. Mourad G. Federico S. Rigotti P. Sparacino V. Bosmans J.-L. Perico N. Ruggenenti P. Lancet (2004) 364:9433 (503–512). Date of Publication: 7 Aug 2004

165. Follow-up of colorectal cancer patients after resection with curative intent—The GILDA trial. Grossmann E.M. Johnson F.E. Virgo K.S. Longo W.E. Fossati R. Surgical Oncology (2004) 13:2–3 (119–124). Date of Publication: August/November 2004

166. Randomised controlled trial comparing single agent paclitaxel vs epidoxorubicin plus paclitaxel in patients with advanced ovarian cancer in early progression after platinum-based chemotherapy: An Italian Collaborative Study from the 'Mario Negri' Institute, Milan, G.O.N.O. (Gruppo Oncologico Nord Ovest) group and I.O.R. (Istituto Oncologico Romagnolo) group. Buda A. Floriani I. Rossi R. Colombo N. Torri V. Conte P.F. Fossati R. Ravaioli A. Mangioni C. British Journal of Cancer (2004) 90:11 (2112–2117). Date of Publication: 1 Jun 2004

167. Effect of oral or transdermal hormone replacement therapy on homocysteine levels: A randomized clinical trial. Bruschi F. Dal Pino D. Fiore V. Parazzini F. Di Pace R. Cesana B.M. Melotti D. Crosignani P.G. Maturitas (2004) 48:1 (33–38). Date of Publication: 28 May 2004

168. Randomized trial of intraportal and/or systemic adjuvant chemotherapy in patients with colon carcinoma. Labianca R. Fossati R. Zaniboni A. Torri V. Marsoni S. Nitti D. Boffi L. Scatizzi M. Tardio B. Mastrodonato N. Banducci S. Consani G. Pancera G. Journal of the National Cancer Institute (2004) 96:10 (750–758). Date of Publication: 19 May 2004

169. The effect of a structured intervention on caregivers of patients with dementia and problem behaviors: A randomized controlled pilot study. Nobili A. Riva E. Tettamanti M. Lucca U. Liscio M. Petrucci B. Porro G.S. Alzheimer Disease and Associated Disorders (2004) 18:2 (75–82). Date of Publication: April/June 2004

170. In renal transplantation blood cyclosporine levels soon after surgery act as a major determinant of rejection: Insights from the MY.S.S. Trial. Perico N. Ruggenenti P. Gotti E. Gaspari F. Cattaneo D. Valente U. Salvadori M. Segoloni G. Donati D. Sandrini S. Ganeva M. Dimitrov B.D. Remuzzi G. Kidney International (2004) 65:3 (1084–1090). Date of Publication: March 2004

171. Cisplatin versus carboplatin in combination with mitomycin and vinblastine in advanced non small cell lung cancer. A multicenter, randomized phase III trial. Paccagnella A. Favaretto A. Oniga F. Barbieri F. Ceresoli G. Torri W. Villa E. Verusio C. Cetto G.L. Santo A. De Pangher V. Artioli F. Cacciani G.C. Parodi G. Soresi F. Ghi M.G. Morabito A. Biason R. Giusto M. Mosconi P. Sileni V.C. Lung Cancer (2004) 43:1 (83–91). Date of Publication: January 2004

172. Improving sun protection behaviour in children: Study design and baseline results of a randomized trial in Italian Elementary Schools: The 'Sole Si Sole No GISED' Project. Naldi L. Di Landro A. Zinetti C. Chatenoud L. La Vecchia C. Cellini A. Simonetti O. Goglio M. Caridi N. Zaccaria E. Morena M. Pinna A.L. Atzori L. Pezzarossa E. Fenizi G. Quarta G. Congedo M. Aurilia A. Tripodi Cutri F. Stanganelli I. Magi S. Ingordo V. Cantoro V.M. Barba A. Tessari G. Rebora A. Gian-netti A. Peserico A. Liberati A. La Vecchia C. Dermatology (2003) 207:3 (291–297). Date of Publication: 2003

173. Adjunctive therapy versus alternative monotherapy in patients with partial epilepsy failing on a single drug: A multicentre, randomised, pragmatic controlled trial. Beghi E. Gatti G. Tonini C. Ben-Menachem E. Chadwick D.W. Nikanorova M. Gromov S.A. Smith P.E.M. Specchio L.M. Perucca E. Epilepsy Research (2003) 57:1 (1–13). Date of Publication: November 2003

174. Treatment of asymptomatic bacterial vaginosis to prevent pre-term delivery: A randomised trial. Guaschino S. Ricci E. Franchi M. Del Frate G. Tibaldi C. De Santo D. Ghezzi F. Benedetto C. De Seta F. Parazzini F. European Journal of Obstetrics Gynecology and Reproductive Biology (2003) 110:2 (149–152). Date of Publication: 10 Oct 2003

175. Randomized study of adjuvant chemotherapy for completely resected stage I, II, or IIIA non-small-cell lung cancer. Scagliotti G.V. Fossati R. Torri V. Crino L. Giaccone G. Silvano G. Martelli M. Clerici M. Cognetti F. Tonato M. Liguori G. Nittolo G. Vasta M. Curcio C. Borasio P. Dogliotti L. Scagliotti G.V. Angeletti C.A. Conte P.F. Laddaga M. Rebecchini S. Spagnesi S. Lewinski T. Salvati F. De Marinis F. Altieri A. Giordano F. Puglisi G. Cipriani A. Favaretto A. Fiorentino M. Giampaglia G. Loreggian L. Zuin R. Jassem J. Ukmar R. Buffoni A. Puricelli C. Talmassons G. Morelli A. Boidi Trotti A. Bretti S. Maggi G. Mussa A. Sannazzari G.L. Baldi S. Ricardi U. Ruffini E. Bruni G. Gridelli C. Checcaglini F. Latini P. Maranzano E. Todisco T. Tonato M. Santo Antonio A. Terzi A. Pavia G. Sartirana A. Ottoni D. Fontanili M. Sturani C. Aiello L.M. Barbera S. Baracco F. Cinquegrana A. Felletti R. Scolaro T. Serrano J. Felci U. Manente P. Drings P. Zannini P. Villa E. Bordone N. Tordiglione M. Bandera M. Fioretti M. Roviaro G. Bianco A.R. Ferrante G. Rossi A. Sodano A. Boni C. Covacev L. Lodini V. Espana P. Belloni P.A. Soresi E. Borghini U. Cimino G. Leoni M. Ravini M. Luporini G. Todeschini G. Campioni N. Cognetti F. Facciolo F. Clini V. Journal of the National Cancer Institute (2003) 95:19 (1453–1461). Date of Publication: 1 Oct 2003

176. Sustained reduction of aldosterone in response to the angiotensin receptor blocker Valsartan in patients with chronic heart failure: Results from the Valsartan heart failure trial. Cohn J.N. Anand I.S. Latini R. Masson S. Chiang Y.-T. Glazer R. Circulation (2003) 108:11 (1306–1309). Date of Publication: 16 Sep 2003

177. Off-pump coronary artery bypass surgery technique for total arterial myocardial revascularization: A prospective randomized study. Muneretto C. Bisleri G. Negri A. Manfredi J. Metra M. Nodari S. Dei Cas L. Bradley S.M. Sundt T. Arom K. Calhoon J.H. Annals of Thoracic Surgery (2003) 76:3 (778–783). Date of Publication: 1 Sep 2003

178. The BErgamo NEphrologic DIabetes Complications Trial (BENEDICT): Design and baseline characteristics. Perna A. Controlled Clinical Trials (2003) 24:4 (442–461). Date of Publication: August 2003

179. Short-term effects of two integrated, non-pharmacological body weight reduction programs on coronary heart disease risk factors in young obese patients.

Sartorio A. Lafortuna C.L. Marinone P.G. Tavani A. La Vecchia C. Bosetti C. Diabetes, Nutrition and Metabolism—Clinical and Experimental (2003) 16:4 (262–265). Date of Publication: August 2003

180. Cetirizine modulates adhesion molecule expression in a double-blind controlled study conducted in psoriatic patients. Pestelli E. Floriani I. Fabbri P. Caproni M. International Journal of Tissue Reactions (2003) 25:1 (1–8). Date of Publication: 2003

181. Retarding progression of chronic renal disease: The neglected issue of residual proteinuria. Ruggenenti P. Perna A. Remuzzi G. Kidney International (2003) 63:6 (2254–2261). Date of Publication: 1 Jun 2003

182. Effect of valsartan on hospitalization: Results from Val-HeFT. Carson P. Tognoni G. Cohn J.N. Journal of Cardiac Failure (2003) 9:3 (164–171). Date of Publication: June 2003

183. Predicting end-stage renal disease: Bayesian perspective of information transfer in the clinical decision-making process at the individual level. Dimitrov B.D. Perna A. Ruggenenti P. Remuzzi G. Kidney International (2003) 63:5 (1924–1933). Date of Publication: 1 May 2003

184. Is total arterial myocardial revascularization with composite grafts a safe and useful procedure in the elderly? Muneretto C. Negri A. Bisleri G. Manfredi J. Terrini A. Metra M. Nodari S. Cas L.D. European Journal of Cardio-thoracic Surgery (2003) 23:5 (657–664). Date of Publication: 1 May 2003

185. Safety and usefulness of composite grafts for total arterial myocardial revascularization: A prospective randomized evaluation. Muneretto C. Negri A. Manfredi J. Terrini A. Rodella G. ElQarra S. Bisleri G. Sundt T.M. Dion R.A. Brodman R.F. Calafiore A.M. Smith C.R. Journal of Thoracic and Cardiovascular Surgery (2003) 125:4 (826–835). Date of Publication: 1 Apr 2003

186. Comparison between the efficacy of dimeric and monomeric non-ionic contrast media (iodixanol vs iopromide) in urography in patients with macroscopic haematuria. Stacul F. Cova M. Pravato M. Floriani I. European Radiology (2003) 13:4 (810–814). Date of Publication: 1 Apr 2003

187. Changes in brain natriuretic peptide and norepinephrine over time and mortality and morbidity in the Valsartan Heart Failure Trial (Val-HeFT). Anand I.S. Fisher L.D. Chiang Y.-T. Latini R. Masson S. Maggioni A.P. Glazer R.D. Tognoni G. Cohn J.N. Circulation (2003) 107:9 (1278–1283). Date of Publication: 11 Mar 2003

188. Renal transplantation: Can we reduce calcineurin inhibitor/stop steroids? Evidence based on protocol biopsy findings. Gotti E. Perico N. Perna A. Gaspari F. Cattaneo D. Caruso R. Ferrari S. Stucchi N. Marchetti G. Abbate M. Remuzzi G. Journal of the American Society of Nephrology (2003) 14:3 (755–766). Date of Publication: 1 Mar 2003

189. Effects of combined ACE inhibitor and angiotensin II antagonist treatment in human chronic nephropathies. Campbell R. Sangalli F. Perticucci E. Aros C. Viscarra C. Perna A. Remuzzi A. Bertocchi F. Fagiani L. Remuzzi G. Ruggenenti P. Kidney International (2003) 63:3 (1094–1103). Date of Publication: 1 Mar 2003

190. A multicentre prospective controlled study to determine the safety of trazodone and nefazodone use during pregnancy. Einarson A. Bonari L. Voyer-Lavigne S. Addis A. Matsui D. Johnson Y. Koren G. Canadian Journal of Psychiatry (2003) 48:2 (106–110). Date of Publication: March 2003

191. Renal and metabolic effects of insulin lispro in type 2 diabetic subjects with overt nephropathy. Ruggenenti P. Flores C. Aros C. Ene-Iordache B. Trevisan R.

Ottomano C. Remuzzi G. Diabetes Care (2003) 26:2 (502–509). Date of Publication: 1 Feb 2003

192. International collaborative ovarian neoplasm trial 1: A randomized trial of adjuvant chemotherapy in women with early-stage ovarian cancer. Colombo N. Guthrie D. Chiari S. Parmar M. Qian W. Swart A.M. Torri V. Williams C. Lissoni A. Bonazzi C. Journal of the National Cancer Institute (2003) 95:2 (125–132). Date of Publication: 15 Jan 2003

193. Premature ovarian failure: Frequency and risk factors among women attending a network of menopause clinics in Italy. Parazzini F. De Aloysio D. Di Donato P. Giulini N.A. Bacchi Modena A. Cicchetti G. Comitini G. Gentile G. Cristiani P. Careccia A. Esposito E. Gualdi F. Golinelli S. Berga-mini E. Masellis G. Rastelli S. Gigli C. Elia A. Marchesoni D. Sticotti F. Del Frate G. Zompicchiatti C. Marino L. Costa M.R. Pinto P. Dodero D. Storace A. Spinelli G. Quaranta S. Bossi C.M. Ollago A. Omodei U. Vaccari M. Luerti M. Repetti F. Zandonini G. Raspagliesi F. Dolci F. Gambarino G. De Pasquale B. Polizzotti G. Borsellino G. Alpi-nelli P. Natale N. Colombo D. Belloni C. Viani A. Cecchini G. Vinci G.W. Samaja B.A. Pasinetti E. Penotti M. Ognissanti F. Pesando P. Malanetto C. Gallo M. Dolfin G. Tartaglino P. Mossotto D. Pistoni A. Tarani A. Rattazzi P.D. Rossaro D. Campanella M. Arisi E. Gamper M. Salvatores D. Bocchin E. Stellin G. Meli G. Azzini V. Tirozzi F. Buoso G. Fraioli R. Mar-soni V. Cetera C. Sposetti R. Candiotto E. Pignalosa R. Del Pup L. Bellati U. Angeloni C. Buonerba M. Garzarelli S. Santilli C. Mucci M. Di Nisio Q. Cappa F. Pierangeli I. Cordone A. Falasca L. Ferrante D. Serra G.B. Cirese E. Todaro P.A. Romanini C. Spagnuolo L. Lanzone A. Donadio C. BJOG: An International Journal of Obstetrics and Gynaecology (2003) 110:1 (59–63). Date of Publication: 1 Jan 2003

194. Occlusive wrap dressing reduces infection rate in saphenous vein harvest site. Rosenfeldt F.L. Negri J. Holdaway D. Davis B.B. Mack J. Grigg M.J. Miles C. Esmore D.S. Annals of Thoracic Surgery (2003) 75:1 (101–105). Date of Publication: 1 Jan 2003

195. Locoregionally advanced carcinoma of the oropharynx: Conventional radiotherapy vs. accelerated hyperfractionated radiotherapy vs. concomitant radiotherapy and chemotherapy—A multicenter randomized trial. Olmi P. Crispino S. Fallai C. Torri V. Rossi F. Bolner A. Amichetti M. Signor M. Taino R. Squadrelli M. Colombo A. Ardizzoia A. Ponticelli P. Franchin G. Minatel E. Gobitti C. Atzeni G. Gava A. Flann M. Marsoni S. International Journal of Radiation Oncology Biology Physics (2003) 55:1 (78–92). Date of Publication: 1 Jan 2003

196. Risks and benefits of early treatment of acute myocardial infarction with an angiotensin-converting enzyme inhibitor in patients with a history of arterial hypertension: Analysis of the GISSI-3 database. Avanzini F. Ferrario G. Santoro L. Peci P. Giani P. Santoro E. Franzosi M.G. Tognoni G. American Heart Journal (2002) 144:6 (1018–1025). Date of Publication: 1 Dec 2002

197. Spinal versus peripheral effects of adjunct clonidine: Comparison of the analgesic effect of a ropivacaine-clonidine mixture when administered as a caudal or ilioinguinal-iliohypogastric nerve blockade for inguinal surgery in children. Ivani G. Conio A. De Negri P. Eksborg S. Lonnqvist P.A. Paediatric Anaesthesia (2002) 12:8 (680–684). Date of Publication: 2002

198. Multicenter prospective randomized placebo controlled study to evaluate efficacy and safety of idebenone in the management of age associated cognitive impairment. Mangone C. Giannaula R. Negri A.L. Muchnik S. Sica R. Kaplan R. Prensa Medica Argentina (2002) 89:9 (797–803). Date of Publication: 2002

199. Effects of valsartan on circulating brain natriuretic peptide and norepinephrine in symptomatic chronic heart failure: The valsartan heart failure trial (Val-HEFT). Latini R. Masson S. Anand I. Judd D. Maggioni A.P. Chiang Y.-T. Bevilacqua M. Salio M. Cardano P. Dunselman P.H.J.M. Holwerda N.J. Tognoni G. Cohn J.N. Circulation (2002) 106:19 (2454–2458). Date of Publication: 5 Nov 2002

200   Effects of valsartan on morbidity and mortality in patients with heart failure not receiving angiotensin-converting enzyme inhibitors. Maggioni A.P. Anand I. Gottlieb S.O. Latini R. Tognoni G. Cohn J.N. Journal of the American College of Cardiology (2002) 40:8 (1414–1421). Date of Publication: 16 Oct 2002

201. Fluoxetine dose and outcome in antidepressant drug trials. Barbui C. Hotopf M. Garattini S. European Journal of Clinical Pharmacology (2002) 58:6 (379–386). Date of Publication: 2002

202. Effect of acetate-free biofiltration and bicarbonate hemodialysis on neutrophil activation. Todeschini M. Macconi D. Fernandez N.G. Ghilardi M. Anabaya A. Binda E. Morigi M. Cattaneo D. Perticucci E. Remuzzi G. Noris M. American Journal of Kidney Diseases (2002) 40:4 (783–793). Date of Publication: 1 Oct 2002

203. Prospective evaluation of a new sternal closure method with thermoreactive clips. Negri A. Manfredi J. Terrini A. Rodella G. Bisleri G. El Quarra S. Muneretto C. European Journal of Cardio-thoracic Surgery (2002) 22:4 (571–575). Date of Publication: October 2002

204. Valsartan benefits left ventricular structure and function in heart failure: Val-HeFT echocardiographic study. Wong M. Staszewsky L. Latini R. Barlera S. Volpi A. Chiang Y.-T. Benza R.L. Gottlieb S.O. Kleemann T.D. Rosconi F. Vandervoort P.M. Cohn J.N. Journal of the American College of Cardiology (2002) 40:5 (970–975). Date of Publication: 4 Sep 2002

205. Atorvastatin and thrombogenicity of the carotid atherosclerotic plaque: The ATROCAP Study. Cortellaro M. Confrancesco E. Arbustini E. Rossi F. Negri A. Tremoli E. Gabrielli L. Camera M. Thrombosis and Haemostasis (2002) 88:1 (41–47). Date of Publication: 2002

206. Fecal occult blood screening for colorectal cancer: Open issues. La Vecchia C. Annals of Oncology (2002) 13:1 (31–34). Date of Publication: 2002

207. Comparison of amlodipine and enalapril in the treatment of isolated systolic hypertension in the elderly: An open-label, randomized, parallel-group study. Bendersky M. Negri A.L. Nolly H. Arnolt M. Re A. Wasserman A. Current Therapeutic Research—Clinical and Experimental (2002) 63:2 (153–164). Date of Publication: 2002

208. Long-term vitamin E supplementation fails to reduce lipid peroxidation in people at cardiovascular risk: Analysis of underlying factors. Chiabrando C. Avanzini F. Rivalta C. Colombo F. Fanelli R. Palumbo G. Roncaglioni M.C. Pioltelli M.B. Capra A. Cristofari M. Rossi S. Current Controlled Trials in Cardiovascular Medicine (2002) 3 Article Number: 5. Date of Publication: 19 Mar 2002

209. A double blind-placebo controlled study on melatonin efficacy to reduce anxiolytic benzodiazepine use in the elderly. Cardinali D.P. Gvozdenovich E. Kaplan M.R. Fainstein I. Shifis H.A. Lloret S.P. Albornoz L. Negri A. Neuroendocrinology Letters (2002) 23:1 (55–60). Date of Publication: 2002

210. Randomized controlled trial of single-agent paclitaxel versus cyclophosphamide, doxorubicin, and cisplatin in patients with recurrent ovarian cancer who responded to first-line platinum-based regimens. Cantu M.G. Buda A. Parma G. Rossi R. Floriani I. Bonazzi C. Dell'Anna T. Torri V. Colombo N. Journal of Clinical Oncology (2002) 20:5 (1232–1237). Date of Publication: 1 Mar 2002

211. Angiotensin-converting-enzyme inhibition therapy in altitude polycythaemia: A prospective randomised trial. Plata R. Cornejo A. Arratia C. Anabaya A. Perna A. Dimitrov B.D. Remuzzi G. Ruggenenti P. Lancet (2002) 359:9307 (663–666). Date of Publication: 23 Feb 2002

212. Cyproterone acetate versus a continuous monophasic oral contraceptive in the treatment of recurrent pelvic pain after conservative surgery for symptomatic endometriosis. Vercellini P. De Giorgi O. Mosconi P. Stellato G. Vicentini S. Crosignani P.G. Fertility and Sterility (2002) 77:1 (52–61). Date of Publication: 2002

213. A randomized trial of the angiotensin-receptor blocker valsartan in chronic heart failure. Cohn J.N. Tognoni G. New England Journal of Medicine (2001) 345:23 (1667–1675). Date of Publication: 6 Dec 2001

214. Medicines for children in Europe at the beginning of the new millennium. Bonati M. Impicciatore P. Pandolfini C. Paediatric and Perinatal Drug Therapy (2001) 4:3 (82–84). Date of Publication: 2001

215. Reperfusion therapy for acute myocardial infarction with fibrinolytic therapy or combination reduced fibrinolytic therapy and platelet glycoprotein IIb/IIIa inhibition: The GUSTO V randomised trial. Franzosi M.G. Italian Heart Journal Supplement (2001) 2:9 (1034–1036). Date of Publication: 2001

216. Effects of losartan on renal and cardiovascular outcomes in patients with type 2 diabetes and nephropathy. Brenner B.M. Cooper M.E. De Zeeuw D. Keane W.F. Mitch W.E. Parving H.-H. Remuzzi G. Snapinn S.M. Zhang Z. Shahinfar S. New England Journal of Medicine (2001) 345:12 (861–869). Date of Publication: 20 Sep 2001

217. Haemolysis due to active venous drainage during cardiopulmonary bypass: Comparison of two different techniques. Cirri S. Negri L. Babbini M. Latis G. Khlat B. Tarelli G. Panisi P. Mazzaro E. Bellisario A. Borghetti B. Bordignon F. Ferrara M. Pavan H. Meco M. Perfusion (2001) 16:4 (313–318). Date of Publication: 2001

218. The dose-response relationship for clonidine added to a postoperative continuous epidural infusion of ropivacaine in children. De Negri P. Ivani G. Visconti C. De Vivo P. Lonnqvist P.-A. Anesthesia and Analgesia (2001) 93:1 (71–76). Date of Publication: 2001

219. The main results of Pentose Phosphate Pathway PPP. Roncaglioni M.C. Ricerca e Pratica (2001) 17:1 (6–20). Date of Publication: 2001

220. Low-dose aspirin and vitamin E in people at cardiovascular risk: A randomised trial in general practice. Roncaglioni M.C. Lancet (2001) 357:9250 (89–95). Date of Publication: 13 Jan 2001

221. Inhibition of the sodium-hydrogen exchanger with cariporide to prevent myocardial infarction in high-risk ischemic situations: Main results of the GUARDIAN trial. Theroux P. Chaitman B.R. Danchin N. Erhardt L. Meinertz T. Schroeder J.S. Tognoni G. White H.D. Willerson J.T. Jessel A. Circulation (2000) 102:25 (3032–3038). Date of Publication: 19 Dec 2000

222. Metformin effects on clinical features, endocrine and metabolic profiles, and insulin sensitivity in polycystic ovary syndrome: A randomized, double-blind, placebo-controlled 6-month trial, followed by open, long-term clinical evaluation. Moghetti P. Castello R. Negri C. Tosi F. Perrone F. Caputo M. Zanolin E. Muggeo M. Journal of Clinical Endocrinology and Metabolism (2000) 85:1 (139–146). Date of Publication: 2000

223. Pretreatment blood pressure reliably predicts progression of chronic nephropathies. Ruggenenti P. Perna A. Lesti M. Pisoni R. Mosconi L. Arnoldi F. Ciocca I.

Gaspari F. Remuzzi G. Kidney International (2000) 58:5 (2093–2101). Date of Publication: 2000

224. Evaluation of ropivacaine 0.2% vs bupivacaine 0.25% for pediatric regional anesthesia. De Negri P. Visconti C. Ivani G. Borrelli F. De Vivo P. Revista de la Sociedad Espanola del Dolor (2000) 7:2 (88–91). Date of Publication: 2000

225. A controlled multicenter pediatric study in the treatment of acute respiratory tract diseases with the aid of a new specific compound, erdosteine (IPSE, Italian Pediatric Study Erdosteine). Titti G. Lizzio A. Termini C. Negri P. Fazzio S. Mancini C. International Journal of Clinical Pharmacology and Therapeutics (2000) 38:8 (402–407). Date of Publication: 2000

226. Effects of low-dose aspirin on clinic and ambulatory blood pressure in treated hypertensive patients. Avanzini F. Palumbo G. Alli C. Roncaglioni M.C. Ronchi E. Cristofari M. Capra A. Rossi S. Nosotti L. Costantini C. Pietrofeso R. American Journal of Hypertension (2000) 13:6 I (611–616). Date of Publication: 2000

227. Lisinopril and mortality in diabetics with acute MI. Zuanetti G. Maggioni A.P. Latini R. Cardiology Review (2000) 17:1 (11–16). Date of Publication: 2000

228. Paclitaxel and cisplatin in ovarian cancer [1]. Torri V. Harper P.G. Colombo N. Sandercock J. Parmar M.K.B. Journal of Clinical Oncology (2000) 18:11 (2349). Date of Publication: 2000

229. Chronic proteinuric nephropathies: Outcomes and response to treatment in a prospective cohort of 352 patients with different patterns of renal injury. Ruggenenti P. Perna A. Gherardi G. Benini R. Remuzzi G. American Journal of Kidney Diseases (2000) 35:6 (1155–1165). Date of Publication: 2000

230. Effects of Vitamin E on clinic and ambulatory blood pressure in treated hypertensive patients. Palumbo G. Avanzini F. Alli C. Roncaglioni M.C. Ronchi E. Cristofari M. Capra A. Rossi S. Nosotti L. Costantini C. Cavalera C. American Journal of Hypertension (2000) 13:5 I (564–567). Date of Publication: 2000

231. Nifedipine administered in pregnancy: Effect on the development of children at 18 months. Bortolus R. Ricci E. Chatenoud L. Parazzini F. British Journal of Obstetrics and Gynaecology (2000) 107:6 (792–794). Date of Publication: 2000

232. Clinical effects of early angiotensin-converting enzyme inhibitor treatment for acute myocardial infarction are similar in the presence and absence of aspirin. Latini R. Tognoni G. Maggioni A.P. Baigent C. Braunwald E. Chen Z.-M. Collins R. Flather M. Franzosi M. Kjekshus J. Kober L. Liu L.-S. Peto R. Pfeffer M. Pizzetti F. Santoro E. Sleight P. Swedberg K. Tavazzi L. Wang W. Yusuf S. Journal of the American College of Cardiology (2000) 35:7 (1801–1807). Date of Publication: June 2000

233. Registering clinical trials (multiple letters). Bonati M. Impicciatore P. Pandolfini C. Scroccaro G. Venturini F. Alberti C. Alberti M.P. Caliumi F. British Medical Journal (2000) 320:7245 (1339–1340). Date of Publication: 13 May 2000

234. Randomized trial of candesartan cilexetil in the treatment of patients with congestive heart failure and a history of intolerance to angiotensin-converting enzyme inhibitors. Granger C.B. Ertl G. Kuch J. Maggioni A.P. McMurray J. Rouleau J.-L. Stevenson L.W. Swedberg K. Young J. Yusuf S. Califf R.M. Bart B.A. Held P. Michelson E.L. Sellers M.A. Ohlin G. Sparapani R. Pfeffer M.A. American Heart Journal (2000) 139:4 (609–617). Date of Publication: 2000

235. Antibiotic prophylaxis in intensive care units: Meta-analyses versus clinical practice. Liberati A. D'Amico R. Pifferi S. Telaro E. Intensive Care Medicine, Supplement (2000) 26:1 (S38–S44). Date of Publication: February 2000

236. The effectiveness of desensitization versus rechallenge treatment in HIV-positive patients with previous hypersensitivity to TMP-SMX: A randomized multicentric study. Bonfanti P. Pusterla L. Parazzini F. Libanore M. Cagni A.E. Franzetti M. Faggion I. Landonio S. Quirino T. Biomedicine and Pharmacotherapy (2000) 54:1 (45–49). Date of Publication: February 2000

237. A randomized controlled trial of recombinant interferon beta-1a in ALS. Beghi E. Chio A. Inghilleri M. Mazzini L. Micheli A. Mora G. Poloni M. Riva R. Serlenga L. Testa D. Tonali P. Neurology (2000) 54:2 (469–474). Date of Publication: 25 Jan 2000

Notes

Introduction

1. Silverman M, Lee PR. *Pills, Profits, and Politics*. Berkeley: University of California Press; 1974.
2. Silverman M, Lee PR, Lydecker M. *Prescriptions for Death: The Drugging of the Third World*. Berkeley: University of California Press; 1982. Silverman M. *The Drugging of the Americas: How Multinational Drug Companies Say One Thing about Their Products to Physicians in the United States and Another Thing to Physicians in Latin America*. Berkeley: University of California Press; 1976.
3. Braithwaite J. *Corporate Crime in the Pharmaceutical Industry*. London: Routledge & Kegan Paul; 1984.
4. Public Citizen Health Research Group. *Rapidly Increasing Criminal and Civil Monetary Penalties Against the Pharmaceutical Industry: 1991–2010*. Washington DC: Public Citizen Health Research Group; 2010.
5. Moore T, Psaty B, Furberg C. Time to act on drug safety. *JAMA*. 1998;279(1571–1573); Moore T. *Prescription for Disaster*. New York: Simon & Schuster; 1998; Moore T. *Deadly Medicine: Why Tens of Thousands of Heart Patients Died in America's Worst Drug Disaster*. New York: Simon & Schuster; 1995.
6. Angell M. *The Truth about the Drug Companies: How They Deceive Us and What to Do about It*. New York: Random House; 2004; Relman A, Angell M. America's other drug problem: how the drug industry distorts medicine and politics. *The New Republic*. 2002 (16 Dec)(4,587):27–36.
7. Healy D. *Pharmageddon*. Berkeley: University of California Press; 2012; Petersen M. *Our Daily Meds: How the Pharmaceutical Companies Transformed Themselves into Slick Marketing Machines and Hooked the Nation on Prescription Drugs*. New York: Sarah Crichton/Farrar, Straus and Giroux; 2008; Avorn J. *Powerful Medicines: The Benefits, Risks, and Costs of Prescription Drugs*. Rev. and updated, 1st Vintage Books ed. New York: Vintage Books; 2005.
8. Goldacre B. *Bad Pharma: How Drug Companies Mislead Doctors and Harm*. London: Faber & Faber; 2012.
9. Light D, Lexchin J. Pharmaceutical R&D—What do we get for all that money? *BMJ*. 2012;344:e4348.
10. Angell, *Truth about Drug Companies*; Healy, *Pharmageddon*; Healy D. Did regulators fail over selective serotonin reuptake inhibitors? *BMJ*. 2006;333:92–95; Avorn J. *Powerful Medicines: The Benefits, Risks, and Costs of Prescription Drugs*. New York: Knopf; 2004; Brody H, Light DW. The inverse benefit law: how drug marketing undermines patient safety and public health. *American Journal of Public Health*. 2011;101(3):399–404.

11. Steinman MA, Bero LA, Chen M-M, Landerfeld CS. Narrative review: The promotion of Gabapentin: an analysis of internal industry documents. *Annals of Internal Medicine*. 2006;145(4):284–293; Sismondo S. Ghost management. *PLoS Medicine*. 2007;4(9):1429–1433; Ross JS, Hill KP, Egilman DS, Krumholz HM. Guest authorship and ghostwriting in publications related to rofecoxib. *JAMA*. 2008;299(15):1800–1812; Hart B, Lundh A, Bero L. Effect of reporting bias on meta-analyses of drug trials: reanalysis of meta-analyses. *BMJ*. 2012;344; Lexchin J. Those who have the gold make the evidence: how the pharmaceutical industry biases the outcomes of clinical trials of medications. *Science and Engineering Ethics*. 2011;18(2):247–261.

12. Light DW, Lexchin J, Darrow J. Institutional Corruption of Pharmaceuticals and the Myth of Safe and Effective Drugs. *Journal of Law, Medicine, & Ethics*. 2013;41(3):590–600.

13. Wright E. *Envisioning Real Utopias*. New York: Verso; 2010.

14. Big Pharma is defined as companies with sales exceeding $10 billion in 2013.

15. Kassirer JP. *On the Take: How Medicine's Complicity with Big Business Can Endanger Your Health*. New York: Oxford University Press; 2005; Bok D. *Universities in the Marketplace*. Princeton, NJ: Princeton University Press; 2003; Brennan TA, Rothman DJ, Blank L, Blumenthal D, et al. Health industry practices that create conflicts of interest: a policy proposal for academic medical centers. *Journal of American Medical Association*. 2006;295:429–433.

16. Brazil Chamber of Deputies. *Brazil's Patent Reform: Innovation Towards National Competitiveness*. Brasilia: Brazil Documentation and Information Center; 2013.

17. Relman and Angell, America's other drug problem; Brennan et al., Health industry practices.

18. Beauchamp T, Childress J. *Principles of Bioethical Ethics, Fifth Edition*. New York: Oxford University Press; 2001.

19. Menzel P, Light DW. A conservative case for universal access to health care. *The Hastings Center Report* 2006;(July):2–11.

20. Waxman HA. *The Marketing of Vioxx to Physicians*. Washington DC: United States House of Representatives, Committee on Government Reform; 5 May 2005; Mathews AW, Martinez B. Warning signs: e-mails suggest Merck knew Vioxx's dangers at early stage. *Wall Street Journal*. 2004 (Nov 1): A1; FDA. *FDA Advisory Committee Briefing Document, NDA 21-042, s007, VIOXX Gastrointestinal Safety*. Washington DC: US Food and Drug Administration; 8 Feb 2001 (8 Feb); Therapeutics Initiative. COX-2 inhibitors update: do journal publications tell the full story? *The Therapeutics Initiative*. 2001 (Nov) 1–2.

21. Public Citizen Health Research Group, *Rapidly Increasing Criminal*; Gøtzsche P. *Deadly Medicines and Organized Crime: How Big Pharma Has Corrupted Healthcare*. Oxford: Radcliffe Medical Press; 2013.

22. Garattini S, Bertele V. How can we regulate medicines better? *BMJ*. 2007;335:803–805; Garattini S, Bertele V. Non-inferiority trials are unethical because they disregard patients' interests. *Lancet*. 2007;370:1875–1877.

23. Light and Lexchin, Pharmaceutical R&D; Lexchin J. New drugs and safety: what happened to new active substances approved in Canada between 1995 and 2010? *Archives of Internal Medicine*. 2012;172(21):1680–1681.

24. Garattini and Bertele, Non-inferiority trials.

25. Light D, Lexchin J, Darrow J. Institutional corruption of pharmaceuticals and the myth of safe and effective drugs. *Journal of Law, Medicine & Ethics*. 2013;41(3):590–600.

26. Healy, *Pharmageddon*; Le Fanu J. *The Rise and Fall of Modern Medicine*. London: Basic; 2002, Ch3.

27. Jasanoff S. *Designs on Nature: Science and Democracy in Europe and the United States*. Princeton, NJ: Princeton University Press; 2005, 207.

28. Ibid.

29. Ibid., 205.

30. Ibid., 207; Winner L. *The Whale and the Reactor: A Search for Limits in an Age of High Technology*. Chicago: University of Chicago Press; 1986.

31. Sismondo S. *An Introduction to Science and Technology Studies, 2nd Edition*. London: Wiley-Blackwell; 2009.

32. Latour B, Woolgar S. *Laboratory Life: The Social Construction of Scientific Facts*. Beverly Hills, CA: Sage; 1979.

33. Knorr-Cetina KD. *The Manufacture of Knowledge: An Essay on the Constructivist and Contextual Nature of Science*. Oxford: Pergamon; 1981.

34. Mathews and Martinez, Warning signs.

35. Ibid.

36. Waxman, *Marketing of Vioxx*.

37. FDA. *HFD-550, medical officer review, Vioxx (rofecoxib), NDA 21-042/052*. Washington DC: US Food and Drug Administration 1999; Topol EJ. Failing the public health—rofecoxib, Merck, and the FDA. *New England Journal of Medicine*. (21 Oct) 2004;351:1707–1709; correspondence 2875–1778; Krumholz H, et al. What have we learnt from Vioxx? *BMJ*. 2007;334:120–123.

38. Bessen J, Meurer M. *Patent Failure: How Judges, Bureacrats and Lawyers Put Innovation at Risk*. Princeton: Princeton University Press; 2008; Heller MA, Eisenberg RS. Can patents deter innovation? The anticommons in biomedical research. *Science*. 1998;280(5364):698–701.

39. Light and Lexchin, Pharmaceutical R&D; Schondelmeyer S, Purvis L. *Rx Price Watch Report*. Washington DC: American Association of Retired Persons 2012; Apolone G, Joppi R, Bertele V, Garattini S. Ten years of marketing approvals of anti-cancer drugs in Europe: regulatory policy and guidance documents need to find a balance between different pressures. *Br J Cancer*. Sep 5 2005;93(5):504–509; Joppi R, Bertele V, Garattini S. Disappointing biotech. *BMJ*. Oct 15 2005;331(7521):895–897.

40. Light DW. Basic Research Funds to Discover Important New Drugs: Who Contributes How Much? In: Burke MA, ed. *Monitoring the Financial Flows for Health Research 2005: Behind the Global Numbers*. Geneva: Global Forum for Health Research; 2006:27–43; Light DW, Warburton RN. Extraordinary claims require extraordinary evidence. *Journal of Health Economics*. 2005;24:1030–1033.

41. Light DW, Warburton RN. Demythologizing the high cost of pharmaceutical research. *Biosocieties*. 2011 (Win):1–17.

42. Light, Lexchin, and Darrow, Institutional corruption of pharmaceuticals; Gagnon M-A. Corruption of pharmaceutical markets: addressing the misalignment of financial incentives and public policy reform. *Journal of Law, Medicine & Ethics*. 2013;41(3).

43. Menzel and Light, conservative case.

44. Page I. Forward. In: Garattini S, Valzelli L, eds. *Serotonin*. Amsterdam, London: Elsevier; 1965: v–vi.

45. Colombo F, Shapiro S, Slone D, Tognoni G, eds. *Epidemiological Evaluation of Drugs*. Amsterdam/London: Elsevier/North Holland Biomedical Press; 1977.

46. Catholic Charities U.S.A. *Code of Ethics*. Alexandria, Virginia: Catholic Charities U.S.A.; 2007.

47. Light D, ed. *The Risks of Prescription Drugs*. New York: Columbia University Press; 2010.
48. *Nature* editors. American inspiration in Milan: Mario Negri pharmacology institute. *Nature*. 1983 (May 12);303:124–125.
49. Healy, *Pharmageddon*; Light, *The Risks of Prescription Drugs*.
50. *Nature* editors, American inspiration in Milan.

Chapter 1

1. Wagstaff A. Masterpiece: The people's pharmacologist. *Cancer World*. 2008; (May):28–33.
2. Ibid.
3. Fox R. Medical scientists in a château. *Science*. 1962;136(11 May):476–483.
4. Clark B. *Academic Power in Italy: Bureaucracy and Oligarchy in a National University System*. Chicago: University of Chicago Press; 1977.
5. Healy D. The role of independent science in psychopharmacology: Silvio Garattini. In: Healy D, ed. *The Psychopharmacologists*. London: Chapman & Hall; 1996:135–158.
6. Garattini S, Ghetti V, eds. *Psychotropic Drugs*. Amsterdam: Elsevier; 1957.
7. Healy, role of independent science.
8. Ibid.
9. Hollister L, Garattini S. In: Silser F, ed. *An Oral History of Neuropsychopharmacology Vol 3 Neuropharmacology*. Brentwood, TN: American College of Psychopharmacology 1995:204.
10. Wagstaff, Masterpiece.
11. Ibid.
12. Garattini S, Paoletti R, eds. *Drugs Affecting Lipid Metabolism* Amsterdam: Elsevier; 1961.
13. Hollister and Garattini, *Oral History of Neuropsychopharmacology*.
14. Ibid.
15. Carrara M, Arduini S. *Storie di ordinaria filantropia*. Milano: Gruppo24ore;2011: 110.
16. Hollister and Garattini, *Oral History of Neuropsychopharmacology*.
17. Anon. Italy gets independent research foundation: nonprofit Mario Negri Pharmacological Institute will do research in chemotherapy and pharmacology. *Chemical and Engineering News*. 1962 (July 9);40(28):54–56.
18. Ibid.

Chapter 2

1. Schein E. *Organizational Culture and Leadership*. 4th ed. San Francisco: Jossey-Bass; 2010: 11, 36.
2. Ibid., Ch 5.
3. Lessig L. *Institutional Corruptions*. Cambridge, MA: Research in Action Working Papers, Edmond J. Safra Center for Ethics, Harvard University; 2013.
4. Angell M. *The Truth about the Drug Companies: How They Deceive Us and What to Do about It*. New York: Random House; 2004; Goldacre B. *Bad Pharma: How Drug Companies Mislead Doctors and Harm*. London: Faber & Faber; 2012; Healy D. *Pharmageddon*. Berkeley: University of California Press; 2012; Light DW.

Reducing Global Health Disparities through Vaccines: Rhetorics and Realities of Advanced Market Commitments. *Dean's Colloquium, UC Berkeley School for Public Health*. Berkeley, CA 2010 (4 Nov).

5. Leonardi A, Baggott J, Pantarotto C. The Mario Negri Institute for Pharmacological Research. *Pharmacy International*. 1980(Sept):170–173.

6. Wright E. *Envisioning Real Utopias*. New York: Verso; 2010.

7. Brody H. The commercialization of medical decisions: physicians and patients at risk. In: Light DW, ed. *The Risks of Prescription Drugs*. New York: Columbia University Press; 2010:70–90; Stults C, Conrad P. Medicalization and Risk Scares: The Case of Menopause and HRT. In: Light DW, ed. *The Risks of Prescription Drugs*. New York: Columbia Unviersity Press; 2010:116–139; NPR. How a bone disease grew to fit the prescription. 2009; file:///Users/dlight/Documents/Safra-Pharm-Osteopenia%20-new%20disease%20NPR.webarchive; Moynihan R, Cassels A. *Selling Sickness: How the World's Biggest Pharmaceutical Companies Are Turning Us All Into Patients*. New York: Nation Books; 2005.

8. Garattini S. *Fa bene o fa male? Salute, ricerca e farmaci: tutto quello che bisogna sapere (Is it healthy or not? Health, research and pharmaceuticals: all you need to know)*. Milano: Sperling & Kupfer; 2013.

9. Knorr-Cetina K. *Epistemic Cultures: How the Sciences Make Knowledge*. Cambridge, MA: Harvard University Press; 1999.

10. Hollister L, Garattini S. In: Silser F, ed. *An Oral History of Neuropsychopharmacology Vol 3 Neuropharmacology*. Brentwood, Tennessee: American College of Psychopharmacology 1995:206.

11. Ibid., 207.

12. Pfeffer J, Salancik G. *The External Control of Organizations: A Resource Dependence Perspective*. Stanford, CA: Stanford University Press; 2003: 1.

13. Christakis N, Fowler J. *Connected: The Amazing Power of Social Networks and How They Shape Our Lives*. New York: Harper Press; 2000.

14. Pfeffer and Salancik, *External Control of Organizations*, 23.

15. Leonardi A. Etica e politica dell'Istituto "Mario Negri." *Negri News*. Milano: The Mario Negri Institute for Pharmacological Research; 1995 (June):41–42.

16. Istituto di Ricerche Farmacologiche Mario Negri. *1963–1968: 6 Anni de Attivita*. Milano: Istituto di Ricerche Farmacologiche Mario Negri; 1969.

17. Istituto di Ricerche Farmacologiche Mario Negri. *20 Anni di Attivita 1963–1983*. Milano: Istituto di Ricerche Farmacologiche Mario Negri; 1983.

18. The Apple-1 machine was first marketed in 1976. They were priced at $666.66 back then. In 2013, one was sold for $640,000 at auction. (S Lohr, "Used computer, $116,000 or best offer" *The New York Times*. May 24, 2013: B1,B4.)

19. Light DW. Basic Research Funds to Discover Important New Drugs: Who Contributes How Much? In: Burke MA, ed. *Monitoring the Financial Flows for Health Research 2005: Behind the Global Numbers*. Geneva: Global Forum for Health Research; 2006:27–43.

20. Bessen J, Meurer M. *Patent Failure: How Judges, Bureacrats and Lawyers Put Innovation at Risk*. Princeton: Princeton University Press; 2008; Heller MA, Eisenberg RS. Can patents deter innovation? The anticommons in biomedical research. *Science*. 1998;280(5364):698–701.

21. Pfeffer and Salancik, *External Control of Organizations*.

22. Istituto di Ricerche Farmacologiche Mario Negri, *1963–1968*.

23. Istituto di Ricerche Farmacologiche Mario Negri. *Foundzione Privata al Servizio della Salute Umana*. Milano: Istituto di Ricerche Farmacologiche Mario Negri 1990.

24. Istituto di Ricerche Farmacologiche Mario Negri, *1963–1968*.

25. Istituto di Ricerche Farmacologiche Mario Negri, *20 Anni di Attivita 1963–1983*.
26. Istituto di Ricerche Farmacologiche Mario Negri, *Foundzione Privata al Servizio*.
27. Leonardi, Baggott, and Pantarotto, The Mario Negri Institute.
28. Istituto di Ricerche Farmacologiche Mario Negri, *Foundzione Privata al Servizio*.
29. Donati M, de Gaetano G. Bio-medical research and search for personhood: a 40-year project. *Journal of Medicine and the Person*. 2012;10:114–125.
30. The Liceo Classico "Giuseppe Parini" was the most prestigious secondary school in Milan.
31. What made it impossible is that the number needed was based on careful calculations of the minimum number needed for statistical power to get valid results, not a number the researcher felt she needed. Reducing the number by 20 percent made no scientific sense and invalidated the study. Heads of departments were sometimes referred to as "Barons."

Chapter 3

1. Maturo A. Health care delivery system: Italy. In: Cockerham W, Dingwall R, Quah S, eds. *The Wiley Blackwell Encyclopedia of Health, Illness, Behavior, and Society*. London: John Wiley & Sons, Ltd; 2014:823–829.
2. Consorzio Mario Negri SUD. Consorzio Mario Negri SUD. In: SUD CMN, ed: Consorzio Mario Negri SUD; 1998.
3. Iacoviello L, Di Castelnuovo A, De Knijff P, et al. Polymorphisms in the coagulation factor VII gene and the risk of myocardial infarction. *New England Journal of Medicine*. 1998;338(2):79–85.
4. Sandel M. *What Money Can't Buy: The Moral Limits of Markets*. New York: Farrar, Straus and Giroux; 2012.
5. Rodwin M. Conflicts of interest, institutional corruption, and Pharma: an agenda for reform. *Journal of Law, Medicine & Ethics*. 2012;40(Fall):511–522; Rodwin M. *Conflicts of Interest and the Future of Medicine*. New York: Oxford University Press; 2011.
6. AMD. *Improving the Quality of Diabetes Care in Italy*: Associazione Medici Diabetologi; 2012.
7. Nicolucci A, Rossi M, Arcangeli A, Ciminot A, et al. Four-year impact of a continuous quality improvement effort implemented by a network of diabetes outpatient clinics: the AMD-Annals initiative. *Diabetic Medicine*. 2010; DOI:10.1111:1041-1048.
8. De Berardis G, Sacco M, Strippoli G, et al. Aspirin for primary prevention of cardiovascular events in people with diabetes: meta-analysis of randomised controlled trials. *BMJ*. 2010 (Nov 6):b4531.
9. De Berardis G, Lucisano G, D'Ettore A, et al. Association of aspirin use with major bleeding in patients with and without diabetes. *Journal of the American Medical Association*. 2012;307(21):2286–2294.
10. Landolfi R, Marchioli R, Kutti J, Gisslinger H, Tognoni G, et al. Efficacy and safety of low-dose aspirin in polycythemia vera. *New England Journal of Medicine*. 2004;350(2):114–124.
11. Marchioli R, Finazzi G, Specchia G, Cacciola R, et al. Cardiovascular events and intensity of treatment in polycythemia vera. *New England Journal of Medicine*. 2013; (Jan 3) 368(1):22–33.
12. Wikipedia. 2009 L'Aquila earthquake. 2013; http://en.wikipedia.org/wiki/2009_L'Aquila_earthquake.

13. Donati M, de Gaetano G. Bio-medical research and search for personhood: a 40-year project. *Journal of Medicine and the Person.* 2012;10:119.

14. Bonaccio M, Iacoviello L, de Gaetano G, Moli-Sani Investigators. The Mediterranean diet: the reasons for a success. *Thrombosis Resarch.* 2012;129(3):401–404; Costanzo S, Di Castelnuovo A, Donati M, Iacoviello L. Alcohol consumption and mortality in patients with cardiovascular disease: a meta-analysis. *Journal of the American College of Cardiology.* 2010;55:1339–1347.

15. Remuzzi G, Mecca G, Cavenaghi A, Donati M, De Gaetano G. Prostacyclin-like activity and bleeding in renal failure *The Lancet.* 1977;310(8050):1195–1197.

16. Remuzzi G, De Gaetano G, Mecca G, eds. *Hemostasis, Protaglandins, and Renal Disease.* New York: Raven Press; 1980. Garattini S, ed. Monographs of the Mario Negri Institute for Pharmocological Research.

17. Bertani T, Poggi A, Pozzoni R, Delaini F, et al. Adriamycin-induced nephrotic syndrome in rats: sequence of pathologic events. *Lab Investigations.* 1982;46(1):16–23.

18. Benigni A, Gregorini G, Frusca T, Chiabrando C, Ballerini S, et al. Effect of low-dose aspirin on fetal and maternal generation of thromboxane by platelets in women at risk for pregnancy-induced hypertension. *New England Journal of Medicine.* 1989;321(6):357–362.

19. The GISEN Group (Gruppo Italiano di Studi Epidemiologici in Nefrologia). Randomised placebo-controlled trial of effect of ramipril on decline in glomerular filtration rate and risk of terminal renal failure in proteinuric, non-diabetic nephropathy. *Lancet.* 1997;349(9069):1857–1863.

20. The GISEN Group (Gruppo Italiano di Studi Epidemiologici in Nefrologia). Renal function and requirement for dialysis in chronic nephropathy patients on long-term ramipril: REIN follow-up trial. *Lancet.* 1998;352(9136):1252–1256.

21. The Remission Clinic Task Force. The Remission Clinic approach to halt the progression of kidney disease. *Journal of Nephrology.* 2011;24(3):274.

22. Ruggenenti P, Fassi A, Ilieva A, Bruno S, Bergamo Nephrologic Diabetes Complications Trial (BENEDICT) Investigators. Preventing microalbuminuria in type 2 diabetes. *New England Journal of Medicine.* 2004;351(19):1941–1951.

23. Remuzzi G, Grinyò J, Ruggenenti P, Beatini M, et al. Early experience with dual kidney transplantation in adults using expanded donor criteria. Double Kidney Transplant Group (DKG) *Journal of the American Society of Nephrology.* 1999;12:2591–2598.

24. Remuzzi G, Cravedi P, Perna A, Dimitrov B, et al. Dual Kidney Transplant Group. Long-term outcome of renal transplantation from older donors. *New England Journal of Medicine.* 2006;354(4):343–352.

25. Cravedi P, Ruggenenti P, Remuzzi G. Old donors for kidney transplantation: how old? *Gerontology.* 2011;57(6):13–20.

26. Lim W, Clayton P, Wong G, Campbell S, et al. Outcome of kidney transplantation from older living donors. *Transplantation.* 2013;95(1):106–113.

27. Benigni A, Morigi M, Rizzo P, Gagliardini E, et al. Inhibiting angiotensin-converting enzyme promotes renal repair by limiting progenitor cell proliferation and restoring the glomerular architecture. *American Journal of Pathology.* 2011;179(2):628–638.

28. Xinaris C, Benedetti V, Rizzo P, Abbate M, et al. *In vivo* maturation of functional renal organoids formed from embryonic cell suspensions. *Journal of the American Society of Nephrology.* 2012;11:1857–1868.

29. Remuzzi G, Benigni A, Finkelstein O, Grunfeld J-P, et al. Kidney failure: aims for the next 10 years and barriers to success. *The Lancet.* 2013;382:353–360.

30. Donati M, Balconi G, Remuzzi G, Borgia R, Morasca L, de Gaetano G. Skin fibroblasts from a patient with Glanzmann's thrombasthenia do not induce fibrin clot retraction. *Thrombosis Research*. 1977;10(1):173–174.
31. See http://www.euscreen.eu/play.jsp?id=EUS_4630CE93797E44BEAF8DB50B20 BEBC65.
32. Legendre C, Light C, Muus P, Greenbaum L, et al. Terminal complement inhibitor eculizumab in atypical hemolytic-uremic syndrome. *New England Journal of Medicine*. 2013;368:2169–2181.
33. Editors. Italian biomedical research under fire. *Nature Neuroscience*. 2013 (Nov 22);16(1709):doi:10.1030/nn.3595.
34. Saraceno B. Il progetto dell'Instituto "Mario Negri": salute mentale in American Latina. *Epidemiologia e Psichiatria Sociale*. 1994;3(1):49–58.
35. Plata R, Silva C, Yahuita J, Perez L, Schieppati A, Remuzzi G. The first clinical and epidemiological programme on renal disease in Bolivia: a model for prevention and early diagnosis of renal diseases in the developing countries. *Nephrology Dialysis Transplantation*. 1998;13(12):3034–3036; Tognoni G. The global burden of disease and the challenge of invisibility. *Nephrology Dialysis Transplantation*. 1998;13(12):3016–3018.
36. Crevedi P, Sharma S, Bravo R, Islam N, et al. Preventing renal and cardiovascular risk by renal function assessment: insights from a cross-sectional study in low-income countries and the USA. *BMJ Open* 2012;2: e001357;doi:001310.001136.
37. Feehally J, Couser W, Dupuis S, Finkelstein F, et al. Nephrology in developing countries: the ISN's story. *Lancet*. 2014;383:1271–1272.

Chapter 4

1. Maturo A. *Sociologia della Malattia*. Milano: FrancoAngeli; 2007.
2. Shim J. Cultural health capital. A theoretical approach to understanding health care interactions and the dynamics of unequal treatments. *Journal of Health and Social Behavior*. 2010;51(1):1–15.
3. Cipolla C. *Perché non possiamo non essere eclettici. Il sapere sociale nella web society* Milano: FrancoAngeli; 2012.
4. Mosconi P, Colombo C. Fostering a strategic alliance between patients' associations and health care professionals. *Journal of Ambulatory Care Management*. 2010;33(3):223–230.
5. Mosconi P, Colombo C, Villani W, Liberati A, Satolli R. PartecipaSalute: a research project and a training program tailored on consumers and patients. In: Albolino S, ed. *Healthcare Systems Ergonomics and Patient Safety*. London: Taylor & Francis; 2011:71–76.
6. Mosconi P, Colombo C, Satolli R, Liberati A. PartecipaSalute, an Italian project to involve lay people, patients' associations and scientific-medical representatives in the health debate. *Health Expectations*. 2006;10:194–204.
7. Fadden R, Powers M. A social justice framework for health and social policy. *Cambridge Quarterly of Healthcare Ethics*. 2011;20:596–604.
8. Richards T, Montori V, Godlee F, Lapsley P, Paul D. Let the patient revolution begin. *BMJ* 2013;346:f2614.
9. Maturo A. Network governance as a response to risk society's dilemmas: a proposal from sociology of health. *Topoì—International Review of Philosophy*. 2004;23(II):195–202.

10. Segall S. Is health care (still) special? *Journal of Political Philosophy.* 2007;4(2):242–263.

11. Bloom SW. *The Doctor and His Patient.* New York: Russell Sage Foundation; 1963.

12. Maturo A. The medicalization of education: ADHD, human enhancement, and academic performance. *Italian Journal of Sociology of Education.* 2013;5(3):178–188.

13. Maturo A. The shifting borders of medicalization: perspective and dilemmas of human enhancement. In: Maturo A, Conrad P, eds. *The Medicalization of Life, Salute e Società.* Vol. VIII. Bologna 2009:13–30.

14. Bonati M. Reducing overdiagnosis and disease mongering in ADHD in Lombardy. *BMJ.* 2013;347:f7474.

15. Affaritaliani. Garattini contro omeopatia e agopuntura negli ospedali: "A quando maghi e fattucchieri?" *Affar Italiani:* Affaritaliani.It; 2011 (Apr 26).

16. Invernizzi G. *Fumo di tabacco e salute respiratoria nella donna: il ruolo del medico di famiglia.* Milano: Rivista della Società Italiana di Medicina Generale; 2010; Gallus S, Murisic B, La Vecchia C. *Anti-smoking campaigns in Italy: the role of the Mario Negri Institute for Pharmacological Research.* Milano: Mario Negri Institute for Pharmacological Research; 2013.

17. Gallus, Murisic, and La Vecchia, *Anti-smoking campaigns in Italy.*

18. La Vecchia C, Garattini S. Italy—attitudes to legislation on restriction of smoking. *The Lancet.* 1987;329(8545):1310.

19. Gallus S, Zuccaro P, Colombo P, et al. Effects of new smoking regulations in Italy. *Annals of Oncology.* 2006;17:346–347.

20. American Cancer Society. Di Belli Therapy. 2008; http://www.cancer.org/treatment/treatmentsandsideeffects/complementaryandalternativemedicine/pharmacologicalandbiologicaltreatment/di-bella-therapy.

21. Italian Study Group for the Di Bella Multitherapy Trials. Evaluation of an unconventional cancer treatment (the Di Bella multitherapy): results of phase II trials in Italy. *BMJ* 1999;318:224.

22. American Cancer Society, Di Belli Therapy, 2008.

23. Bocci M. Intervista a Silvio Garattini, "Una terapia non si approva per sentenza". *la Repubblica.* 2012 (Sept 1):17.

24. Gualtani A, De Francesco L, Garattini S. Reduced use of laboratory animals in research institute. *The Lancet.* 1997; 349 (9064):1557–58.

25. Garattini S. Forward: The necessity of animal experimentation. In: Garattini S, van Bekkum D, eds. *The Importance of Animal Experimentation for Safety and Biomedical Research.* Dordrecht: Kluwer Academic Publishers; 1990:vii–3.

26. Editors. Italian biomedical research under fire. *Nature Neuroscience.* 2013 (Nov 22);16(1709):doi:10.1030/nn.3595.

27. Ibid.

28. Tulli dF. Garattini, S. "Non chiamatela vivisezione." *Left.* Rome 2013 (30 Nov).

29. Rosati E. "Umberto Veronesi e Silvio Garattini, due scienziati a confronto." *OGGI.* 2012 (March).

30. Sztompka P. *Trust: A Sociological Theory.* Cambridge, UK: Cambridge University Press; 1999.

31. Leonardi A. Interview with Alfredo Leonardi, Ricercatori formati sul campo di battaglia. *Negri News.* Vol XIII. Milano: Mario Negri Institute for Pharmacological Research; 1981.

32. Schein EH. *Organizational Culture and Leadership.* 3rd ed. San Francisco: Jossey-Bass; 2004.

33. Kelley R, Caplan J. How Bell Labs creates star performers. *Harvard Business Review.* Jul–Aug 1993;71(4):128–139.
34. Jori A. Quarantaquattro anni dopo. *MarioNegri News.* 2005: 3–5.
35. Bendotti C. "Studio come vincere la SLA. Intanto ho vinto il mio tumore" (I study how to beat SLA and meantime defeated my cancer.). *L'Eco di Bergamo.* 2011 (Oct 11).
36. Cowan A, Ghezzi D, Samanin R. Effect of midbrain raphe lesion and 6-hydroxy-dopamine on the antinociceptive action of buprenorphine in rats. *Archives Internationales de Pharmacodynamie et de Therapie* 1974;208:302–305.
37. Adler MW, Manara L, Samanin R, eds. *Factors Affecting the Action of Narcotics.* New York: Raven 1978. In Garattini S, ed. The Mario Negri Monograph Series.
38. The Open University Research Degrees Committee. *Affiliated Research Centre Programme Report on the Visit to Istituto di Ricerche Farmacologiche Mario Negri.* London: The Open University; 2013 (June).

Chapter 5

1. Hay A. *The Chemical Scythe: Lessons of 2, 4, 5-T, and Dioxin.* New York: Plenum Press; 1982: Ch 9.
2. Fanelli R, Chiabrando C, Bonaccorsi A. TCDD contamination in the Seveso incident. *Drug Metabolism Reviews.* 1982;13(3):407–422.
3. Manara L, Garattini S. Seveso: premature optimism. *Nature.* 1978;276(7):556.
4. Morgan SG, Bassett KL, Wright JM, et al. "Breakthrough" drugs and growth in expenditure on prescription drugs in Canada. *BMJ.* 2005;331(7520):815–816.
5. Light D, Lexchin J, Darrow J. Institutional corruption of pharmaceuticals and the myth of safe and effective drugs. *Journal of Law, Medicine & Ethics.* 2013;41(3):590–600.
6. MistraPharma. *Collaborating to Reduce the Environmental Risks of Pharmaceuticals.* Stockholm: Elanders Sverige; 2011; A leading policy group that brings together industry and government leaders to address medicines as environmental hazards is the Swedish organization, MistraPharma. They have written a series of informative short monographs: *A Healthy Future—Pharmaceuticals in a Sustainable Society* (2009), *Towards Sustainable Pharmaceuticals in a Health Society* (2010), *Collaborating to Reduce the Environmental Risks of Pharmaceuticals* (2011), and *Pharmaceuticals in a Health Environment* (2012).
7. Hay, *Chemical Scythe*, Ch 9.
8. Jefferson T, Doshi P, Thompson M, Heneghan C. Ensuring safe and effective drugs: who can do what it takes? *BMJ.* 2011;342:c7258; Doshi P, Jones M, Jefferson T. Rethinking credible evidence synthesis. *BMJ.* 2012;344:d7898; Sismondo S, Doucet M. Publication ethics and the ghost management of medical publication. *Bioethics.* 2010;24(6):273–283; Rodwin M. Conflicts of interest, institutional corruption, and Pharma: an agenda for reform. *Journal of Law, Medicine & Ethics.* 2012;40(Fall):511–522.
9. Hay, *Chemical Scythe*, 199.
10. Bonaccorsi A, Fanelli R, Tognoni G. In the wake of Seveso. *Ambro.* 1978;7:237.
11. Fanelli, Chiabrando, and Bonaccorsi, TCDD contamination.
12. Ibid.
13. Bonaccorsi, Fanelli, and Tognoni, In the wake of Seveso, 234.

14. European Commission. *Directive of the European Parliament and of the Council on control of major-accident hazards involving dangerous substances.* Brussels: European Commission; 2010(21.12); Schecter A. *Dioxins and Health: Including Other Persistent Organic Pollutants and Endocrine Disruptions, 3rd Edition.* Hoboken, NJ: John Wiley & Sons; 2012.

15. Markowitz G, Rosner D. *Deceit and Denial: The Deadly Politics of Industrial Pollution.* Berkeley: University of California Press; 2002.

16. Hay, *Chemical Scythe.*

17. Fanelli R. Interview. Milano: Mario Negri Institute; 2012 (May 8).

18. Bonaccorsi, Fanelli, and Tognoni, In the wake of Seveso.

19. Fanelli, Chiabrando, and Bonaccorsi, TCDD contamination.

20. Mocarelli P, Gerthoux P, Brambilla P, Marocchi A, et al. Dioxin health effects on humans twenty years after Seveso: a summary. In: Ballarin-Denti A, Berazzi P, Facchetti S, Fanelli R, Mocarelli P, eds. *Chemistry, Man and Environment: The Seveso Accident 20 Years On.* Amsterdam: Elsevier; 1999:41–51.

21. Morcarelli P, Brambill P, Patterson DJ, Needham L. Change in sex ratio with exposure to dioxin. *The Lancet.* 1996;348(9024):409.

22. Axelson O. The epidemiologic evidence of health effects of TCDD in human beings. In: Mocarelli P, Gerthoux P, Brambilla P, Marocchi A, et al., eds. *Chemistry, Man and Environment: The Seveso Accident 20 Years On.* Amsterdam: Elsevier; 1999:29–38.

23. Delaney J. *First X, Then Y, Now Z: An Introduction to Landmark Thematic Maps.* Princeton, NJ: Princeton University Press for Firestone Library; 2012: 119–121; You can see his detailed map at http://libweb5.princeton.edu/visual_materials/maps/websites/thematic-maps/quantitative/medicine/medicine.html#Lancisi. Lancisi also analyzed fetid air in Rome and designed measures to reduce it. He is also regarded as the founder of cardiovascular pathology and described in detail angina pectoris half a century before William Heberden published his account of it. At the request of Clement XI, he analyzed an epidemic of sudden deaths in 1705, based on autopsies of the victims, and published a monograph on their causes.

24. Bonati M, Tognoni G. Has clinical pharmacology lost its way? *The Lancet.* 1984;323(8376):556–558.

25. Mariani G, Benfenati E, Fanelli R. Concentrations of PCDD and PCDF in different points on a modern refuse incinerator. *Chemosphere.* 1990;21:507–517.

26. Bittman M. Opinionator: Breeding bacteria on factory farms. *The New York Times.* 2013 (July 9).

27. Kessler D. Antibiotics and the meat we eat. *The New York Times.* 2013 (Mar 27).

28. Zuccato E, Calamari D, Natangelo M, Fanelli R. Presence of therapeutic drugs in the environment. *The Lancet.* 2000;355(9217):1789–1790.

29. WHO. *Pharmaceuticals in Drinking-water.* Geneva: The World Health Organization; 2011.

30. MistraPharma, *Collaboration to reduce*; Shah S. *As Pharmaceutical Use Soars, Drugs Taint Water and Wildlife.* New Haven, CT: Yale University; 2010.

31. Bienkowski B. Fish on Prozac: anxious, anti-social, aggressive. *Environmental News.* 2013 (June 12).

32. MistraPharma, *Collaboration to reduce.*

33. Associated Press National Investigative Team. Drugs in the drinking water (14 parts). *Drugs in the drinking water* New York: Associated Press; 2012.

34. Lexchin J. New drugs and safety: what happened to new active substances approved in Canada between 1995 and 2010? *Archives of Internal Medicine.* 2012;172(21):1680–1681.
35. Light, Lexchin, and Darrow, Institutional corruption of pharmaceuticals.
36. Kaiser Family Foundation. *Prescription Drug Trends.* Palo Alto, CA: Kaiser Family Foundation; 2010.
37. Zuccato E, Castiglioni S, Fanelli R, et al. Pharmaceuticals in the environment in Italy: causes, occurence, effects, and control. *Environmental Science & Pollution Research.* 2006;13(1):15–21.
38. Prescrire International editors. Drugs in wastewater: incomplete removal by treatment plants. *Prescrire International.* 2013 (feb);22(135):52–54.
39. Calamari D, Zuccato E, Castiglioni S, Fanelli R. Strategic survey of therapeutic drugs in the rivers Po and Lambro in northern Italy. *Environmental Science & Technology.* 2003;37(1241–48).
40. Zuccato E, Chaibrando C, Castiglioni S, et al. Cocaine in surface water: a new evidence-based tool to monitor community drug abuse. *Environmental Health.* 2005;4(14):1–7.
41. Khamsi R. Sewage study spots cocaine users. *Nature News;* 2005 (Aug 5).
42. Zuccato E, Castiglioni S, Bagnati R, Fanelli R. Estimating community drug abuse by wastewater analysis. *Environmental Health Perspectives.* 2008;116(8):1027–1032.
43. Castiglioni S, Zuccato E. Occurrence of illicit drugs in wastewater and surface water in Italy. In: Castiglioni S, Zuccato E, Fanelli R, eds. *Illicit Drugs in the Environment.* Hoboken, NJ: John Wiley & Sons; 2011:137–151.
44. Castiglioni S, Zuccato E, Fanelli R, eds. *Illicit Drugs in the Environment.* Hoboken, NJ: John Wiley & Sons; 2011.
45. Panawennage D, Castiglioni S, Zuccato E, Davoli E, Chiarelli M. Measurement of illicit drug consumption in small populations: prognosis for noninvasive drug testing of student populations. In: Castiglioni S, Zuccato E, Fanelli R, eds. *Illicit Drugs in the Environment.* Hoboken, NJ: John Wiley & Sons; 2011:321–331.

Chapter 6

1. Editors. What is the purpose of medical research? *The Lancet.* 2013 (Feb 2);381(9864):doi:10.1016/S0140-6736(1013)60149-X.
2. Chalmers I, Glasziou P. Avoidable waste in the production and reporting of research evidence. *The Lancet.* 2009;374(9683):86–89.
3. Tognoni G, Bonati M. Second-generation clinical pharmacology. *The Lancet.* 1986;328(8514):1028–1029.
4. Goldacre B. *Bad Pharma: How Drug Companies Mislead Doctors and Harm.* London: Faber & Faber; 2012.
5. Major P, Kocen A, Vasu A. *Pharmaceuticals: Changing the R&D Debate.* London: Redburn Partners; 2011; Munos B. *Open Scientific Collaboration for Innovation in Global Health (OpenSCI).* Durham, NC: DukeSanfordSchool; 2012 (May 2).
6. Chalmers I. Biomedical research: are we getting value for money? *Significance.* 2006;3(4):172–175; Garattini S, Chalmers I. Patients and the public deserve big changes in evaluation of drugs. *BMJ.* 2009 (31 Mar);338:b1025.
7. Goldacre, *Bad Pharma.*
8. Light DW. Reducing Global Health Disparities through Vaccines: Rhetorics and Realities of Advanced Market Commitments. *Dean's Colloquium, UC Berkeley School for Public Health.* Berkeley, CA; 2010 (4 Nov).

9. Braunwald E. Happy birthday, GISSI! *American Heart Journal.* 2004;1(48):187.
10. Tognoni G, Fresco C, Maggioni A, Turazza F. The GISSI story (1983–1996). *Journal of Interventional Cardiology.* 1997;10(1):3–28.
11. Tognoni G, Franzosi M, Garattini S, Maggioni A. The case of GISSI in changing the attitudes and practice of Italian cardiologists. *Statistics in Medicine.* 1990;9:17–27.
12. Peto R, Pike M, Armitage P, Breslow N, et al. Design and analysis of randomized clinical trials requiring prolonged observation of each patient. *British Journal of Cancer.* 1976;34:587.
13. When someone says a drug is "significantly better," it may not mean it has an important or substantial benefit because "significant" refers to statistical significance, the likelihood that the difference is not due to chance. For example, a drug that increases a benefit from merely 1.0 percent to 1.5 percent can be shown to be "significantly better" by mounting a large trial that proves the difference is not due to chance. A company can also say, "Our new drug is 50 percent better," though the absolute benefit is small. Large commercial trials can be a sign that drugs that make little difference to patients are being proven to be "statistically significant"— a great waste of money and time to mislead patients and their doctors.
14. Yusuf S, Collins R, Peto R. Why do we need some large, simple, randomized trials? *Statistics in Medicine.* 1984;3:409–420.
15. Maroo A, Topol E. The early history and development of thrombolysis in acute myocardial infarction. *Journal of Thrombosis and Haemostasis.* 2004;2:1867–1870.
16. Tognoni et al., Case of GISSI.
17. Tognoni G, Ferrario L, Inzalaco M. Progestagens in threatened abortion. *The Lancet.* 1980 (Dec 6)(1519):1242–1243.
18. Sleight P. We could all learn from the Italian cardiologists. *American Heart Journal.* 2004;148:188–189.
19. Tavazzi L, Maggioni A, Tognoni G. Participation versus education: the GISSI story and beyond. *American Heart Journal.* 2004;148(2):222.
20. Yusuf S. Transforming the scientific, health care, and sociopolitical culture of an entire country through clinical research: the story of GISSI. *American Heart Journal.* 2004;148(2):194.
21. Taylor J. The evolution of GISSI during the last 30 years. *CardioPulse: European Heart Journal.* 2010;31:1027–1029.
22. Gruppo Italiano per lo studio della streptochinasi nell'infarto miocardico (GISSI). Effectiveness of intravenous thrombolytic treatment of acute myocardial infarction *The Lancet.* 1986;327(8478):398.
23. Ibid.
24. Tognoni et al., Case of GISSI, 21.
25. Ibid.
26. Light DW, Warburton RN. Demythologizing the high cost of pharmaceutical research. *Biosocieties.* 2011;6:34–50.
27. Tognoni et al., Case of GISSI, 21.
28. Ibid., 18.
29. Tognoni G, Geraci E. Approaches to informed consent. *Controlled Clinical Trials.* 1997;18:623.
30. Gruppo Italiano per lo studio della streptochinasi nell'infarto miocardico (GISSI). Long-term effects of intravenous thrombolytic treatment of acute myocardial infarction: final report of the GISSI study. *The Lancet.* 1987;328:871–874.
31. Franzosi M, Santoro E, DeVita C, Geraci E, et al. Ten-year follow-up of the first megatrial testing thrombolytic therapy in patients with acute myocardial infarction. *Circulation.* 1998;98:2659.

32. Waitzkin H. A Marxian interpretation of the growth and development of coronary care technology. *American Journal of Public Health*. 1979;69(12):1260.
33. Yusuf, Transforming the scientific, 193.
34. Braunwald, Happy birthday, GISSI!
35. Tognoni et al., Case of GISSI.
36. Goldacre, *Bad Pharma*; Gøtzsche P. *Deadly Medicines and Organized Crime: How Big Pharma Has Corrupted Healthcare*. Oxford: Radcliffe Medical Press; 2013; Healy D. *Pharmageddon*. Berkeley: University of California Press; 2012; Light D, ed. *The Risks of Prescription Drugs*. New York: Columbia University Press; 2010.
37. "Generic" is a misleading and unfortunate term. They are not "generic" but specific copies of well-established postpatent drugs. The correct term would be "drugs with the generic name," because it is the name that is generic, not the drug. By the same token, branded drugs are "drugs with the name of fantasy," but their effects are not fantasy. It would be most accurate to call generics "established postpatent drugs" because they were once patented as innovative and we know much more about how they affect patients.
38. Fleming T, DeMets D. Surrogate end points in clinical trials: are we being misled? *Annals of Internal Medicine*. 1996;125(7):605–612.
39. Angell M. *The Truth about the Drug Companies: How They Deceive Us and What to Do about It*. New York: Random House; 2004.
40. Light D, Lexchin J, Darrow J. Institutional corruption of pharmaceuticals and the myth of safe and effective drugs. *Journal of Law, Medicine & Ethics*. 2013;41(3):590–600; Light D, Lexchin J. Pharmaceutical R&D—What do we get for all that money? *BMJ*. 2012;344:e4348.
41. Garattini S. Non-inferiority trials are unethical because they disregard patients' interests. *Lancet*. 2007;370:1875–1877; Bertele V, Banzi R, Gluud C, Garattini S. EMA's reflection on placebo does not reflect patients' interests. *European Journal of Clinical Pharmacology*. 2012;68:877–879; Garattini S, Bertele V, Banzi R. Placebo? No thanks, it might be bad for me! *European Journal of Clinical Pharmacology*. 2013 (Mar);69(3):711–714.
42. Fisher JA. Institutional mistrust in the organization of pharmaceutical clinical trials. *Medicine, Health Care and Philosophy*. 2008;11:403–413; Fisher JA. *Medical Research for Hire: The Political Economy of Pharmaceutical Clinical Trials*. New Brunswick: Rutgers University Press; 2009.
43. Lexchin J. Sponsorship bias in clinical research. *The International Journal of Risk and Safety in Medicine*. 2012;24(4):233–242.
44. Sismondo S. Ghost management: how much of the medical literature is shaped behind the scenes by the pharmaceutical industry? *PLoS Medicine*. 2007;4(9):1429–1433; Sismondo S. How pharmaceutical industry funding affects trial outcomes: causal structures and responses. *Social Science & Medicine*. 2008;66:1909–1914; Lexchin J, Grootendorst P. *The effects of prescription drug user fees on drug and health services use and health status in vulnerable populations: a systematic review of the evidence*. Toronto: unpublished mss; 2003; Spurling G, Mansfield P, Montgomery B, et al. Information from pharmaceutical companies and the quality, quantity and cost of physicians' prescribing: a systematic review. *PLoS Medicine*. 2010;7(10):e1000352; Bero L. Impact of reporting bias on information about drugs . . . Or what you don't know won't help you or could hurt you. Paper presented at: ISDB General Assembly2012 (Mar 25); Loon Lake, Vancouver, CA; Rising K, Bacchetti P, Bero L. Reporting bias in drug trials submitted to the Food

and Drug Administration: review of publication and presentation. *PLoS Medicine.* 2008 (Nov);5(11):e217.

45. Tognoni et al., GISSI story (1983–1996).
46. Chase M. Genentech's shares are taking a pounding from analysts's leak of study on clot drug. *Wall Street Journal.* 1988 (May 31).
47. Gruppo Italiano per lo studio della streptochinasi nell'infarto miocardico (GISSI-2). A factorial randomised trial of alteplase versus strepokinase and aspirin versus no aspirin among 12,490 patients with acute myocardial infarction. *The Lancet.* 1990;336:65–71.
48. Chase M. Old heart drug works as well as costly TPA in study. *Wall Street Journal (Mar 9)*1990: B1, B4.
49. Michaels D. *Doubt Is Their Product: How Industry's Assault on Science Threatens Your Health.* New York: Oxford University Press; 2008.
50. (GISSI-2), Factorial randomised trial.
51. ISIS-2 (Second International Study of Infarct Survival) collaborative group. Randomised trial of intravenous strepokinase, oral aspirin, both, or neither among 17,187 cases of suspected acute myocardial infarction: ISIS-2. *The Lancet.* 1988:349–360.
52. Ibid., 350.
53. Topol E, Califf R. Answers to complex questions cannot be derived from "simple" trials. *British Heart Journal.* 1992;68:348–351.
54. Gruppo Italiano per lo studio della streptochinasi nell'infarto miocardico (GISSI). GISSI-3: effects of lisinopril and transdermal glyceryl trinitrate singly and together on 6-week mortality and ventricular function after acute myocardial infarction. *The Lancet.* 1994;343:1115–1122.
55. Taylor, Evolution of GISSI.
56. GISSI-AF Investigators. Valsartan for prevention of recurrent atrial fibrillation. *New England Journal of Medicine.* 2009;360:1606–1617.
57. Ibid., 1614.
58. GISSI-Prevenizone Investigators. Dietary supplementation with n-3 polyunsaturated fatty acids and vitamin E after myocardial infarction: results of the GISSI-Prevenzione trial. *The Lancet.* 1999;354:447–455.
59. GISSI-HF investigators. Effect of n-3 polyunsaturated fatty acids in patients with chronic heart failures (the GISSI-HF trial): a randomised, double-blinded, placebo-controlled trial. *The Lancet.* 2008;372:1223–1228.
60. GISSI-AF Investigators, Valsartan for prevention.
61. Sleight, We could all learn.
62. GISSI-HF investigators, Effect of n-3, 1226.
63. Lexchin, Sponsorship bias; Lexchin J. Those who have the gold make the evidence: how the pharmaceutical industry biases the outcomes of clinical trials of medications. *Science and Engineering Ethics.* 2011;18(2):247–261.
64. Pandolfini C, Bonati M. Clinical trial registries: from an omen to a common and disclosed practice. Milan: Mario Negri Institute; 2013:1–6.
65. ISGC. Genome-wide association study identifies a variant in HDAC9 associated with large vessel ischemic stroke. *Nature Genetics.* 2012;44:328–333.
66. ICAI Study Group. Prostanoids for chronic critical leg ischemia. *Annals of Internal Medicine.* 1999;130:412–421.
67. Tognoni G, Alli C, Bettelli G, et al. Randomised clinical trials in general practice: lessons from a failure. *BMJ.* 1991;303:969–970.

68. Tognoni G, Caimi V, Tombesi M, Visentin G, et al. Primary care as a permanent setting for research. *Primary Health Care Research & Development.* 2012;13:1–9.
69. Anecchino C, Fanizza C, Roni C, Castellani L, et al. Epidemiology and outcome of depression in Italian general practice: a large prospective outcome cohort study Mario Negri—Sud; 2013.
70. Liberati A, Colombo F, Franceschi S, et al. Quality of breast-cancer care in Italian general hospitals. *The Lancet.* 1982 (Jul 31);320(8292):258–260.
71. GIVIO (Interdisciplinary Group for Cancer Care Evaluation). Reducing diagnostic delay in breast cancer. *Cancer.* 1986;58:1756–1761.
72. GIVIO (Interdisciplinary Group for Cancer Care Evaluation). What doctors tell patients with breast cancer about diagnosis and treatment. *British Journal of Cancer.* 1986;54(2):319–326.
73. GIVIO (Interdisciplinary Group for Cancer Care Evaluation). Impact of follow-up testing on survivial and health-related quality of life in breast cancer patients: a multicenter randomized controlled trial. *Journal of the American Medical Association.* 1994;271(20):1587–1592.
74. Ibid.
75. CTT. Lack of effect of lowering LDL cholesterol on cancer. *PloS One.* 2012; 7(1):e29849.
76. Garassino M, Martelli O, Broggini M, Farina G, et al. Erlotinib versus docetaxel as second-line treatment of patients with advanced non-small-cell lung cancer and wild-type EGFR tumours (TAILOR): a randomised controlled trial. *The Lancet—Oncology.* 2013 (July 22):1–8.
77. Sollecito W, Johnson J. *McLaughlin and Kaluzny's Continuous Quality Improvement in Health Care, 4th Edition.* New York: Jones & Bartlett; 2011.
78. Wikipedia. W. Edwards Deming. 2013; http://en.wikipedia.org/wiki/W._Edwards_Deming Accessed Spet 17, 2013.
79. Nolte E, McKee CM. Measuring the health of nations: updating an earlier analysis. *Health Affairs.* 2008;27(1):58–71.
80. Gawande A. Big med. New York: *The New Yorker.* 2012 (Aug 13).
81. Lundh A, Sismondo S, Lexchin J, Busuioc O, Bero L. *Industry sponsorship and research outcome.* London: The Cochrane Library; 2012:15.

Chapter 7

1. Young JH. *The Toadstool Millionaires: A Social History of Patent Medicines in America Before Federal Regulation.* Princeton, NJ: Princeton University Press; 1961; Garattini S. *Pharmaceutical Companies in Italy.* Milano: The Mario Negri Institute for Pharmacological Research 2012 (Sept 12).
2. Young, *Toadstool Millionaires.*
3. Tognoni G, et al. A drug information system for an Italian community hospital. In: Anderson J, Fosthe J, eds. *Medinfo 74.* Amsterdam: North-Holland; 1975:895–899.
4. Tognoni G. A therapeutical formulary for Italian general practitioners. *The Lancet* (June 24). 1978:1352–1353.
5. Ibid.
6. Ibid.
7. Tognoni et al., Drug information system.
8. n.a. *The Selection of Essential Drugs.* Geneva: World Health Organization; 1977.
9. Light D, Lexchin J. Pharmaceutical R&D—What do we get for all that money? *BMJ.* 2012;344:e4348.

10. Hilts PJ. *Protecting America's Health: The FDA, Business and One Hundred Years of Regulation*. New York: Alfred A. Knopf; 2003:Ch 8.
11. Farina M, Levati A, Tognoni G. A multicenter study of ICU drug utilization. *Intensive Care Medicine*. 1981;7(3):125–131.
12. WHO Expert Committee. *The Selection of Essential Drugs*. Geneva: World Health Organization 1977; WHO. *Essential Drugs Monitor*. Geneva: World Health Organization, Essential Drugs Monitor; 2003.
13. WHO, *Essential Drugs Monitor*, 1.
14. Ibid., 12.
15. Le Fanu J. *The Rise and Fall of Modern Medicine: revised edition*. New York: Basic Books; 2012.
16. Antezana F, Seuba X. *Thirty Years of Essential Medicines: The Challenge*. Amsterdam: HAI Europe; 2009.
17. Ibid.
18. Morgan SG, Bassett KL, Wright JM, et al. "Breakthrough" drugs and growth in expenditure on prescription drugs in Canada. *BMJ*. 2005;331(7520):815–816.
19. Fattore G, Jommi C. The new pharmaceutical policy in Italy. *Health Policy*. 1998;46:26.
20. Garattini S. The cultural shift in Italy's pharmaceutical policy in 1994: a case history. *Journal of Ambulatory Care Management*. 2004;27(2):120–126.
21. Fattore and Jommi, New pharmaceutical policy.
22. Garattini, Cultural shift.
23. Light and Lexchin, Pharmaceutical R&D.
24. Garattini, Cultural shift.
25. Ibid.
26. Fattore and Jommi, New pharmaceutical policy.
27. Fattore G, Jommi C. The last decade of Italian pharmaceutical policy: instability of consolidation? *Pharmacoeconomics*. 2008;26(1):5–15.
28. Barbui C, Campomori A, Mezzalira L, Lopatriello S, Da Cas R, Garattini S. Psychotropic drug use in Italy, 1984–1999: the impact of a change in reimbursement status. *International Clinical Psychopharmacology*. 2001;16:227–233.
29. Fattore and Jommi, Last decade.
30. Garattini S, Garattini L. Pharmaceutical prescriptions in four European countries. *The Lancet*. 1993;342:1191–1192.
31. Garattini, Pharmaceutical companies in Italy.
32. Ibid.
33. Light and Lexchin, Pharmaceutical R&D; Munos B. Lessons from 60 years of pharmaceutical innovation. *Nature Reviews/ Drug Discovery*. 2009;8:959–968; Adamini S, Maarse H, Versluis E, Light DW. Policy making on data exclusivity in the European Union: from industrial interests to legal realities. *Journal of Health Politics, Policy and Law*. 2009;34:979–1010.
34. Joppi R, Bertele' V, Garattini S. Disappointing biotech. *BMJ*. Oct 15 2005;331(7521):895–897; Hopkins MM, Martin PA, Nightingale P, Kraft A, Mahdi S. The myth of the biotech revolution: an assessment of technological, clinical, and organizational change. *Research Policy*. 2007;36:566–589; Palmer B. Where are all the miracle drugs? *Slate*; 2013 (Sept 30).
35. Goldacre B. *Bad Pharma: How Drug Companies Mislead Doctors and Harm*. London: Faber & Faber; 2012:x.
36. Mundy A. *Dispensing with the Truth: The Victims, the Drug Companies, and the Dramatic Story behind the Battle Over Fen-Phen*. New York: St. Martin's Press; 2001.

37. Mullard A. World report: Mediator scandal rocks French medical community. *The Lancet.* 2011;377:891.
38. Sayare S. Scandal over Mediator, a French weight-loss drug, prompts calls for wide changes. *The New York Times.* 2011 (Dec 11).
39. Jessop N. 2012: A good, bad, and ugly year for France's Servier. *Pharmaceutical Technology Europe.* 2012;(Feb 1):Vol 24.
40. Mullard, World report.
41. Italian Medicines Agency (AIFA) Research & Development Working Group. Feasibility and challenge of independent research on drugs: the Italian Medicines Agency (AIFA) experience. *European Journal of Clinical Investigation.* 2010;40(1):69–86.
42. Ibid.
43. Robbins R. Profiles in medical courage: evidence-based medicine and Archie Cochrane. *Southwest Journal of Pulmonary and Critical Care.* 2012;5:65–72.
44. Cochrane A. *Effectiveness and Efficiency: Random Reflections on Health Service.* London: Nuffield Provincial Hospitals Trust; 1972.
45. Chalmers I, Dickersin K, Chalmers T. Getting to grips with Archie Cochrane's agency: a register of all randomized controlled trials. *BMJ.* 1992;3005:786–788.
46. Colombo F, Shapiro S, Slone D, Tognoni G, eds. *Epidemiological Evaluation of Drugs.* Amsterdam/London: Elsevier/North Holland Biomedical Press; 1977; (http://www.jameslindlibrary.org/illustrating/records/epidemiological-evaluation-of-drugs/title_pages).
47. Himel H, Liberati A, Gelber R, Chalmers T. Adjuvant chemotherapy for breast cancer: a pooled estimate based on results from published randomized trials. *JAMA.* 1986;256:1148–1159; (http://www.jameslindlibrary.org/illustrating/records/adjuvant-chemotherapy-for-breast-cancer-a-pooled-estimate-based/key_passages).
48. See the interview with her in Chapter 2.
49. Pecoraro V, Allen C, Banzi R, et al. The Italian Contribution to the Cochrane Collaboration and to the Dissemination of Evidence-Based Healthcare. Milan; 2009.
50. Ibid.
51. Welch H, Schwartz L, Woloshin S. *Overdiagnosed: Making People Sick in the Pursuit of Health.* Boston: Beacon; 2012; Brownlee S. *Overtreated: Why Too Much Medicine Is Making Us Sicker and Poorer.* New York: Bloomsbury; 2007; Moynihan R, Cassels A. *Selling Sickness: How the World's Biggest Pharmaceutical Companies Are Turning Us All Into Patients.* New York: Nation Books; 2005.
52. Pecoraro et al., Italian contribution; n.a. Alessandro Liberati. 2013; http://en.wikipedia.org/wiki/Alessandro_Liberati Accessed Dec 6, 2013.
53. Colombo C, Moja L, Gonzalez-Lorenzo M, Liberati A, Mosconi P. Patient empowerment as a component of health system reform: rights, benefits and vested interests. *International Emergency Medicine.* 2012;7:183–187.
54. Ibid.
55. Mosconi P, Colombo C, Satolli R, Liberati A. PartecipaSalute, an Italian project to involve lay people, patients' associations and scientific-medical representatives in the health debate. *Health Expectations.* 2006;10:194–204.
56. Chalmers I, Glasziou P. Avoidable waste in the production and reporting of research evidence. *The Lancet.* 2009;374(9683):86–89.
57. Liberati A. Need to realign patient-oriented and commercial academic research. *The Lancet.* 2011;378:1777–1778.
58. Gartlehner G, Flamm M. *Is the Cochrane collaboration prepared for the era of patient-centered outcomes research?* The Cochrane Library; 2013 (Mar 28).

59. Pecoraro et al., Italian contribution.
60. Gøtzsche P. *Deadly Medicines and Organized Crime: How Big Pharma Has Corrupted Healthcare.* Oxford: Radcliffe Medical Press; 2013; Gøtzsche P, Jorgensen A. Opening up data at the European Medicines Agency. *BMJ.* 2011;342: d2686.

Chapter 8

1. Lessig L. *Republic, Lost: How Money Corrupts Congress—and a Plan to Stop It.* New York: Twelve/Hachette; 2011; Lessig L. *Institutional Corruptions.* Cambridge, MA: Research in Action Working Papers, Edmond J. Safra Center for Ethics, Harvard University; 2013.
2. The Committee was then the Committee for Proprietary Medicinal Products (CPMP), but later renamed CHMP or the Committee for Human Medicinal Products. Garattini S, Bertele' V. Policing the European pharmaceutical market's priorities. *European Journal of Clinical Pharmacology.* 2000;56:441–443; EEC Council Reguation. No 2309/93. 1993 (July 22); http://ec.europa.eu/health/files/eudralex/vol-1/reg_1993_2309/reg_1993_2309_bg.pdf 2013.
3. EEC Council Reguation, No 2309/93.
4. Gøtzsche P. *Deadly Medicines and Organized Crime: How Big Pharma Has Corrupted Healthcare.* Oxford: Radcliffe Medical Press; 2013.
5. Silverman M, Lee PR, Lydecker M. *Prescriptions for Death: The Drugging of the Third World.* Berkeley: University of California Press; 1982; Silverman M, Lee PR. *Pills, Profits, and Politics.* Berkeley: University of California Press; 1974; Braithwaite J. *Corporate Crime in the Pharmaceutical Industry.* London: Routledge & Kegan Paul; 1984.
6. Wikipedia. Center for Drug Evaluation and Research. 2013; http://en.wikipedia.org/wiki/Center_for_Drug_Evaluation_and_Research.
7. Lexchin J. New drugs and safety: what happened to new active substances approved in Canada between 1995 and 2010? *Archives of Internal Medicine.* 2012;172 (21):1680–1681.
8. Garattini and Bertele', Policing European pharmaceutical.
9. Garattini S. EMEA: for patients or for industry? *Pharmacoeconomics.* 2005;23(3): 207–208.
10. Ibid.
11. Bassi L, Bertele' V, Garattini S. European regulatory policies on medicines and public health needs. *European Journal of Public Health.* 2003;13:246–251.
12. Ujeyl M, Schlegel C, Walter S, Gundert-Remy U. New drugs: evidence relating to their therapeutic value after introduction to the market. *Deutsches Arzteblatt International.* 2012;109(7):117–123.
13. Garattini and Bertele', Policing European pharmaceutical.
14. Garattini, EMEA.
15. Bassi, Bertele', and Garattini, European regulatory policies.
16. Fugh-Berman A, Ahari S. Following the script: how drug reps make friends and influence doctors. *PLoS Medicine.* 2007;4(4):e150; Mintzes B, Lexchin J, Sutherland J, et al. Pharmaceutical sales representatives and patient safety: a comparative prospective study of information quality in Canada, France and the United States. *Journal of General Internal Medicine.* 2013;28(10):1368–1375.
17. Garattini and Bertele', Policing European pharmaceutical.

18. Garattini S, Bertele' V. Efficacy, safety, and cost of new anticancer drugs. *BMJ.* 2002;325(7358):269–271, 1303; Apolone G, Tafuri G, Trotta F, Garattini S. A new anti-cancer drug in the market: good news for investors or for patients? *European Journal of Cancer.* 2008;44:1786–1788.

19. Light DW, Kantarjian H. Market spiral pricing of cancer drugs. *Cancer.* 2013 (Nov);119(22):3900–3902.

20. Garattini S, Bertele' V. The European Commission should require better medicines, not just faster reimbursements. *European Journal of Internal Medicine.* 2013;24:e1.

21. Morgan SG, Bassett KL, Wright JM, et al. "Breakthrough" drugs and growth in expenditure on prescription drugs in Canada. *BMJ.* 2005;331(7520):815–816.

22. Garattini S, Bertele' V, Banzi R. Placebo? No thanks, it might be bad for me! *European Journal of Clinical Pharmacology.* 2013 (Mar);69(3):711–714.

23. Chalmers I, Bracken M, Djulbegovic B, Garattini S, et al. Research: increasing value, reducing waste 1: how to increase value and reduce waste when research priorities are set. *The Lancet.* 2014;383:156–165.

24. Garattini S, Bertele' V. Rosiglitazone and the need for a new drug safety agency. *BMJ.* 2010 (Oct 9) 341:781.

25. Light DW. Pricing pharmaceuticals in the USA. In: Temple NJ, Thompson A, eds. *Excessive Medical Spending: Facing the Challenge.* Oxford: Radcliffe Publishing; 2006:63–79.

26. Moore TJ. *Deadly Medicine: Why Tens of Thousands of Heart Patients Died in America's Worst Drug Disaster.* New York: Simon & Schuster; 1995.

27. Garattini S, Bertele' V. Anything new in EU pharmacovigilance? *European Journal of Clinical Pharmacology.* 2011;67:1199–1200.

28. Ibid.

29. Eichler H-G, Oye K, Baird L, Abadie E, et al. Adaptive licensing: taking the next step in the evolution of drug approval. *Clinical Pharmacology & Therapeutics.* 2012;91(3):426–437.

30. Light D, Lexchin J, Darrow J. Institutional corruption of pharmaceuticals and the myth of safe and effective drugs. *Journal of Law, Medicine & Ethics.* 2013;41(3):590–600.

31. Gøtzsche, *Deadly Medicines.*

32. Garattini and Bertele', European Commission.

33. Turner EH, Matthews AM, Linardatos E, Tell RA, Rosenthal R. Selective publication of antidepressant trials and its influence on apparent efficacy. *New England Journal of Medicine.* 2008;358:252–260; Lundh A, Sismondo S, Lexchin J, Busuioc O, Bero L. *Industry sponsorship and research outcome.* London: The Cochrane Library; 2012.

34. Lundh et al., *Industry sponsorship*; Sismondo S. How pharmaceutical industry funding affects trial outcomes: causal structures and responses. *Social Science & Medicine.* 2008;66:1909–1914.

35. Hart B, Lundh A, Bero L. Effect of reporting bias on meta-analyses of drug trials: reanalysis of meta-analyses. *BMJ.* 2012;344; Rising K, Bacchetti P, Bero L. Reporting bias in drug trials submitted to the Food and Drug Administration: review of publication and presentation. *PLoS Medicine.* 2008 (Nov);5(11):e217.

36. Lundh et al., *Industry sponsorship*; Rising, Bacchetti, and Bero, Reporting bias; Lexchin J, Bero LA, Djulbegovic B, Clark O. Pharmaceutical industry sponsorship and research outcome and quality: systematic review. *BMJ.* 2003;326(31 May):1167–1170.

37. Garattini, EMEA.
38. Garattini S, Bertele' V. Europe's opportunity to open up drug regulation. *BMJ.* 2010;340(30 Mar):842–843.
39. Ibid.
40. Ibid.
41. Eichler H-G, Petavy F, Pignatti F, Rasi G. Access to patient-level trial data—a boon to drug developers. *New England Journal of Medicine.* 2013;369(17):1577–1579.
42. European Ombudsman. Ombudsman concerned about change of policy at Medicines Agency as regards clinical trial transparency 2014 (16 May); http://www.ombudsman.europa.eu/en/press/release.faces/en/54348/html.bookmark.
43. UK House of Commons CoPA. *Access to clinical trial information and the stockpiling of Tamiflu* London: UK House of Commons, Committee of Public Accounts;2014 (Jan 3).
44. Garattini S, Bertele' V. New approach to clinical trials and drug registration. *BMJ.* 2001;323:341.
45. Garattini S, Bertele' V. Risk: benefit assessment of old medicines. *British Journal of Clinical Pharmacology.* 2004;58:581–586.
46. Garattini and Bertele', Efficacy, safety, and cost; Garattini S, Bertele' V. Efficacy, safety and cost of new drugs acting on the central nervous system. *European Journal of Clinical Pharmacology.* 2002;59:79–84.
47. Yudkin J, Lipska K, Montori V. The idolatry of the surrogate. *BMJ.* 2011;343:d7995.
48. Ottolenghi L, Bertele' V, Garattini S. Limits of add-on trials: antirheumatic drugs. *European Journal of Pharmacology.* 2009;65(1):33–41.
49. Goldacre B. *Bad Pharma: How Drug Companies Mislead Doctors and Harm.* London: Faber & Faber; 2012; Goldacre B. *Bad Science.* UK: Fourth Estate; 2009.
50. Garattini S, Bertele' V. The impact of European regulatory policies on psychotropic drug prescribing patterns. *International Review of Psychiatry.* 2005;17: 199–204.
51. Hart, Lundh, and Bero, Effect of reporting bias on meta-analyses of drug trials: reanalysis of meta-analyses; Bero L, Oostvogel F, Bacchetti P, Lee K. Factors associated with findings of published trials of drug-drug comparisons: why some statins appear more efficacious than others. *PLoS Medicine.* 2007;4(6): e184.
52. Garattini, Bertele', and Banzi, Placebo? No thanks; Bertele' V, Banzi R, Gluud C, Garattini S. EMA's reflection on placebo does not reflect patients' interests. *European Journal of Clinical Pharmacology.* 2012;68:877–879; Garattini S, Bertele' V. How can we regulate medicines better? *BMJ.* 2007;335:803–805; Garattini S. Non-inferiority trials are unethical because they disregard patients' interests. *The Lancet.* 2007;370:1875–1877; Garattini S. Reconsidering the Declaration of Helsinki. *The Lancet.* 2013;382:1247.
53. Bertele' et al., EMA's reflection.
54. Ibid.
55. Garattini, Bertele', and Banzi, Placebo? No thanks; Garattini, Non-inferiority trials.
56. Bertele' et al., EMA's reflection.
57. Ibid.
58. Gluud C, Demotes-Mainard J, Bertele' V, et al. *Proposals for amendments to the draft revision of the Declaration of Helsinki.* 2013 (June 14).
59. Ibid.
60. Joppi R, Bertele' V, Garattini S. Orphan drug development is progressing too slowly. *British Journal of Clinical Pharmacology.* 2006;61(3):355–360.

61. Joppi R, Bertele' V, Garattini S. Orphan drugs, orphan diseases. The first decade of orphan drug legislation in the EU. *British Journal of Clinical Pharmacology.* 2012;69(4):1009–1024.

62. Dupont A, Van Wilder P. Access to orphan drugs despite poor quality of clinical evidence. *British Journal of Clinical Pharmacology.* 2011;71(4):488–496.

63. Light DW. Reducing Global Health Disparities through Vaccines: Rhetorics and Realities of Advanced Market Commitments. *Dean's Colloquium, UC Berkeley School for Public Health.* Berkeley, CA 2010 (4 Nov); Brody H, Light DW. The inverse benefit law: how drug marketing undermines patient safety and public health. *American Journal of Public Health.* 2011;101(3):399–404.

64. Kesselheim AS, Myers J, Solomon D, Winkelmayer W, Levin R, Avorn J. The prevalence and cost of unapproved uses of top-selling orphan drugs. *PloS One.* 2012;7(2):e31894.

65. Garattini and Bertele', European Commission.

66. Garattini S. Financial interests constrain drug development. *Science.* 1997;275(5298):287.

67. Garattini S, Bertele' V. A matter of public interest. *BMJ.* 2010;341:c3721.

68. Ibid.

69. Remuzzi G, Schieppati A, Boissel J-P, Garattini S, Horton R. Independent clinical research in Europe. *The Lancet.* 2004;364:1723–1726.

70. Bassi, Bertele', and Garattini, European regulatory policies.

71. IMI. Innovative Medicines Initiative 2014; http://www.imi.europa.eu.

72. Garattini S, Bertele' V, Bertolini G. A failed attempt at collaboration. *BMJ.* 2013;347:d5354.

Chapter 9

1. Light D, Lexchin J, Darrow J. Institutional corruption of pharmaceuticals and the myth of safe and effective drugs. *Journal of Law, Medicine & Ethics.* 2013;41(3):590–600; Lexchin J. New drugs and safety: what happened to new active substances approved in Canada between 1995 and 2010? *Archives of Internal Medicine.* 2012;172(21):1680–1681; Light DW. Pricing pharmaceuticals in the USA. In: Temple NJ, Thompson A, eds. *Excessive Medical Spending: Facing the Challenge.* Oxford: Radcliffe Publishing; 2006:63–79.

2. Light, Lexchin, and Darrow, Institutional corruption of pharmaceuticals.

3. Gagnon M-A. Corruption of pharmaceutical markets: addressing the misalignment of financial incentives and public policy reform. *Journal of Law, Medicine & Ethics.* 2013;41(3); Davis C, Abraham J. *Unhealthy Pharmaceutical Regulation: Innovation, Politics and Promisory Science.* New York: Palgrave Macmillan; 2013.

4. Goozner M. *The $800 Million Pill: The Truth Behind the Cost of New Drugs.* Berkeley: University of California Press; 2004.

5. Brody H, Light DW. The inverse benefit law: how drug marketing undermines patient safety and public health. *American Journal of Public Health.* 2011;101(3):399–404.

6. Cosgrove L, Krimsky S. A comparison of DSM-IV and DSM-V panel members financial associations with industry: a pernicious problem persists. *PLoS Medicine.* 2012 (Mar 13) 10.1371/journal.pmed.1001190; Cosgrove L, Wheeler E. Drug firms, the codification of diagnostic categories, and bias in clinical guidelines. *Journal of Law, Medicine & Ethics.* 2013;41(3):644–653.

7. Healy D. *Pharmageddon*. Berkeley: University of California Press; 2012.
8. McGoey L. Sequestered evidence and the distortion of clinical practice guidelines. *Perspectives in Biology and Medicine*. 2009;52:203–217; McGoey L, Jackson E. Seroxat and the suppression of clinical trial data: regulatory failure and the uses of legal ambiguity. *Journal of Medical Ethics*. 2009;35:107–112.
9. Every-Palmer S, Howick J. How evidence-based medicine is failing due to biased trials and selective publication. *Journal of Evaluation in Clinical Practice*. 2014 (May):doi:10.1111/jep.12147.
10. Morgan SG, Bassett KL, Wright JM, et al. "Breakthrough" drugs and growth in expenditure on prescription drugs in Canada. *BMJ*. 2005;331(7520):815–816.
11. Davis and Abraham, *Unhealthy Pharmaceutical Regulation*.
12. Olson MK. Are novel drugs more risky for patients than less novel drugs? *Journal of Health Economics*. 2004;23(6):1135–1158; Olson MK. The risk we bear: the effects of review speed and industry user fees on new drug safety. *Journal of Health Economics*. 2008;27(2):175–200; Carpenter D, Chattopadhyay J, Moffitt S, Nall C. The complication of controlling agency time discretion: FDA review deadlines and postmarket drug safety. *American Journal of Political Science*. 2012;56(1):98–114.
13. Ibid.
14. Davis and Abraham, *Unhealthy Pharmaceutical Regulation*, 264.
15. Ibid., 279.
16. Stafford RS. Regulating off-label drug use—rethinking the role of the FDA. *New England Journal of Medicine*. 2008;358:1427–1429; Kesselheim AS, Avorn J. A hemorrhage of off-label use. *Annals of Internal Medicine*. 2011;154(8):566–567; Rodwin M. Five un-easy pieces of pharmaceutical policy reform. *Journal of Law, Medicine & Ethics*. 2013;41(3):581–589.
17. Gøtzsche P. *Deadly Medicines and Organized Crime: How Big Pharma Has Corrupted Healthcare*. Oxford: Radcliffe Medical Press; 2013.
18. Public Citizen Health Research Group. *Rapidly Increasing Criminal and Civil Monetary Penalties Against the Pharmaceutical Industry: 1991–2010*. Washington DC: Public Citizen Health Research Group; 2010.
19. McGoey, Sequestered evidence; McGoey and Jackson, Seroxat and suppression.
20. Braithwaite J. *Corporate Crime in the Pharmaceutical Industry*. London: Routledge & Kegan Paul; 1984; Braithwaite J, Dukes M. *Corporations, Crime and Medicines*. 2015 (forthcoming).
21. Mokhiber R. Corporate crime in the pharmaceutical industry. *CounterPunch*. 2012 (Jan 3).
22. Gøtzsche, *Deadly Medicines*, vii.
23. Light DW, ed. *The Risks of Prescription Drugs*. New York: Columbia University Press; 2010.
24. Light, Lexchin, and Darrow, Institutional corruption of pharmaceuticals; European Commission Enterprise and Industry. *Safe, Innovative and Accessible Medicines: A Renewed Vision for the Pharmaceutical Sector*. Brussels: European Commission Enterprise and Industry; 2008; Lazarou J, Pomeranz BH, Corey PN. Incidence of adverse drug reactions in hospitalized patients. *Journal of American Medical Association*. 1998;279(15):1200–1205.
25. NPR. How a bone disease grew to fit the prescription. 2009; file:///Users/dlight/Documents/Safra-Pharm-Osteopenia%20-new%20disease%20NPR.webarchive.
26. De La Merced M, Gelles D, Abrams R. Seeking the right chemistry, drug makers hunt for mergers. *The New York Times*. 2014 (Apr 22).

27. Goozner, *$800 Million Pill*; Angell M. *The Truth about the Drug Companies: How They Deceive Us and What to Do about It.* New York: Random House; 2004.

28. t' Hoen E. The Global Politics of Pharmaceutical Monopoly Power. Geneva: MSF 2009: http://www.msfaccess.org/content/global-politics-pharmaceutical-monopoly-power.

29. Lundh A, Sismondo S, Lexchin J, Busuioc O, Bero L. *Industry sponsorship and research outcome.* London: The Cochrane Library; 2012; Steinman MA, Bero LA, Chen M-M, Landerfeld CS. Narrative review: the promotion of Gabapentin: an analysis of internal industry documents. *Annals of Internal Medicine.* 2006;145(4):284–293; Rising K, Bacchetti P, Bero L. Reporting bias in drug trials submitted to the Food and Drug Administration: review of publication and presentation. *PLoS Medicine.* 2008 (Nov);5(11):e217; Steinman MA, Harper GM, Chen M-M, Landerfeld CS, Bero LA. Characteristics and impact of drug detailing for Gabapentin. *PLoS Medicine.* 2007;4(4):743–751; Hart B, Lundh A, Bero L. Effect of reporting bias on meta-analyses of drug trials: reanalysis of meta-analyses. *BMJ.* 2012;344; Turner EH, Matthews AM, Linardatos E, Tell RA, Rosenthal R. Selective publication of antidepressant trials and its influence on apparent efficacy. *New England Journal of Medicine.* 2008;358:252–260.

30. Kesselheim AS, Robertson C, Meyers J, et al. A randomized study of how physicians interpret research funding disclosures. *New England Journal of Medicine.* 2012;367:1119–1127.

31. Drazen J. Believe the data. *New England Journal of Medicine.* 2012;367(12):1152–1153.

32. Light DW. How physicians interpret research funding disclosures. *New England Journal of Medicine.* 2012;367:2358–2360.

33. Posner R. Why there are too many patents in America. *The Atlantic.* Boston: The Atlantic; 2012 (Jul 12).

34. Liberati A. Need to realign patient-oriented and commercial academic research. *The Lancet.* 2011;378:1777–1778.

35. Brody and Light, Inverse benefit law; Steinman et al., Narrative review: promotion; Public Citizen Health Research Group. *Pharmaceutical Industry Criminal and Civil Penalties: An Update.* Washington DC: Public Citizen Health Research Group; 2012.

36. McManus R. Vaccine research center celebrates first decade *nih record.* Vol. LXIII. Bethesda, MD; 2011:1–4.

37. Munos B, Chin W. How to revive breakthrough innovation in the pharmaceutical industry. *Science Translational Medicine.* 2011;3(89):1–3; Munos B. *Open Scientific Collaboration for Innovation in Global Health (OpenSCI.)* Durham, NC: DukeSanfordSchool; 2012 (May 2).

38. Maroso M, Balosso S, Ravizza T, et al. Toll-like receptor 4 and high mobility group box-1 are involved in ictogenesis and can be targeted to reduce seizures. *Nature Medicine.* 2010;16:413–419.

39. Lucca U, Garri M, Recchia A, Logroscino G, et al. A population-based study of dementia in the oldest old: the Monzino 80-plus study. *BMC Neurology.* 2011;11:54–68.

40. Lucca U, Nobili A, Riva E, Tettamanti M. Cholinesterase inhibitor use and age in the general population. *Archives of Neurology.* 2006;63:134–135.

41. Nobili A, Garattini S, Mannucci P. Multiple disease and polypharmacy in the elderly: challenges for the internist of the third millennium. *Journal of Comorbidity.* 2011;1:28–44.

42. Ghibelli S, Marengoni A, Djade C, Nobili A, et al. Prevention of inappropriate pre-scribing in hospitalized older patients using a computerized prescription support system. *Drugs Aging.* 2013 (Aug 14):DOI:1007/s40266-40013-40109-40265.

43. Kantarjian HM, Steensma D, Sanjuan JR, Elshaug A, Light D. High cancer drug prices in the United States: reasons and proposed solutions. *Journal of Oncology Practice.* 2014 (May); Light DW, Kantarjian H. Market spiral pricing of cancer drugs. *Cancer.* 2013 (Nov);119(22):3900–3902.

44. Healy, *Pharmageddon*; Gøtzsche, *Deadly Medicines*; Kassirer JP. *On the Take: How Medicine's Complicity with Big Business Can Endanger Your Health.* New York: Oxford University Press; 2005.

45. Bok D. *Universities in the Marketplace.* Princeton, NJ: Princeton University Press; 2003.

46. Graedon J. Are drug companies bankrupting healthcare? *The People's Pharmacy Newsletter.* 2014 (Sept 25). http://www.peoplespharmacy.com/2014/09/22/are-drug-companies-bankrupting-healthcare/; Rother J. Abusive specialty drug pricing threatens healthcare system. *The Hill.* 2014 (June 3). http://thehill.com/blogs/congress-blog/healthcare/207929-abusive-specialty-drug-pricing-threatens-healthcare-system.

Appendix 1

1. Hollister L, Garattini S. In: Silser F, ed. *An Oral History of Neuropsychopharmacol-ogy, Vol. 3 Neuropharmacology.* Brentwood, TN: American College of Psychop-harmacology 1995:203–216.

2. Healy D. *The Anti-depressant Era.* Cambridge, MA: Harvard University Press; 1997.

Index